T0266275

ENDOCRINE DISRUPTORS IN THE ENVIRONMENT

ENDOCRINE DISRUPTORS IN THE ENVIRONMENT

SUSHIL K. KHETAN

WILEY

For general information on our other products and services or for technical support, please contact our
Customer Care Department within the United States at (800) 762-2974, outside the United States at
(317) 572-3993 or fax (317) 572-4002.

Wiley also publishes its books in a variety of electronic formats. Some content that appears in print
may not be available in electronic formats. For more information about Wiley products, visit our web
site at www.wiley.com.

Library of Congress Cataloging-in-Publication Data:

Khetan, Sushil K.
  Endocrine disruptors in the environment / Sushil K. Khetan.
    pages cm
  Includes bibliographical references and index.
  ISBN 978-1-118-85293-4 (cloth)
  1. Endocrine-disrupting chemicals–Environmental aspects. 2. Endocrine-disrupting
chemicals–Toxicity testing. 3. Endocrine toxicology. I. Title.
  RA1224.2.K48 2014
  614.5′94–dc23

                                                        2013047840

ISBN: 9781118852934

10 9 8 7 6 5 4 3 2 1

CONTENTS

FOREWORD

Why should people concern themselves with endocrine disruptors (EDs)? And why should scientists, and especially green chemists, rank endocrine disruption as the single most important problem space for their work in reducing/eliminating chemical hazards? These are key questions that Dr. Sushil Khetan seeks to answer through the scholarly journey he undertakes in this bravely and conscientiously constructed book entitled *Endocrine Disruptors in the Environment*.

I write "bravely" because *Endocrine Disruptors in the Environment* integrates aspects of physiology, biology, genetics, epigenetics, endocrinology, toxicology, ecotoxicology, public policy, and green chemistry into a concise and coherent picture of the challenges that endocrine disruption poses. Dr. Khetan was trained as an organic chemist, and spent much of his working career in the pesticides industry at the interfaces of chemistry with biology and toxicology. Thereafter, he joined the Institute for Green Science (IGS) of Carnegie Mellon University and spent many years working to help advance this emerging field. Green science has as its core goals the challenges of helping to conceive, articulate, and build the scientific dimension of a sustainable civilization. Dr. Khetan has a keen sense for what is of great importance to the positive advancement of science, especially chemistry. He enthusiastically adopted the IGS insight that to be effective in the pursuit of sustainability, green chemists have to find ways to understand endocrine disruption well enough to be able to avoid EDs by design in the commercialized products and processes of the future. One of Dr. Khetan's great accomplishments in these years was to read and interpret for the IGS the literature on pharmaceuticals in the environment. His efforts resulted the *Chemical Reviews* article, "Human Pharmaceuticals in the Aquatic Environment: A Challenge to Green Chemistry," which we coauthored in 2007. Many pharmaceuticals are developmental disruptors and are ecotoxic at environmentally relevant concentrations, typically in wastewater from low parts per billion and to even as low as subparts per trillion, consistent with the endocrine system being targeted. Dr. Khetan's work helped to underpin the IGS development of technologies based on TAML activator/hydrogen peroxide oxidation catalysis that possess high technical, environmental, and cost performances for degrading excreted and adventitious pharmaceuticals in wastewater before the water is released to the environment.

Over the last several years, Dr. Khetan has thrown himself heart and soul into writing *Endocrine Disruptors in the Environment* as a way of finding answers to the following questions which involve us all and which have tectonic significance to whether or not the chemical enterprise can become a positive force in the pursuit of a sustainable civilization:

- What can each of us do to build a safer world upon becoming aware that everyday commercial chemicals are disrupting the hormonal control of cellular development and signaling to change the way life develops and evolves?
- What should those scientists who are designing the technologies of the future do in light of the mountain of evidence which prescribes that the ever-expanding adverse effects of low doses of EDs are potentially ruinous of any meaningful quest for a sustainable future?
- What must society do given that some EDs are high production volume chemicals that are integral to myriad products and processes across the material fabric of our civilization but result in the endemic exposure of living things to both individual EDs and mixtures of EDs?
- How can scientists resolve the obvious dilemmas with certain existing EDs that society would wish to keep for valuable benefits – where and how through the full lifecycles can these EDs be intercepted so that the benefits can be maintained while the collateral adverse effects are avoided? Some chemicals have been designed and/or deployed to take advantage of endocrine disruption properties; the steroid components of the birth control pill are examples in point.

Why have I posed these questions in such dramatic terms? To me, the scientific case is indisputable that endocrine disruption turns the whole meaning of chemicals to the advancement of our civilization on its head. In the light of endocrine disruption, nothing in the chemical enterprise can ever look quite the same. The very idea that infinitesimal traces of commercial chemicals could be altering the way life develops and evolves is shocking. The chemicals we use in food, in agriculture, in our homes, in personal cares products, in pharmaceuticals, in fact across the entire landscape of our highly chemical civilization were never meant to disrupt development. But now we understand that some of them clearly do as an almost inescapable consequence of the way the endocrine system works to control cellular development and signaling. So every chemical has to be reexamined to see whether our appreciation of it is upside down – to learn whether short-term benefits are accompanied by longer-term penalties which society absolutely must avoid. And we must know whether new chemicals have uncontrollable endocrine disruption properties. An Everest of scientific information now has the potential to require the chemical industry to re-evaluate, reposition, and even abandon lucrative products as a prerequisite for a sustainable future. This reality further highlights Dr. Khetan's courage in writing this book.

The above underlying questions are of immediate relevance to anyone who wants our civilization to last. Dr. Khetan skillfully describes how the questions are being approached by researchers and their supporters who have led in developing our understanding of EDs, by government officials who evaluate and regulate against toxic chemicals, by commentators and advocates who raise public awareness about chemical hazards, by corporation owners and stockholders who have the power to insist that chemical producing and/or using companies chart courses away from endocrine disruptors, by corporate executives who hold the responsibility for developing practical company policies and dynamics that do not expand but instead reduce public and environmental exposures to EDs, by researchers who are responsible for learning how to avoid EDs, and by educators who are responsible for teaching future generations about the dangers of EDs. In fact, everyone at some level shares the responsibility for ensuring that the chemical sector of our civilization finds a new path forward that frees living things from ED exposures.

Dr. Khetan's highly informative book can be of assistance to anyone who is working to advance the economy while protecting the future from endocrine disruption. Its publication comes at a time when government officials and informed members of the public are scrutinizing EDs' adverse effects on wildlife and people with growing conviction that regulatory control is unavoidable. At the same time, segments of the chemical industry and its trade associations are lobbying to convince the powers that be that chemicals are safe once they have passed the classical toxicological screening we have relied on for decades. This screening does not adequately recognize the peculiarities of how the endocrine system works by using small concentrations of hormones to control the fate of cellular development. Unfortunately, even at low doses, EDs disrupt these hormone signals that are exquisitely programmed by healthy organisms in both time and space. Dr. Khetan's combining of the science with the policy issues and remediation efforts rounds out his treatise to deliver a multidisciplinary, cross-sectoral, and trans-cultural domain as is required for understanding and coping with endocrine disruption to advance sustainability. Dr. Khetan also makes a special attempt to show how positive paths forward are deriving from green chemistry.

In conclusion, in writing *Endocrine Disruptors in the Environment*, Dr. Khetan has embarked on a courageous exercise to scan the broad literature of endocrine disruption and to explore whether he, in his own person, can provide an example of the challenging journey that the science of chemistry and the chemical enterprise must undertake. What has resulted is a treasure trove of well-organized information covering the things that readers would want to know about endocrine disruption but did not know how or whom to ask. Ultimately, this is an immensely positive book because, as we are learning about EDs and how to identify them, we are also learning about how to avoid them by design and even to how to eliminate some of them after they have been used for beneficial purposes, but before collateral negative effects can be manifested. And, it is my fervent hope that the fruits of Dr. Khetan's labor of interest and conviction will advance the ability of chemists to build a chemical world that is free of endocrine disruption.

TERRENCE J. COLLINS

Teresa Heinz Professor of Green Chemistry and Director
Institute for Green Science
Carnegie Mellon University
Pittsburgh, PA

PREFACE

The last two decades have seen an increase in the number of reports on organic chemicals that pollute the aquatic environment and in turn our drinking water supplies. Aquatic ecosystems are especially susceptible to exposure to compounds with endocrine-disrupting activity, because a great variety of substances exhibiting such activity are eventually introduced into the surface waters. Environmental contaminants called *endocrine disruptors* (EDs), a diverse group of chemicals and heavy metals, are now widely reported to affect the reproductive and developmental health of animals, experimental as well as wild, and are considered to be the developmental basis of many diseases, including obesity in humans. These chemicals mimic the function of various hormones and induce an imbalance in the natural hormonal milieu. Plasticizers, such as phthalates, that can block the functioning of male sex hormones, and basic chemicals for plastics, such as bisphenol A, that act like female hormones have been found in the blood and urine of most people in the United States.

Traditional toxicology testing has largely missed endocrine disruption in the first place and overlooked chemicals that could penetrate the womb environment and interfere with the development of the embryo and fetus. The idea that the dose makes the poison is overly simplistic. The latest research results clearly demonstrate that biology is affected by low doses of chemicals, often within the range of general population exposure, and reveals the sensitivity of the developing individual to the slightest chemical perturbation during development. It has been demonstrated that exposure to a biologically active chemical within the range in which free hormones operate can have an effect. And exposure to the chemical leads to an entirely different suite of effects that change during progressive stages of development than when the same chemical is administered in high doses after an individual has fully developed. These studies have also confirmed that endocrine effects are time specific, chemical and/or hormone specific, and also dose related.

The very idea that some man-made chemicals are the cause of unintended physiological and environmental effects is worrisome. Chemists often primarily see the beneficial and useful aspects of synthetic substances. And as scientists, they may be skeptical about claims that specific synthetic chemicals cause harm. This has led to the introduction of consumer products that unintentionally contain harmful chemicals such as EDs, and to the subsequent replacement of these products. One reason is that most chemists have no training in basic toxicology or an understanding of the science around endocrine-disrupting substances. Therefore, it is crucial that they have access to this science in order to understand the basis of the problem in a language they can absorb and thus enable them to offer viable solution(s). There are many areas where scientists can effectively contribute. For example, some of the most severe examples of endocrine disruption in fish have been found adjacent to sewage treatment plants and near the discharge of effluents from pulp and paper mills. The participation of scientists from interrelated disciplines will yield solutions to various problems arising out of environmental sources of endocrine disruption. Some of the areas include looking at life-cycle effects of chemicals introduced in new products, finding safe substitutes of problematic chemicals, designing of safer chemicals, employing green catalytic processes for remediation of endocrine-disrupting contaminants, and providing inputs to policy and regulatory issues of chemicals.

While specialists in different scientific disciplines such as endocrinology, toxicology, molecular and developmental biology, physiology, and others have peered into the subject, focusing on human health endpoints in the literature in the last decade, there is a distinct lack of a holistic view due to the difficulty in comprehension of this interdisciplinary area. One of the prime objectives of this book is to fill this gap by synthesizing current knowledge relevant to endocrine disruption and reviewing well-studied environmental contaminants. Endocrine toxicology science requires expertise in environmental chemistry, green chemistry, and toxicology including ecotoxicology, endocrinology, developmental biology, epidemiology, and risk assessment. Of course, no one discipline can cover all of these areas, so progress in endocrine disruption science will require collaborations across disciplinary boundaries. Therefore, I hope that this book would be of interest to professionals in these disciplines working or participating in research across the boundary of their specific discipline. It is also my hope that this book would interest scientists in academia and the chemical industry, regulators, as well as environmentalists and policy makers.

Endocrine disruption, which is considered an esoteric science topic, much like global warming was a decade earlier, has lately become mainstream headline news in the media. There were great many skeptics in the linkage of global warming to the generation of CO_2 from anthropogenic sources then, but few can deny this linkage today (with atmospheric CO_2 concentrations reaching 400 ppm versus norm of 275 ppm level) and it is now too late to avoid the negative impacts of climate change, resulting in a steadily warming climate, melting glaciers and the Arctic

Sea, and rapidly spreading droughts. Analogously, for most of the last decade, the science of endocrine disruption has evolved with more definitive evidences of its damaging potential to health and environment. Endocrine disruption can have devastating population-level effects with a potential to change human gender ratio, early puberty, reproductive disruption, infertility, abortions, and life-threatening diseases such as breast cancer in women, prostate cancer in men, and thyroid cancer. Increasingly, science is able to provide the mechanistic basis of multigenerational deleterious effects of low levels exposure to endocrine disruptors.

As in the case of global warming, there is a section of society that has adopted the precautionary approach and moved towards things such as organic foods, avoiding plastic bottles for infant feeding, and so on. Nonetheless, there remains a vast gap in knowledge and awareness of the risks. A February 2013 United Nations report declared EDs a "global threat" to wildlife and humans, particularly infants and children, with close to 800 chemicals known or suspected to disrupt hormone function, but thousands in use that have never been tested. Therefore, it has become imperative to involve a large swath of scientific community to urgently work toward the prevention and cure of its effects. Exposure to EDCs and their effects on human and wildlife health is a global problem that will require global solutions. There is also a need to stimulate new adaptive approaches that break down institutional and traditional scientific barriers and foster collaboration and stimulate interdisciplinary and multidisciplinary team science. I hope that this book would help to contribute toward these goals. For updates on the book contents, please visit www.sushilkhetan.com.

ACKNOWLEDGEMENTS

I am grateful to many of my colleagues in academia and industry who have made useful suggestions for improving this book as a reference source. My special thanks are to Prof. Terry Collins, who inspired me to review the subject from a chemical perspective and graciously wrote the foreword for this book. I especially recognize Dr. Anurag Khetan, Dr. Rick Stahlhut, and Dr. Naseer Ali for offering their critical comments and useful suggestions during various stages of the planning, researching, and writing of this book.

Finally, I would like to acknowledge the constant support of my wife, Manju, who endured countless hours of working on the manuscript. Without her forbearance and understanding, this venture could never have been accomplished.

Sushil K. Khetan

ACRONYMS

ADI	Acceptable daily intake
AGD	Anogenital distance
A^{vy}	Agouti viable yellow
AhR	Arylhydrocarbon receptor
AOP	Advanced oxidation process
AR	Androgen receptor
ARE	Androgen response elements
AST	Accessory sex tissues
BBP	Butyl benzyl phthalate
BDE	Brominated diphenyl ether
BDE-209	Decabromo diphenyl ether
BMI	Body mass index
BPs	Biotransformation products
BPA	Bisphenol A
BPS	Bisphenol A sulfate
BPAF	Hexafluoro-bisphenol A
CA	Concentration addition, also known as dose addition (DA)
cAMP	Cyclic adenosine monophosphate
CAR	Constitutive androstane receptor
CpG	Cytosine–phosphate–guanine sites
CDC	Center for Disease Control and Prevention
CDPH	California Department of Public Health

CHO	Chinese hamster ovary
CGI	CpG island
ChIP	Cromatin immunoprecipitation
CYP450	Cytochrome $P450$ enzyme
p, p′-**DDE**	2,2-Bis(*p*-chlorophenyl)-1,1-dichloroethene
o, p′-**DDT**	2-(*o*-Chlorophenyl)-2-(*p*-chlorophenyl)-1,1,1-trichloroethane
p, p′-**DDT**	2,2-Bis(*p*-chlorophenyl)-1,1,1-trichloroethane
DBAD	Developmental basis of adult disease
DBP	Di-*n*-butyl phthalate
DCDD	Dichlorodibenzo-*p*-dioxin
DE	Diphenyl ether
DEHP	Di(2-ethylhexyl) phthalate
DES	Diethylstilbestrol
DHT	5α-Dihydrotestosterone
DNA	Deoxyribonucleic acid
DNMT	DNA methyltransferase
DOP	Di-*n*-octyl phthalate
dsRNA	Double-stranded RNA
DWTP	Drinking water treatment plant
ECs	Emerging contaminants
E1	Estrone
E2	17β-Estradiol
EE2	17α-Ethinylestradiol
EGF	Epidermal growth factor
ED	Endocrine disruptor
EDC	Endocrine disrupting chemical
EDSP	Endocrine disruptor screening program
EDSTAC	Endocrine Disruptor Screening and Testing Advisory Committee
ER	Estrogen receptor
mER	Membrane-associated ER
ERR	Estrogen-related receptor
ESC	Embryonic stem cell
EU	European Union
F0	Mother (F0 generation)
F1	Developing embryo (first generation)
Fn	*n*th generation
FDA	Food and Drug Administration
Fe-TAML	Iron-tetraamido macrocyclic ligand
FeTsPc	Iron-tetrasulfophthalocyanine
FQPA	Food Quality Protection Act

FSH	Follicle stimulating hormone
GD	Gestational day
GLP	Good laboratory practice
GnRH	Gonadotropin-releasing hormone
GPR30	G-Protein-coupled receptor 30
GR	Glucocorticoid receptor
HAA	Hormonally active agents
HAT	Histone acetyltransferase
HDAC	Histone deacetylase
HOMO	Highest occupied molecular orbital
HPA	Hypothalamus–pituitary–adrenal
HPG	Hypothalamus–pituitary–gonadal
HPT	Hypothalamus–pituitary–thyroidal
HPTE	Bis(*p*-hydroxy phenyl)-1,1,1-trichloroethane (a metabolite of methoxychlor)
HRE	Hormone response elements
HRP	Horseradish peroxidase
HTS	High throughput screen
IA	Independent action
IGF	Insulin-like growth factor
IPCS	International Program on Chemical Safety
LH	Luteinizing hormone
LUMO	Lowest unoccupied molecular orbital
M1	Vinclozolin metabolite 1
M2	Vinclozolin metabolite 2
MBC	Methylbenzylidene camphor
MBR	Membrane bioreactor
MCF-7	Human breast cancer cell line, the acronym refers to the institute where the cell line was established
MCL	Maximum contaminant level
MEHP	Mono-2-ethylhexyl phthalate
MMA	Monomethyl arsenite
MOA	Mechanism of action
mRNA	Messenger RNA
miRNA	MicroRNA
NADPH	Nicotinamide adenine dinucleotide phosphate
ncRNA	Noncoding RNA
NIH	National Institute of Health
NIS	Sodium–iodine symporter
NOAEL	No observed adverse effect level

NOEC	The highest tested dose of a substance that has been reported to have no harmful (adverse) health effects
NPE	Nonylphenol ethoxylate
NRs	Nuclear hormone receptors
NIEHS	National Institute of Environmental Health Sciences
NOEL	No observed effect level
NPs	Nonylphenols
NPEOs	Nonylphenol polyethoxylates
NTP	National Toxicology Program
NR	Nipple retention
OC	Organochlorine
OECD	Organization for Economic Cooperation and Development
4-OHT	4-Hydroxy tamoxifen (an antagonist of ERs)
OMC	Octylmethoxy-cinnamate
OP	Organophosphorus
PBDE	Polybrominated diphenyl ether
PCBs	Polychlorinated biphenyls
PCDD	Polychlorinated dibenzodioxins
PCDF	Polychlorinated dibenzofurans
PET	Polyethylene terephthalate
PFOA	Perfluorooctanoate
PFCs	Perfluorinated compounds
PFOS	Perfluorooctane sulfonate
PHAHs	Polyhalogenated aromatic hydrocarbons
PPARs	Peroxisome-proliferator-activated receptors
PPCPs	Pharmaceuticals and personal care products
PND	Postnatal day
PNEC	Predicted-no-effect concentration
POM	Polyoxometallate
PVC	Polyvinyl chloride
QSAR	Quantitative structure–activity relationship
RBA	Relative binding affinity
REACH	Registration, evaluation, authorization, and restriction of chemicals
RISC	RNA-induced silencing complex
RNA	Ribonucleic acid
RO	Reverse osmosis
ROS	Reactive oxygen species
RXR	Retinoid X receptor
SDWA	Safe Drinking Water Act

siRNA	Small interfering RNA
STP	Sewage treatment plant
SULT	Sulfotransferase enzyme
TBT	Tributyltin
T	Testosterone
T3	Deiodinized thyroxine
T4	Thyroxine
TBBPA	3,3′,5,5′-Tetrabromo-bisphenol A
TCs	Trace contaminants
TCBPA	3,3′,5,5′-Tetrachloro-bisphenol A
TCDD	Tetrachlorodibenzo-p-dioxin
TDCs	Thyroid disrupting chemicals
TDI	Tolerable daily intake
TDS	Testicular dysgenesis syndrome
TH	Thyroid hormone
TiPED	Tiered protocol for endocrine disruption
TSCA	Toxic Substances Control Act
TR	Thyroid hormone receptor
TRE	Thyroid hormone responsive element
TRH	Thyrotropin-releasing hormone
TSH	Thyroid-stimulating hormone
TTC	Threshold of toxicological concern
TTR	Transthyretin
TEF/TEQ	TCDD equivalency factor – TCDD equivalents
UGTs	UDP-gucuronosyltransferases
USGS	United States Geological Survey
UV	Ultraviolet
VTG	vitellogenin
VZ	Vinclozolin
WFD	Water Framework Directive
WHO	World Health Organization
WWF	World Wildlife Federation
WWTP	Waste water treatment plant
YES	Yeast estrogen screen – *in vitro* assay for xenoestrogens using yeast cells
ZEN	Zearalenone
ZVAl	zero-valent aluminum
ZVI	zero-valent iron

GLOSSARY

Additive effect
A biologic response to exposure to multiple substances that equals the sum of responses of all the individual substances added together.

Adipocyte
A cell specialized in storage of fat.

Adverse effect
A change in morphology, physiology, growth, reproduction, development, or lifespan of an organism that results in impairment of functional capacity or impairment of capacity to compensate for additional stress or increased susceptibility to the harmful effects of other environmental influences.

Agonist
A ligand that binds to and activates a receptor and elicits a physiological response.

Allosteric
Activity of an enzyme that results from combination with a substance at a point other than the chemically active site.

Androgen
A sex steroid hormone that stimulates or controls the development and maintenance of male characteristics in vertebrates by binding to androgen receptors, for example, testosterone.

Anogenital distance
The distance from the anus to the genitalia, the base of the penis or vagina.

Antagonist
Any ligand that blocks binding of endogenous agonists to the receptor, thereby modulating receptor activity.

Antiandrogen	Chemicals that acts as an antagonist at the androgen receptor or otherwise interferes with the effects of endogenous androgens.
Bioaccumulation	Accumulation of a toxic substance in various tissues of a living organism. Bioaccumulation occurs when the rate of intake of a substance is greater than the rate of excretion or metabolic transformation of that substance.
Cell division	Separation of a cell into two daughter cells – in higher eukaryotes, it involves division of the nucleus (mitosis) and the cytoplasm (cytokinesis); mitosis often is used to refer to both nuclear and cytoplasmic division.
Chromatin	A DNA–protein complex consisting of chromosomes. Histones are the primary protein components of chromatin that serve to compact the tightly coiled DNA.
Cryptorchidism	Testicular nondescent (failure of testicular descent into the scrotum).
Developmental toxicity	Any adverse effect induced prior to attainment of adult life including effects induced or manifested in the embryonic or fetal period and those induced or manifested postnatally.
DNA methylation	A key epigenetic mechanism involving the biochemical process of the conversion of cytosine (within a CpG dinucleotide) into 5-methyl cytosine in DNA, which has the effect of reducing gene expression.
End point	Measurable parameter that indicates a preceding exposure or the effect of a chemical; it constitutes one of the target observations of the trial.
Epidemiology	Study of disease distribution in defined populations, and of factors that influence the occurrence of disease including environmental and personal characteristics.
Epididymis	A coiled tube through which sperm exits the testes.
Epigenetics	The study of factors that influence heritable changes to gene expression without alterations to the underlying DNA sequence, mostly mediated by DNA methylation and histone modifications.
Endogenous	Naturally occurring or produced within an organism.

E-Screen	Human breast cancer cell proliferation assay that measures growth of MCF-7 cells *in vitro* in response to endocrine substances.
Exogenous	Not naturally occurring or produced within an organism.
Fertility	Reproductive competence.
Gametes	Reproductive cells that unite during sexual reproduction to form a new cell called a *zygote*. In humans, male gametes are sperm and female gametes are ova (eggs).
Gametogenesis	Germ-line-specific epigenetic reprogramming.
Germ cells	The spermatozoa and their precursors in males or the ova [eggs] and their precursors in females.
Gonad	Ovaries in females, testes in males; an organ that produces cells and hormones necessary for reproduction.
Histone	A family of simple proteins, abundant in the cell nucleus and constituting a substantial part of the protein-and-DNA complex known as *chromatin*.
Hormone	Any extracellular substance that induces specific responses in target cells. Coordinate the growth, differentiation, and metabolic activities of various cells, tissues, and organs in multicellular organisms.
Homeostasis	Physiological processes that maintain the internal environment of the body in balance.
Hoxa10	An estrogen-regulated gene necessary for uterine development and pregnancy.
Hypospadias	Penile malformations (an abnormality of development of the penis in which the urethra does not open at the tip of the organ).
Hypothalamus–pituitary–gonadal axis	The reproductive system of vertebrates, comprising the hypothalamus at the base of the brain, the anterior pituitary gland, and the gonads (ovary or testis).
Imposex	A type of intersexuality, in which females develop male sexual organs.
Imprinting	A process by which one allele of a gene is expressed from the parental genome. Specifically, one allele of a gene is silenced by epigenetic mechanisms, resulting in expression of only the paternal or maternal allele of a gene. These epigenetic patterns are determined in the germ cells and inherited in the next generation.

Inheritance	Transmission of information between generations of an organism.
In utero	An event occurring within the uterus of a mammal during pregnancy; describes the state of an embryo or fetus.
In vitro	Biological study outside of a living organism, in a controlled environment such as in a cell culture or in cells grown in a petri dish.
In vivo	Experimentation using a whole living organism.
Lydig cell	The testosterone producing cells of the testis.
Malformation	A permanent alteration (abnormality) in which there is a morphologic defect of an organ or a larger region of the body, resulting from an abnormal developmental process and/or will adversely affect survival, growth, or development of functional competence.
MicroRNA (miRNA)	Small lengths of RNA that are not translated into proteins.
Narcosis	A disturbance in the cell membrane permeability by hydrophobic chemicals.
Neonatal	The newborn infants.
Nuclear receptor	General term for intracellular receptors whose members reside in the nucleus that bind lipid-soluble hormones (e.g., steroid hormones); they can bind directly to DNA, either activating or repressing gene expression. Nuclear receptors are therefore transcription factors.
Parabens	*p*-Hydroxybenzoates – preservatives.
Perinatal	Period leading up to birth and after.
Plasma membrane	The membrane surrounding a cell that separates the cell from its external environment, consisting of a phospholipid bilayer and associated proteins.
Pleiotropic	Producing more than one effect.
Precautionary principle	Where there are threats of serious or irreversible damage, lack of full scientific certainty shall not be used as a reason for postponing cost-effective measures to prevent environmental degradation.
Preputial separation	Separation of the foreskin of the penis from the glans penis.
Puberty	Bodily changes of sexual maturation, such as vaginal opening or balanopreputial separation.

Receptor (cell receptor)   A protein molecule, embedded in either the plasma membrane or the cytoplasm of a cell that binds a specific extracellular signaling molecule (ligand) and then initiates a cellular response. Receptors for steroid hormones, which diffuse across the plasma membrane, are located within the cell; receptors for water-soluble hormones, peptide growth factors, and neurotransmitters are located in the plasma membrane with their ligand-binding domain exposed to the external medium.

RNA interference   A mechanism that inhibits gene expression at the stage of translation or by hindering the transcription of specific genes. This method has been referred to as post-transcriptional gene silencing and is an important tool for gene expression.

Reproductive toxicity   Structural and/or functional alterations that may affect reproductive competence in sexually mature males and females, manifested as impairment of fertility, parturition, or lactation.

Signal transduction   Conversion of a signal from one physical or chemical form into another. In cell biology, it commonly refers to the sequential process initiated by binding of an extracellular signal to a receptor and culminating in one or more specific cellular responses.

Seminal vesicles   Pouches located above the prostate that store semen.

Spermatogenesis   The process initiated in the male testis with the beginning of puberty of sperm cell development.

Steroidogenesis   The biological synthesis of steroid hormones.

Sustainability   Attaining a society and environment that can meet its current needs while preserving the ability of future generations to meet their needs (Brundtland Commission)

Testicular dysgenesis syndrome   Spectrum of reproductive disorders that originate in male fetal life including poor sperm quality (impaired spermatogenesis), cryptorchidism, hypospadias, and testicular cancer.

Totipotent   A single cell that has the capability of developing into any kind of cell. In mammals, the zygote and the embryo during early stages of development are totipotent.

Transcription   A protein that binds directly to a recognized DNA sequence, thereby factor playing a role in gene regulation. Transcription factors called *activators* may increase a gene's expression, while repressors may decrease expression.

Translation   The process that converts an mRNA sequence into a string of amino acids that form a protein. Translation follows transcription.

Transgenic   A term describing an organism containing genetic material from a source other than its parents.

Transgenerational effects   Effects that are observed not only in an exposed organism but also in that organism's offspring and future generations.

Vas deferens   A part of the male anatomy of many vertebrates; they transport sperm from the epididymis in anticipation of ejaculation.

Vitellogenin   An egg yolk protein present in female fish but generally absent in male fish.

Water resources   A general term encompassing all water types that may include groundwater, lakes, streams, rivers, wetlands, drinking water, estuaries, coastal waters, and marine waters.

Wolffian duct   A duct in the embryo that becomes the vas deferens in the male and forms the urinary duct in the female.

Xenobiotic   A substance, typically a synthetic chemical, that is foreign to an ecological system or to the body.

Xenoestrogen   Synthetic chemicals with estrogenic properties.

Zygote   A fertilized egg; diploid cell resulting from fusion of a male and female gamete.

As the tide of chemicals born of the Industrial Age has arisen to engulf our environment, a drastic change has come about in the nature of the most serious public health problems.

Rachel Carson, Silent Spring, 1962

It is now clear that a single chemical can have an impact on multiple systems, via several exposure pathways and via a number of modes of action, and expressed in multiple ways over the period of a lifetime. These findings, that traditional toxicology continues to miss, have dire implications for public and environmental health.

Theo Colborn, 2009

1

ENVIRONMENTAL ENDOCRINE DISRUPTORS

1.1 INTRODUCTION

Many man-made chemicals used in industrial and agricultural applications are now widely dispersed as contaminants in the environment. The original uses of these include as pesticides, plasticizers, antimicrobials, and flame-retardants. These chemicals are typically stable in the environment and most are present at small concentrations. The population is exposed to these chemicals in air, water, food, and also sometimes as ingredients in consumer and personal care products. Some of these chemicals have a significant potential to interfere with normal biological functions and cause adverse health effects. Ubiquitously present in the environment, these chemicals may interfere with our bodies' complex and carefully regulated hormonal messenger systems by mimicking or antagonizing the actions of the endogenous hormones. These chemicals as a group are referred to as *endocrine disruptor chemicals (EDCs)*. As most synthetic compounds have been present in our biosphere since recently in human and vertebrate evolutionary history, biological evolution has not had enough time to evolve mechanisms against their potential adverse effects.

1.1.1 The Endocrine System

Endocrine system and nervous system constitute the two main regulatory systems in mammalian physiology. The endocrine system regulates biological processes in the body from conception through adulthood, including general growth and the development of the brain and nervous system, the growth and function of the reproductive system, and metabolism and blood-sugar levels. The human endocrine system

Endocrine Disruptors in the Environment, First Edition. Sushil K. Khetan.
© 2014 John Wiley & Sons, Inc. Published 2014 by John Wiley & Sons, Inc.

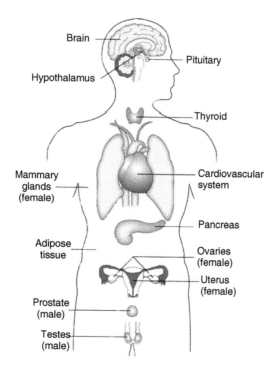

Figure 1.1   Endocrine systems include brain and hypothalamic neuroendocrine systems, pituitary, thyroid, cardiovascular system, mammary gland, adipose tissue, and pancreas; ovary and uterus in females; and testes and prostate in males. All these hormone-sensitive physiological systems are vulnerable to EDCs. Source: Adapted from Diamanti-Kandarakis et al., 2009. Reproduced with permission of Endocrine Society.

is an extensive network of hormone-producing glands comprising hypothalamus, pituitary, thyroid, and organs such as female ovaries, male testes, and pancreas as major constituents (Fig. 1.1). These endocrine glands and organs produce and secrete carefully measured amounts of different types of hormones that perform different functions. Hormones are transported throughout the body via the bloodstream exerting physiological effects on their target cells. The target cells for each hormone are characterized by the presence of certain docking molecules, a class of proteins known as receptors. The interaction between the hormone and its receptor triggers a cascade of biochemical reactions in the target cell that eventually modify the cell's function or activity.

Hormones act at very low blood concentrations and are characterized by their specificity of action on certain tissues and organs. The timing of the hormonal secretion and delivery is critical and carefully orchestrated to maintain the body's homeostasis (the body's ability to maintain itself in the presence of external and internal changes), and to the body's ability to control and regulate reproduction, development, and/or behavior. Human health depends on a well-functioning endocrine system to regulate the release of certain hormones that are essential for functions such as metabolism, growth and development, and sleep and mood. Some substances known as *endocrine disruptors* (EDs) can change the function(s) of this hormonal system increasing the risk of adverse health effects.

1.1.2 Endocrine Disrupting Chemicals (EDCs)

EDCs mostly act as mimetic to natural hormones, but some of the EDCs can antagonize the action or modify the synthesis, metabolism, and transport of the endogenous hormones, producing a range of developmental, reproductive, neurological, immune, or metabolic diseases in humans and wildlife. According to the U.S. Environmental Protection Agency (EPA), EDCs have been described as exogenous agents that interfere with the production, release, transport, metabolism, binding, or elimination of the natural hormones in the body responsible for the maintenance of homeostasis and the regulation of developmental processes (Kavlock et al., 1996). The European Union and WHO definition proposes an ED as "an exogenous substance that causes adverse health effects in an intact organism, or its progeny, consequent to changes in endocrine function" (Damstra et al., 2002). There appear to be significant differences between the EPA and European definition, as the EPA merely requires interference with the endocrine system, the European definition explicitly requires *in vivo* evidence that a substance actually causes harm to the organism. However, these two definitions can be considered complementary, as both indicate that the effects induced by EDs probably involve mechanisms relating in some way to hormonal homeostasis and action (Cravedi et al., 2007). A recent Endocrine Society statement stipulated the ability of a chemical to interfere with hormone action as a clear predictor of adverse outcome, endorsing the EPA definition of EDC that focuses on its ability to interfere with hormone action rather than stipulate adverse outcome (Zoeller et al., 2012). Thus, ED was described in the statement more simply as "an exogenous chemical, or mixture of chemicals, that interferes with any aspect of hormone action" (Zoeller et al., 2012). Earlier, a panel constituted by the National Academy of Sciences, chose to describe such compounds as *hormonally active agent (HAA)*, as it was feared that the language of disruption unjustifiably encourages the notion that any interference or influence on the endocrine system is harmful or "disruptive" (NRC, 1999).

The concept of endocrine disruption, the inappropriate modulation of the endocrine system by dietary and environmental chemicals, as a mode of action for xenobiotic chemicals in animals first burst into prominence with the publication of *Our Stolen Future* by Theo Colborn, Dianne Dumanoski and John Peterson Myers, which is often credited for garnering major public attention to the concern about the hazards posed by EDCs (Colborn et al., 1996). It brought up the issue of man-made chemicals threatening the reproductive capability and intelligence of future generations of humans and wildlife. She and other authors proposed that many EDCs elicited effects at doses far lower than toxicities caused by other modes of action and thus required special regulation (Colborn et al., 1993; Colborn et al, 1996). Since then, the topic has generated considerable controversy. Much of this controversy centers on determining what chemicals cause detectable adverse effects at exposure levels typically experienced by humans or animals.

EDCs comprise a broad-class of exogenous substances, many man-made chemicals that are widely dispersed in the environment and compounds that can bind steroid hormone receptors. Some chemicals with endocrine disrupting effects are legacy pollutants, such as pesticides and heavy metals, and many are emerging contaminants (Fig. 1.2). Many of these newer compounds are industrial contaminants, such as phthalates (used in the manufacture of plastics to make it pliable), bisphenol A (BPA; used in plastics to make it harder, clearer, and more resistant to heat stress), alkyl phenols (present in detergents and surfactants), polychlorinated biphenyls (PCBs; formerly used in electrical equipment), dioxins (released from incinerators), organochlorine pesticides and organohalogens (used as flame-retardants), and triazine herbicides (atrazine and simazine). There also are pharmaceuticals purposely designed to have hormonal activity, such as diethylstilbestrol (DES), contraceptive agents, and others that are used in the treatment of diseases such as osteoporosis. These xenobiotic compounds have a wide range of chemical structures but all of them have the capacity to disrupt normal hormonal actions. Even though the intended use of pesticides, plasticizers, antimicrobials, and flame-retardants is beneficial, effects on human health are a global concern. Some naturally occurring EDCs can also be found in plants or fungi, such as the so-called phytoestrogens: genistein, daidzein, or the mycoestrogen zearalenone.

1.1.3 Sources of EDCs in the Environment

EDCs can originate from numerous sources and enter the environment by many routes. From the air, soil, and water, EDCs enter the food chain, and because some of these compounds are lipophilic and persistent, they have the potential to bioaccumulate and become a part of a plant's or animal's body burden and biomagnify in higher trophic levels.

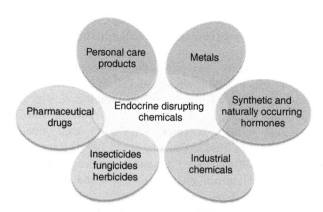

Figure 1.2 Grouping of chemicals of some potential endocrine disruptors.

Discharges from municipal wastewater treatment plants (WWTPs) have been identified as significant contributors of EDCs to surface waters (Kolpin et al., 2002; Legler et al., 2002; Snyder et al., 2003). The actual sources are upstream discharges to the treatment facilities, which include natural hormones and pharmaceutical estrogens excreted by humans flushed down home toilets, pharmaceuticals and personal care products (PPCPs) excreted or washed from the body, plant material, items treated with fire retardants, other household cleaning products, and pesticides (Staples et al., 1998; Ying et al., 2002; Snyder et al., 2003). WWTPs might also receive effluents from industrial processes that use cleaners containing nonylphenols and plastics containing BPA or hospital and storm water runoff streams that contain EDCs (Boyd et al., 2004) (Fig. 1.3).

However, WWTP effluents and reclaimed water are not the only sources of EDCs to the environment. Discharges from fish hatcheries and dairy facilities (Kolodziej et al., 2004), fish spawning in natural waters (Kolodziej et al., 2004), runoff from agricultural fields and livestock feeding operations (Orlando et al., 2004; Soto et al., 2004), and land amended with biosolids or manure (Hanselman et al., 2003; Khanal et al., 2006) also contribute as nonpoint sources for EDCs in the aquatic environment. In addition, the potential exists for agricultural runoff containing pesticides and fertilizers to contain the estrogenic surfactants (e.g., nonylphenol ethoxylates) that make up the chemical formulation (Staples et al., 1998; Ying et al., 2002). Other potential sources include private septic systems (Swartz et al., 2006), untreated stormwater flows and urban runoff (Boyd et al., 2004), industrial effluents (Kosaka et al., 2007), landfill leachate (Coors et al., 2003), and atmospheric deposition. Human exposure can occur via the ingestion of food, dust and water, inhalation of gases and particles in the air, and skin contact.

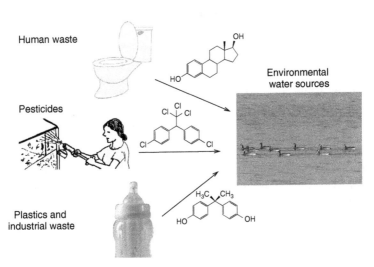

Figure 1.3 Sources of EDCs in environmental waters.

1.1.4   Deleterious Effects of EDCs on Wildlife and on Humans

Exposure to EDCs in water has been associated with a range of reproductive impacts, particularly in fish, including the induction of intersex (presence of both male and female sex organs) (Jobling et al., 1998), lowered hormone levels (Folmar et al. 1996), and reduced gamete production and fertilization capability (Jobling et al., 2002). WWTP effluents contain a mixture of known or potential EDCs. In most cases researchers have been unable to pinpoint the specific chemicals responsible for effects indicating endocrine disruption in exposed fish. Estradiol, estrone, ethinylestradiol, nonylphenol, octylphenol, alkylphenol ethoxylates, and BPA have been identified as likely causes (Purdom et al., 1994; Damstra et al., 2002) based on their concentrations in wastewater effluents and their potency in laboratory studies.

The adverse effects of EDCs have become an important issue drawing public attention, especially since the link between synthetic birth control pharmaceuticals (e.g., ethinylestradiol) and their toxicological impact on fish was reported (Nash et al., 2004). These concerns have primarily been related to adverse effects observed in wildlife. In wildlife, EDCs are suspected in the decline of certain species (e.g., possible increased sterility in the American alligator), change of sex in fish and shellfish (Vos et al., 2000), eggshell thinning in birds and reptiles, and other problems. As hormone receptor systems function similarly in humans and animals, these observations have raised concern of potential human health effects.

With regard to humans, evidence is limited and inconsistent to clearly establish a causal inference; however, accumulating data is circumstantial evidence linking EDCs to reproductive disorders and disturbed thyroid homeostasis. Key data are the increased incidences of malformations of the reproductive organs in newborn boys, early onset of puberty in girls, as well as increased incidence of certain endocrine-related human diseases. Laboratory studies are correlating the developmental exposure to EDCs with a growing list of adverse health consequences in both males and females. In males, EDCs have been associated with decreases in semen quality/sperm count (Li et al., 2011), testicular germ cell cancer (Chia et al., 2010), and urogenital tract malformation (Fernandez and Olea, 2012). Similarly, EDCs are associated with numerous female reproductive disorders, affecting puberty and breast cancer (Crain et al., 2008; Roy et al., 2009).

Recent research has shown that EDCs also affect physiological systems that control fat development, weight gain, and glucose levels. Endocrine control of glucose homeostasis can impact development of diabetes, obesity, and cardiovascular diseases (Thayer et al., 2012; Newbold, 2010). Some EDCs can transmit health problems across generations, so that exposures during pregnancy can create health problems for several generations. Nonetheless, specific mechanisms by which substances disrupt the endocrine systems are very complex, likely due to time of impact and space being extended, and not yet completely understood.

1.1.5   Endocrine Disruption Endpoints

Endocrine disruption end-effect may be a functional change but is not considered to be toxicological endpoints *per se* as is cancer or allergy, but more as a mode of action leading to outcomes such as carcinogenic, reproductive, or developmental effects. These functional changes may or may not lead to an adverse event (Damstra et al., 2002). An adverse effect that is manifested in a physiological outcome in an animal only would be considered as a toxicological endpoint. Primarily reproductive toxicity and impaired development are seen as the well-established endpoints of endocrine disruption. These gross changes observed *in vivo* can offer presumptive evidence of the toxicity of the chemical or compound under study (CSTEE, 2000).

The three major endocrine disruption endpoints studied are estrogenic (compounds that mimic or block natural estrogens), androgenic (compounds that mimic or block natural testosterone), and thyroidal (compounds with direct and/or indirect impacts on the thyroid) (Snyder et al., 2003). However, EDCs can act via more than one mechanism. Some EDCs have mixed steroidal properties. For example, a single EDC may be both estrogenic and antiandrogenic. EDCs may be broken down or metabolized to generate by-products with different properties. For instance, the estrogen agonist DDT is metabolized into the androgen antagonist DDE (Diamanti-Kandarakis et al., 2009).

Finally, many EDCs may have actions via (or independent of) classic actions at cognate steroid receptors. More recently, studies have shown the activity of the retinoid X receptor (RXR), and peroxisome proliferator-activated receptors (PPARs) to be targets for EDC action. EDCs can affect these systems in several different ways; for example, by directly interfering with receptor signaling or by activating other signaling pathways, in particular that of the aryl hydrocarbon receptor (AhR), a receptor involved in the metabolism of many xenobiotic substances. Thus, all members of the nuclear hormone receptor family are potential targets of EDCs. Chemicals also interfere with metabolism, fat storage, bone development, and the immune system, and this suggests that all endocrine systems can and will be affected by EDCs (UNEP/WHO, 2012).

1.2 SALIENT ASPECTS ABOUT ENDOCRINE DISRUPTION

A number of salient points have emerged defining the specific features of endocrine disruption. While EDCs having effects at high dose and low doses are both of concern, in reality the ones active at low doses are the ones that make it past the typical toxicity screens and are thus of most concern. The EDCs generally occur in the environment as complex chemical mixtures, not single compounds; their impacts can vary substantially over the life cycle of an organism and are often particularly severe during gestation and early development, their impacts can occur long after exposure and many EDCs exhibit transgenerational (epigenetic) impacts.

1.2.1 Low-Dose Effects and Nonmonotonic Dose Responses

It is well established that natural hormones act at extremely low serum concentrations, typically in the picomolar to nanomolar range. Because of shared receptor-mediated mechanisms, EDCs that mimic natural hormones have been proposed to follow the same rules and therefore have biological effects at low doses (Welshons et al., 2003).

Low-dose effects, postulated as typical for EDCs, are defined as biologic changes that occur in the range of human exposures or at doses lower than those typically used in the standard testing paradigm of the U.S. EPA for evaluating reproductive and developmental toxicity (Melnick et al., 2002). Risk assessments for virtually all chemicals, except genotoxic chemicals, assume that, for any substance, there exists a threshold dose below which exposure is safe. However, early studies of EDCs in sensitive animal models have established examples in which no lower threshold dose could be detected; that is, effects were already apparent at the lowest doses tested.

The endocrine system is tuned to respond to very low concentrations of hormone. The typical physiological levels of endogenous hormones are in the range of 10–900 pg/ml for estradiol, 300–10,000 pg/ml for testosterone, and 8–27 pg/ml for thyroid hormone (T4) (Vandenberg et al., 2012). Similarly, EDCs that influence in any way the production, metabolism, uptake, or release of hormones also have effects at low doses, because even small changes in hormone concentration can have biologically important consequences (Welshons et al., 2003). There is also evidence that EDCs work additively or even synergistically with other chemicals and natural hormones in the body (Carpenter et al., 2002). Thus, it is plausible that some of the low-dose effects of an EDC are actually effects of that exogenous chemical plus the effects of endogenous hormone (Vandenberg et al., 2012).

Moreover, there are some EDCs whose effects can be seen at low doses but not at high doses, in opposition to the usual dose–response curve familiar to toxicologists, which shows continually increasing responses with increases in dose (vom Saal et al., 1997). Much like endogenous hormones, which exert their physiological actions through receptors and exhibit nonlinear dose–response relationships, EDCs display a general characteristic of a nonlinear relationship between doses and effect where the slope of the curve changes sign somewhere within the range of doses examined (Vandenberg et al., 2012; EPA, 2013). The dose–response curves can be shaped like an inverted U (Fig. 1.4a), in which low doses increase the response with greatest response at intermediate dose levels, and high doses decrease the response, or like a U with a high response at both low and high levels of exposure (Fig. 1.4b). In some cases the slope of the curve reverses sign at multiple points along the curve (Fig. 1.4c), which could reflect different mechanisms of action at different concentrations. These curves do not conform to the traditional expectations of toxicology, which states that an increase in dose is matched by an increase in effect (Welshons et al., 2003).

Two well-known examples of nonmonotonicity are Lupron used to treat reproductive disorders in women and men and tamoxifen (an ER antagonist) used to treat breast cancer, in which low doses stimulate while high doses inhibit disease. A phenomenon known as low dose "flare" occurs for both of these drugs during which there is stimulation of the response that the drug inhibits when the blood level of the drug is at the high clinically effective dose range (for example, testosterone secretion in men with prostate cancer for Lupron, and proliferation of mammary tissue in women with breast cancer for tamoxifen) (Myers et al., 2009).

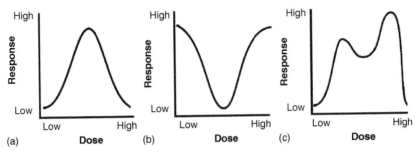

Figure 1.4 Three different types of nonmonotonic dose–response curves. The slope changes sign one or more times in all of these curves (EPA, 2013).

Dose–response relationship for individual endocrine toxicants can be an important piece of evidence in the determination of the risk posed by exposure to the toxicant. If some EDCs act directly on receptors, low levels of exposure, particularly during developmentally critical period, can disrupt hormone actions. If the concentration of EDC is higher, it may inhibit receptor-mediated action by down regulation of receptor levels, in which the body reacts to hormonal overstimulation by reducing the number of hormone receptors it produces (Myers et al., 2009). There is also evidence that nonmonotonic dose–response curves are generated by the integration of two or more monotonic dose–response curves that occur through different pathways affecting a common endpoint with opposing effects (Vandenberg et al., 2009; Soto et al., 1995). A 2007 NIEHS-sponsored review of studies of *in vivo* effects of an estrogenic plastic leachate BPA, for example, identified evidence for effects of low-dose exposure during development on subsequent brain structure, function, and behavior in rats and mice. BPA on low-dose exposure in mice also produces prostate enlargement with an inverted U-shaped dose–response curve (vom Saal et al., 1997).

The endocrine system acts like a thermostat, through self-regulating feedback loops. Receptors typically respond to very low levels of hormone, similarly low levels of an endocrine mimic may activate them, whereas high levels of a chemical may actually cause receptors to shut down altogether, preventing any further response. Very high doses, however, can overwhelm the system and cause damage and even death. It is the body's responses to BPA at very low doses, operating well under traditional toxicology's no observed effect level that has been found to result in deleterious effects on mice (Endocrine Disruption Exchange, 2009). The classic example of lead shows that there is no "safe" dose at which no negative effects are found (Lanphear et al., 2005). Thus, traditional toxicological assumptions based on the monotonic dose–response curve, in which more of the chemical leads to a greater effect, may not be applicable to assess the toxicity of EDCs.

1.2.2 Exposures during Periods of Heightened Susceptibility in Critical Life Stages

In cases of endocrine disruption, exposure levels affect organisms during critical organizational periods of early life stages (Guillette et al. 1995). Endocrine disruption can be profound because of the crucial role hormones play in controlling development (Colborn and Clement, 1992). During development, the genome of the cells that make up tissues and organs become programmed to specify their function in the adult. Because the hormones are naturally present in the body, addition of any hormone-like material from the environment into the body can elicit adverse effects at much lower doses than a toxicant.

There are critical windows of developmental sensitivity to natural or exogenous hormones or hormone-like molecules. In mammals, the late embryonic/early postnatal period is considered a critical period for brain development and sexual differentiation, during which even very short-term exposure to a hormone, or the lack thereof, causes adverse, permanent and irreversible molecular changes in the brain (Gore, 2008). Later in life, in response to increased gonadal steroid hormones during puberty, these organizational effects of hormones on the brain are manifested as appropriate masculine or feminine reproductive physiology and behavior. Adult mammals have feedback mechanisms that can cope with at least some variation in hormone levels. Those mechanisms may not be active during embryonic development, a time at which it is thought animals are most susceptible to the effects of endocrine disrupters. Therefore, EDC exposure during the critical periods of brain development and sexual differentiation is particularly detrimental.

Although hormone signaling is normally reversible and induces dynamic changes in cellular function, during development EDCs can induce permanent effects on gene activity that enable cellular and tissue differentiation. Hormonal effects in the fetus are much more profound because they affect gene expression that governs development of organs as well as lifelong hormonal "set points," such as receptor numbers and hormonal production.

The exquisite sensitivity of the developing fetus and neonate is suggested to be due to numerous factors including undeveloped DNA repair mechanisms, an immature immune system, lack of detoxifying enzymes, primitive liver metabolism, lack of development of the blood/brain barrier, and an increased metabolic rate (Bern, 1992). Numerous studies exist where age of exposure is a known risk factor. Thus, exposure of an adult to an EDC may have very different consequences from exposure to a developing fetus or infant.

The hormonal environment of the developing fetus is protected from endogenous steroids by conjugation to binding proteins produced by the mother and the placenta. In mammals, steroid-hormone-binding globulins regulate the accessibility of sex-steroids to various organs. For example, bound estradiol is unable to pass the blood brain barrier, whereas unbound testosterone has relatively high access to the brain (Pardridge et al. 1980). Little is known about the effects of EDCs on these proteins, or the extent to which they bind. It is therefore not possible to exclude the possibility that some chemicals, because of their particular properties, could more readily gain access to, or accumulate in, the fetus in amounts sufficient to cause effects.

Metabolization of compounds may be faster in children, but detoxification in them is much slow, resulting in greater body burdens due to higher dietary intakes in relation to the body size, compared to adults (Jacobs, 2001). Therefore, at this stage of life, they are sensitive to changes in the hormonal milieu, or chemical exposure, which can result in organizational changes that are permanent. Even very subtle effects on the endocrine system can result in changes in growth, development, reproduction, or neurologically driven behavior that can affect the organism itself, or the next generation. An exposure to the ED does not need to be chronic, as transient exposure at a critical time during development is all that is required (Damstra et al., 2002).

1.2.3 Delayed Dysfunction

Fetal exposure to EDCs at critical time points, especially during early development when cells are differentiating and tissues are developing, will have harmful health effects that do not become evident until puberty and adulthood.

Animal models consistently demonstrate that low-dose exposures of fetuses to EDCs often have no discernible effects at birth, but result in infertility, abnormalities, and cancers much later in life (Welshons et al., 2006). A compelling example comes from humans, as millions of women who took the estrogenic pharmaceutical DES, under physicians' advice to avert miscarriage, inadvertently exposed their fetuses to a potent estrogen. The drug had no observable adverse effect on the mother, and at birth, the infant girls appeared externally normal, but later in life they were found to have a disproportionately high level of reproductive-tract abnormality and increased incidence of development of rare vagino-cervical cancers (Newbold, 2004). Laboratory rodent models of DES are quite consistent with the human data, as fetal DES is associated with the latent development of uterine cancer (Newbold et al., 2006).

The implication is that events in prenatal (embryonic and fetal development) and postnatal (infant) stages can affect disease states in adults (Fig. 1.5), also termed as the *developmental basis of adult disease* (DBAD), leading to the propensity of an individual to develop a disease or dysfunction in later life (Barouki et al., 2012). In other words, the latency between EDC exposure and the emergence of consequential health effects can be considerably long, even decades, and the degree to which gene–environment interactions can produce inter-individual variability is poorly understood. This is especially true for growth and development, processes that are very sensitive to endocrine regulation.

1.2.4 Importance of Mixtures

When it is considered that, in nature, virtually all contamination is in the form of mixtures, the importance of this aspect of endocrine disruption cannot be overestimated. Contamination occurs when the source(s) and nature of the chemicals are man-made. Combinations of EDCs are able to produce significant effect even when each chemical is present at low doses that individually do not induce observable effects. This is true for a variety of endpoints representing a wide range of organizational levels and biological complexity. Some of the contaminants modulate each other's effects which can be additive, but synergistic interactions

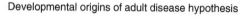

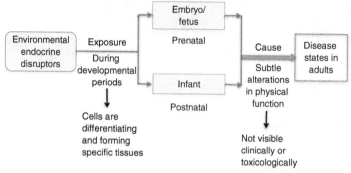

Figure 1.5 Important developmental time periods during which perturbations such as EDC exposure can effect disease states in adults.

among toxic substances have also been known. These typically occur when two or more compounds contribute to the same endpoint through different mechanisms. A case in point is that of a herbicide S-metolachlor (0.1 ppb) that was found to have no adverse effect on its own in amphibians; however, in combination, harmful effects of atrazine such as retarded larval development and growth were multiplied (Hayes et al., 2006). In practice, these two substances are often mixed together in industrial products.

1.2.5 Transgenerational, Epigenetic Effects

Some EDCs are not only potentially capable of having an effect on the individual but can also transmit health problems across generations. These effects might be transmitted by regulatory factors that control gene expression. This is the case with DES, which caused abnormal female sexual development in the granddaughters of patients who were prescribed the drug. Similarly, an endocrine-disrupting fungicide vinclozolin exposure of pregnant rats resulted in latent development of reproductive dysfunctions, infertility, and cancers in their male F1 offspring (Anway and Skinner, 2006). Moreover, if the F1 males mated prior to the development of disease, their F2 male offspring developed a similar physical attributes, or phenotype. It has been demonstrated that this effect carried at least as far as in the F5 offspring, and that the mechanism involves (at least in part) an epigenetic modification caused by a change in methylation patterns to the male germline (Gore and Crews, 2009). For detailed discussion on epigenetic effects, see Chapter 8.

1.3 HISTORICAL PERSPECTIVE OF ENDOCRINE DISRUPTION

The overall understanding that has been achieved on EDCs is the accumulation of evolutionary and revolutionary steps especially over the last half-century. Some of the early milestones in environmental hormone research were identified in the *e.hormone* website of the Tulane University. Recently, a historical perspective on endocrine disruption has also been put together (Marty et al., 2011). Here, we provide a brief history of key events characterizing the development and expansion of the ED hypothesis.

In the 1940s, reports appeared on breeding difficulties in female sheep and cows grazing on pastures rich in red clover (*Trifolium pretense*) species (Bennetts et al., 1946), which later were found to contain estrogenic compounds such as coumestrol (Adams, 1995). In the 1950s, scientists learnt that certain synthetic chemicals could interfere with the hormones that regulate the body's most vital systems. This led to the use of steroidal compounds in the livestock industry to modulate reproductive cycles and to enhance rate and efficiency of body weight gain.

In 1962, concerns about DDT in the environment were publicized in Rachel Carson's book, *Silent Spring*. It described health problems observed in wildlife such as egg-shell thinning, deformities, and population declines linked to pesticides and other synthetic chemicals. Interestingly, Carson intuitively anticipated the ability of certain organochlorines to interfere with reproduction, although at that time the endocrine-disrupting mechanisms were unclear. Studies beginning in the mid-1960s in Lake Michigan suggested that environmental contaminants were adversely affecting hatching success in herring gulls (Keith, 1966). Around 1965–1970, the presence of natural hormones and synthetic estrogens used as birth control agents was noted in wastewater treatment outfalls in the United States (Sumpter, 1995). The first observation of the impact of EDs in humans was done when DES, a "synthetic estrogen," was linked to vaginal cancer in daughters whose mothers had taken the drug during the first three months of pregnancy prescribed to prevent miscarriage (Herbst et al., 1971). As a result, the Food and Drug Administration (FDA) advised physicians to stop prescribing DES to pregnant women.

In 1968, about 2000 people were poisoned by hormonally active PCBs and their pyrolysis products polychlorinated dibenzofurans (PCDFs) following consumption of contaminated rice oil in Japan. A similar poisoning by PCBs occurred in Taiwan in 1979 (Aoki, 2001). Later studies on PCB exposure at low–dose levels have found neurodevelopmental and reproductive effects (Brouwer et al., 1999). In 1976, exposure of the population to an accidental release of tetrachlorodibenzo-*p*-dioxin (TCDD) from a pressure tank in Seveso, Italy, was found to have various developmental and reproductive effects (Baccarelli et al., 2004; Eskenazi et al., 2000). A similar occupational exposure of Vietnam veterans to TCDD has been associated with an imbalance in thyroid hormone and thyroid-stimulating hormone (TSH) levels (Pavuk et al., 2003).

In 1981, tributyltin (TBT), a constituent of marine antifouling paints, was linked to induction of imposex (penis growth in females) in molluscs, when it was shown that the incidence of the condition was highest close to marinas (Smith, 1981). This became the first well-documented, worldwide population-level effect in wildlife caused by an EDC. Public concern due to adverse effects of environmental chemicals led National Institute of Environmental Health Sciences (NIEHS) to organize conferences on Estrogens in the Environment in 1979 (McLachlan, 1980) and

1985 (McLachlan, 1985). Presentations noted the ubiquitous nature of the contaminants, their potency, and their potential impact on public and environmental health.

In 1991, the idea that xenobiotic chemicals could inappropriately modulate the endocrine system thereby causing detrimental effects in wildlife and humans was first articulated in the watershed first World Wildlife Federation (WWF) Wingspread Conference (Colborn and Clement, 1992). The term *endocrine disruptor* was coined in this conference. Some plastics widely used in a variety of consumer products were found leaching estrogenic chemicals in laboratory research, mounting the concerns about the potential for environmental chemicals to alter endocrine physiology (Soto et al., 1991). This was the first time that scientists became aware of hormone-altering chemicals in plastics. In 1993, the link between environmental estrogens and male reproductive problems was hypothesized (Sharpe and Shakkebaek, 1993), and associations were drawn between EDCs and declining sperm counts (Toppari et al., 1996; Swan et al., 1997). In 1995, the National Academy of Sciences and National Research Council sponsored a panel study on Hormone Related Toxicants in the Environment (NRC, 1999).

Awareness of endocrine disruption was intensified by the 1996 publication of the book, *Our Stolen Future*, by Theo Colborn of the World Wildlife Fund and coauthors Dumanoski and Myers, who emphasized on how anthropogenic chemicals have been subtly altering the development, behavior, physiology, and ultimately well being and survival of natural populations, including our own (Colborn et al., 1996). In the same year, a report on male alligators in Florida's Lake Apopka having strikingly low levels of testosterone and abnormally small phallus size was published. Chlorinated pesticide residues in this contaminated lake due to a chemical spill occurred in 1980 was cited to have caused demasculinization of alligators there (Guillette et al., 1996). Also in 1996, the first known North American report of endocrine disruption in fish below wastewater outfalls was published (Bevans et al. 1996). These reports helped to establish the credibility of endocrine disruption science as a discipline. Since then, a number of important milestones followed.

The first European workshop on the impacts of EDs on human health and wildlife was organized in Weybridge, UK (Weybridge, 1996). Concern about endocrine disruption fostered US legislative mandates including the update of the U.S. Safe Drinking Water Act and Food Quality Protection Act requiring U.S. EPA to implement screening and testing program to detect EDCs (FQPA, 1996). Consequently, EPA formed the Endocrine Disruptor Screening and Testing Advisory Committee (EDSTAC) to evaluate protocols and select a subset to comprise a "Tier I" screening battery for biological activity involving the estrogen, androgen, and thyroid hormone systems. The challenge was made complicated by the need to screen for receptor agonists and antagonists, as well as compounds, which act indirectly, including the inhibition of steroid biosynthesis.

In 1997, BPA, a component of polycarbonate plastic, was shown to alter the reproductive development of lab mice at extremely low doses. BPA mimics the natural sex hormone estrogen (vom Saal et al., 1997). In 1998, widespread occurrence of intersex fish in British rivers was reported as a consequence of exposure to STP effluents (Jobling et al. 1998). In 1998, Japanese Environmental Agency presented their Strategic Program on Environmental Endocrine Disruptors. In 2000, a book was published reviewing EDCs becoming a social and political concern (Krimsky, 2000). Reports on low-dose effects of EDCs led to National Toxicology Program (NTP) report on EDs low-dose peer review in 2001, concluding that endocrine effects have been demonstrated for a number of chemicals at doses below their previously determined no-effect levels (Melnick et al. 2002). Low levels of atrazine exposure during development were cited for hermaphroditic and demasculinized frogs (Hayes et al., 2002). A USGS study found low concentrations of human and animal drugs, natural and synthetic hormones, detergents, plasticizers, insecticides, and fire retardants in most of the 139 stream sites sampled in 30 states in the United States during 1999–2000 (Kolpin et al., 2002). WHO/International Program on Chemical Safety (IPCS) issued a global assessment of state-of-the-science of EDs (Damstra et al., 2002). In 2002, Terry Collins pioneered introduction of endocrine disruption in his "introduction to green chemistry" class at Carnegie Mellon University (CMU) and from that year he invited annually leading scientists to deliver prominent lectures on the impacts of endocrine disruption on public health. In 2004, long-term exposure to environmental concentrations of ethinylestradiol was reported to cause reproductive failure in zebrafish (Nash et al., 2004). In the following years, endocrine disruption influence on genes' activity, altering phenotype expression, was recognized to be epigenetic, and transgenerational implications of some EDCs-induced epigenetic alterations were reported (Crews and McLachlan, 2006; Anway and Skinner, 2006; Anway et al., 2005).

In 2009, the Endocrine Society issued a Scientific Statement outlining the scientific evidence supporting the existence and detrimental effects of EDCs and underscoring them as a significant concern for public health (Diamanti-Kandarakis et al., 2009). In the same year, American Medical Association endorsed this statement and called for new federal policies to decrease the public's exposure to EDCs. Eight other scientific bodies then joined the Endocrine Society in a letter of concern published in *Science* in 2011 (Hunt, 2011). In late 2012, a cross-disciplinary team of scientists developed a tiered protocol for endocrine disruption (TiPED) testing to weed out potentially harmful chemicals early in the development (Ritter, 2012). In early 2013, WHO/UNEP published a report on State of the Science of Endocrine Disrupting Chemicals – 2012. It concluded that the speed with which the incidence of endocrine-related diseases increased in recent decades rules out genetic factors as the sole plausible explanation, and points to environmental causes as a contributory factor (WHO/UNEP 2013)). In the summer of 2013, a controversy broke out over the leaked draft proposal of the European Union to regulate EDCs recommending a precautionary approach. The editors of journals of toxicology, endocrinology, and other related fields published combative editorials about how endocrine disrupting chemicals should be regulated (Cressey, 2013).

Table 1.1 shows a summary of various observations of endocrine disrupting effects in wildlife and humans and related progress in understanding their impact

TABLE 1.1   Historical Milestones in Understanding Adverse Impacts of EDCs

Timeline	Observations	Books/Conferences/Reports/Policy Action
1930s–1940s	Reproductive problems in female sheep and cows grazing on pastures rich in certain clover species, later found to contain estrogenic coumestrol	1950s – Sex steroidal compounds use began for modulation of reproductive cycles and body weight gain in livestock and poultry
Evidence of the health impacts of EDCs grew from the 1960s to the 1990s		
1961–1970	Environmental contaminants in Lake Michigan found adversely affecting hatching success in herring gulls (1966)	Rachel Carson's book Silent Spring (1962) describes DDT impact on the health and environment and problems in wildlife
	Presence of natural hormones and synthetic estrogens used as birth control agents observed in wastewater treatment outfalls in the United States	
	Exposure of PCBs and PCDFs in populations in Japan (1968) and Taiwan (1979)	
	Exposure to TCDD in Italy (1976) and Vietnam veterans	
1971–1990	DES linked to vaginal cancer in daughters whose mothers had taken the drug during the first three months of pregnancy (1971)	NIEHS organizes Estrogens in the Environment conferences (1979 and 1985)
	Imposex in molluscs first linked to marine anti-fouling paints containing organotin compound TBT, when it was shown that the incidence of the condition was highest close to marinas (1981)	
1991–1995	Some plastic compounds found leaching estrogenic chemicals in laboratory research (1991), made aware of hormone altering chemicals in plastics	Link between EDCs and declining sperm counts hypothesized (1993)
		Wingspread Conference (1991) proposed first time that xenobiotic chemicals inappropriately modulate the endocrine system causing detrimental effects in wildlife and humans and coined the term endocrine disruptor
		National Academy of Sciences and National Research Council sponsor a panel study on Hormone Related Toxicants in the Environment (1995)

1996	Male alligators in Florida's Lake Apopka found with strikingly low levels of testosterone and abnormally small phallus size (1996). First North American report of endocrine disruption in fish below wastewater outfalls (1996)	Theo Colborn, Dumanoski, and Myers publish *Our Stolen Future* (1996) strongly advocating that EDCs posed a serious threat to humans and wildlife Weybridge (UK) meeting on EDCs (1996) first time discussed the problem of EDCs in Europe. OECD established a special activity on endocrine disruptor testing and assessment (1996) U.S. Safe Drinking Water Act Amendments (1996) and Food Quality Protection Act (1996) enacted. U.S. Congress mandates EPA to implement screening and testing to detect EDCs EDSTAC formed to evaluate protocols and select a subset to comprise a "Tier I" screening battery for activity of the estrogen, androgen, and thyroid hormone systems
1997–2000	BPA shown to alter the reproductive development of lab mice at extremely low doses (1997) Widespread occurrence of intersex fish in British rivers reported as a consequence of exposure to STP effluents (1998)	Japanese Environmental Agency presented Strategic Program on Environmental Endocrine Disruptors (1998) Reports on increases in breast cancer, cryptorchidism and hypospadias and developmental abnormalities in wildlife appeared (1999) A book *Hormone Chaos* (2000) is published reviewing EDCs becoming a social and political concern
2001–2010	Low levels of atrazine exposure during development cited (2002) for hermaphroditic and demasculinized frogs Long-term exposure to environmental concentrations of EE2 reported (2004) to cause reproductive failure in zebrafish EDCs action on genes developmental mechanisms, altering phenotype expression seen as epigenetic and transgenerational action of vinclozolin reported (2005)	NTP report on EDs low-dose peer review (2001), found effects for a number of EDCs at doses below their previously determined no-effect levels USGS study (2002) finds low concentrations of human and animal drugs, natural and synthetic hormones, detergents, plasticizers, insecticides, and fire retardants in most of the 139 stream sites sampled in 30 states WHO/IPCS (2002) issued a global assessment of the state-of-the-science of endocrine disruptors

(continued)

TABLE 1.1   (Continued)

	Terry Collins pioneers introduction of endocrine disruption in green chemistry class at CMU (2002), and annually invites leading scientists to deliver prominent lectures.
	Introduction of the European legislation REACH (2007)
	The Endocrine Society issued a scientific statement (2009) outlining the scientific evidence supporting the existence and detrimental effects of EDCs and underscoring them as a significant concern for public health
	American Medical Association endorses Endocrine Society statement (2009) and calls for reduced exposure to EDCs
2011–2013	Eight scientific societies in the fields of reproductive biology, endocrinology, reproductive medicine, genetics, and developmental biology in a letter to *Science* (2011) offer expertise for chemical testing and risk assessment
	A tiered protocol for endocrine disruption (TiPED) testing created for use in the design of new materials to eliminate potentially harmful chemicals early in development (2012)
	WHO/UNEP (2013) publish a report on state of science of EDCs – 2012
	Regulation of EDCs gets mired into controversy on leakage of the European Union draft proposal (2013). The editors of journals of toxicology, endocrinology and other related fields published combative editorials about how EDCs should be regulated (2013)

on reproductive health of humans by information collection, dissemination, and policy initiatives.

1.4   SCOPE AND LAYOUT OF THIS BOOK

The endocrine disruption science has exploded and has seen an exponential growth in the last two decades. This book summarizes research findings of numerous scientists in several inter-related disciplines. It is not planned as a comprehensive compendium but more of a concise reading for non-specialist audience interested in learning about challenges and possible solutions to endocrine disruption phenomena. The inclusion of key references provides resources for those who wish to go into various topics in more depth.

The book is divided in three parts and 14 chapters. An introductory chapter provides an overview of endocrine system, EDs discusses their salient features and a historical perspective of endocrine disruption phenomena. The first part includes seven chapters. It begins with the second chapter on hormone-signaling mechanisms, followed by laying out various broad classes of putative EDs and a brief introduction to environmental epigenetic modifications. Chapters 3 and 4 describe various putative estrogenic chemicals and heavy metals, and antiandrogenic compounds, respectively. Chapter 5 is devoted to thyroid toxicants while Chapter 6 deals with environmental chemicals that disrupt endocrine system via xenobiotic-sensing and other receptors. In real-world scenario, humans and wildlife are not exposed to one chemical at a time, but rather to complex mixtures. Therefore, Chapter 7 reviews mixture effects of estrogenic, androgenic and thyroid hormone disrupting compounds. The Chapter 8 introduces the emerging science of epigenetic modifications and includes examples of ED compounds with transgenerational effects.

The second part focuses on removal processes of various EDCs by biotic and abiotic transformation/degradation. Chapter 9 includes metabolic and/or microbial biotransformations of ED compounds while Chapter 10 covers various chemical (oxidation) processes for the degradation ED compounds.

The third and final part consists of four chapters, embracing themes on finding solutions to environmental EDCs including their detection, regulation, replacement and remediation. Chapter 11 briefly discusses the endocrine disruptor-screening program of US EPA and various Tier 1 screening assays and includes a discussion on the ongoing efforts for development of high throughput assays. Chapter 12 dwells upon water quality sustainability due to impact of environmental trace contaminants, including EDCs. Chapter 13 addresses policy and regulatory issues relevant to EDCs including scientific uncertainty and precautionary policy. Chapter 14 brings forth the use of Green Chemistry principles in avoiding endocrine disruption in the designing and screening for safer chemicals, and remediation of the EDCs in aquatic environment.

Per evolutionary biologists, ancient estrogen receptor was the precursor of a plethora of other specific hormone receptor systems. The initial identification that some of the environmental chemicals affect endocrine system was also related to disruption of endogenous estrogenic activity. Therefore, to date maximum work has been carried out on the activity of various estrogen mimics, including their mechanism(s) of action, low-dose and non-monotonic effects, and adverse impact on health and environment. This would explain, relatively disproportionate space taken in the book by xenoestrogens as compared to other endocrine effects.

The EDCs that have received attention due to their observed effectiveness, abundance or distribution are described in chapters three to six in the book. The reader would keep in mind that hormone actions are pleiotropic (producing more than one effect) – complex endocrine interactions of EDs with other steroids, peptides and lipids are integral to the function of sex-steroids in living vertebrates. Therefore it is critical to consider the enormous range of physiological variation that occurs in vertebrates under "normal" conditions that would be considered "uncontaminated". Using terms like "estrogenic" or "androgenic" to chemicals may limit the reader because androgens and estrogens have well-characterized function in a very small percentage of species. It is important to note that although compounds may be defined based on a given outcome or mechanism of action, almost all chemicals influence multiple physiological systems and influence the way physiological systems interact with each other.

1.5   CONCLUSION

Pollutants pose destructive consequences to our ecosystem and impose negative health effects to wildlife and humans. It is estimated that about 40% of human deaths (62 million per year) are attributed to the exposure of chemical pollutants (Pimentel et al., 2007). These pollutants include legacy and emerging persistent organic pollutants of chronic toxicity that have been shown or suspected to have endocrine-disrupting properties. Concerns about EDCs have come to the forefront of toxicology only in the last 15 years or so. Traditional toxicological testing had missed endocrine disruption in the first place and overlooked chemicals that could penetrate the womb environment and interfere with the development of the embryo and fetus. The idea that the dose makes the poison (Binswanger and Smith, 2000) has turned out to be overly simplistic. The newest research has clearly shown that biology is affected by low doses of chemicals, and revealed the sensitivity of the developing individual to the slightest chemical perturbation during development.

Recent reports have shown that a number of environmental EDs are capable of interfering with the normal endocrine function in a variety of animals. It has been demonstrated that exposure to a biologically active chemical within the range in which free hormones operate can have an entirely different suite of effects that change during progressive stages of development than when the same chemical is administered in high doses after an individual has fully developed. These studies also confirmed that endocrine effects are time specific, chemical and/or hormone specific, and dose related. Timing of exposure to EDs is found to be of equal or greater importance than potency, pointing to the importance of the perinatal environment to long-term outcomes of disease states and human health.

REFERENCES

Adams, N. R. Detection of the effects of phytoestrogens on sheep and cattle, *J. Anim. Sci.* **1995**, 73,1509–1515.

Anway, M. D.; Skinner, M. K. Epigenetic transgenerational actions of endocrine disruptors, *Endocrinology* **2006**, 147(6 Suppl), S43–S49.

Anway, M. D.; Cupp, A. S.; Uzumcu, M.; Skinner, M. K. Epigenetic transgenerational actions of endocrine disruptors, *Science* **2005**, 308(5727), 1466–1469.

Aoki, Y. Polychlorinated biphenyls, polychlorinated dibenzo-p-dioxins, and polychlorinated dibenzofurans as endocrine disrupters what we have learned from Yusho disease, *Environ. Res.* **2001**, 86(1), 2–11.

Baccarelli, A.; Pesatori, A.C.; Masten, S.A.; Patterson, D.G., Jr.; Needham, L.L.; Mocarelli, P.; Caporaso, N.E.; Consonni, D.; Grassman, J.A.; Bertazzi, P.A.; Landi, M.T. Aryl-hydrocarbon receptor-dependent pathway and toxic effects of TCDD in humans: a population-based study in Seveso, Italy, *Toxicol. Lett.* **2004**, 149(1–3), 287–293.

Barouki, R.; Gluckman, P. D.; Grandjean, P.; Hanson, M.; Heindel, J. J. Developmental origins of non-communicable disease: implications for research and public health, *Environ. Health* **2012**, 11, 42.

Bennetts, H. W.; Underwood, E. J.; Shier, F. L. A specific breeding problem of sheep on subterranean clover pastures in Western Australia, *Aust. Vet. J.* **1946**, 22, 2–12.

Bern, H. The fragile fetus, in *Chemically-induced alterations in sexual and functional development: the wildlife/human connection*, Colborn, T.; Clement, C., eds., Princeton, NJ: Princeton Scientific, **1992**, pp. 9 –15.

Bevans, H. E.; Goodbred, S. L.; Miesner, J. F.; Watkins, S. A.; Gross, T. S.; Denslow, N. D.; Schoeb, T. Synthetic organic compounds and carp endocrinology and histology in Las Vegas Wash and Las Vegas and Callville Bays of Lake Mead, Nevada, 1992 and 1995, *Water-Resources Investigations Report 96-4266*, 1996.

Binswanger, H. C.; Smith, K. R. Paracelsus and Goethe: founding fathers of environmental health, *Bull. WHO* **2000**, 78, 1162–1164.

Boyd, G.R.; Palmeri, J. M.; Zhang, S.; Grimm, D. A. Pharmaceuticals and personal care products (PPCPs) and endocrine disrupting chemicals (EDCs) in stormwater canals and Bayou St. John in New Orleans, Louisiana, USA, *Sci. Total Environ.* **2004**, 333(1–3), 137–148.

Brouwer, A.; Longnecker, M. P.; Birnbaum, L. S.; Cogliano, J. Kostyniak, P.; Moore, J.; Schantz, S.; Winneke, G. Characterization of potential endocrine-related health effects at low-dose levels of exposure to PCBs, *Environ. Health Perspect.* **1999**, 107(Suppl 4), 639–649.

Carpenter, D. O.; Arcaro, K.; Spink, D.C. Understanding the human health effects of chemical mixtures, *Environ. Health Perspect.* **2002**, 110 (Suppl 1), 25–42.

Chia, V. M.; Li, Y.; Quraishi, S. M.; Graubard, B. I.; Figueroa, J. D.; Weber, J. P., et al. Effect modification of endocrine disruptors and testicular germ cell tumor risk by hormone-metabolizing genes, *Int. J. Androl.* **2010**, 33(4), 588–596.

Colborn, T.; Clement, C. R. *Chemically-induced Alterations in Sexual and Functional Development: The Wildlife/Human Connection– Proceedings*, Princeton, NJ: Princeton Scientific Pub. Co., **1992**.

Colborn, T.; vom Saal, F. S.; Soto, A. M. Developmental effects of endocrine-disrupting chemicals in wildlife and humans, *Environ. Health Perspect.* **1993**, 101, 378–384.

Colborn, T., Dumanoski, D., and Myers, J. P. Our stolen future: are we threatening our fertility, intelligence and survival? – A scientific Detective Story, New York: Penguin Books USA, **1996**.

Coors, A.; Jones, P. D.; Giesy, J. P.; Ratte, H. T. Removal of estrogenic activity from municipal waste landfill leachate assessed with a bioassay based on reporter gene expression, *Environ. Sci. Technol.* **2003**, 37(15), 3430–3434.

Crain, D. A.; Janssen, S. J.; Edwards, T. M., et al., Female reproductive disorders: the roles of endocrine-disrupting compounds and developmental timing, *Fertil. Steril.* **2008**, 90(4), 911–940.

Cravedi, J. P.; Zalko, D.; Savouret, J. F.; Menuet, A.; Jegou, B. The concept of endocrine disruption and human health, *Med. Sci. (Paris)* **2007**, 23(2), 198–204.

Cressey, D. Journal editors trade blows over toxicology, *Nature* **2013**. DOI: 10.1038/nature.2013.13787.

Crews, D.; McLachlan, J. A. Epigenetics, evolution, endocrine disruption, health, and disease, *Endocrinology* **2006**, 147(6 Suppl.), S4–S10.

CSTEE, Opinion on BKH Consulting Engineers Report, "Towards the establishment of a priority list of substances for further evaluation of their role in endocrine disruption"—Opinion adopted at the 17th CSTEE plenary meeting, Brussels, 5 September, 2000. Available at: http://europa.eu.int/comm/food/fs/sc/sct/out73_en.html (accessed 28 Jan 2014).

Damstra, T.; Barlow, S.; Bergman, A.; Kavlock, R.; Van Der Kraak, G. Global assessment of the state-of-the-science of endocrine disruptors, International Programme on Chemical Safety, WHO/PCS/EDC/02.2. World Health Organization, Geneva, Switzerland, 2002. Available at: http://www.who.int/ipcs/publications/new_issues/endocrine_disruptors/en/print.html.

Diamanti-Kandarakis, E.; Bourguignon, J.P.; Giudice, L.C.; Hauser, R.; Prins, G.S.; Soto, A.M.; Zoeller, R.T.; Gore, A.C. Endocrine-disrupting chemicals: an Endocrine Society scientific statement. *Endocr. Rev.* **2009**, 30(4), 293–342.

EPA, Non-monotonic dose response curves research, low dose effects, April 5, 2013. Available at: http://www.epa.gov/research/endocrinedisruption/non-monotonic.htm.

Eskenazi, B.; Mocarelli, P.; Warner, M.; Samuels, S.; Vercellini, P.; Olive, D.; Needham, L.; Patterson, D.; Brambilla, P. Seveso Women's Health Study: a study of the effects of 2,3,7,8-tetrachloro-dibenzo-*p*-dioxin on reproductive health, *Chemosphere*, **2000**, 40(9–11), 1247–1253.

Fernandez, M. F.; Olea, N. Developmental exposure to endocrine disruptors and male urogenital tract malformations, in *Endocrine Disruptors and Puberty*, Diamanti-Kandarakis E.; Gore A. C., eds, New York: Humana Press, **2012**, pp. 225–239.

Folmar, L. C.; Denslow, N. D.; Rao, V.; Chow, M.; Crain, D. A.; Enblom, J., et al. Vitellogenin induction and reduced serum testosterone concentrations in feral male carp (*Cyprinus carpio*) captured near a major metropolitan sewage treatment plant, *Environ. Health Perspect.* **1996**, 104, 1096–1101.

FQPA, Food Quality Protection Act. Public Law 104-170, 110 STAT. 1489. 1996. Available at: http://www.epa.gov/scipoly/oscpendo/pubs/fqpa.pdf.

Gore, A. C. Developmental programming and endocrine disruptor effects on reproductive neuroendocrine systems, *Front. Neuroendocrinol.* **2008**, 29, 358–374.

Gore, A. C.; Crews, D. Environmental endocrine disruption of brain and behavior, in *Hormones, Brain and Behavior*, 2nd Ed., Vol. 3, Pfaff, D. W., Arnold, A.P., Etgen, A. M., Fahrbach, S. E., Rubin, R. T., eds., San Diego: Academic Press, **2009**, pp. 1789–1816.

Guillette, L. J., Jr.,; Crain, D. A.; Rooney, A. A.; Pickford, D. B. Organization versus activation: the role of endocrine- disrupting contaminants (EDCs) during embryonic development in wildlife, *Environ. Health Perspect.* **1995**, 103(Suppl 7), 157–164.

Guillette, L. J., Jr.,; Pickford, D. B.; Cain, D. A.; Rooney, A. R.; Percival, H. F. Reduction in penis size and plasma testosterone concentrations in juvenile alligators living in a contaminated environment, *Gen. Comp. Endocrinol.* **1996**, 101, 32–42.

Hanselman, T. A.; Graetz, D. A.; Wilkie, A. C. Manure-borne estrogens as potential environmental contaminants: A review, *Environ. Sci. Technol.* **2003**, 37, 5471–5478.

Hayes, T. B., et al. Hermaphroditic, demasculinized frogs after exposure to the herbicide atrazine at low ecologically relevant doses, *Proc. Natl. Acad. Sci. U. S. A.* **2002**, 99(8), 5476–5480.

Hayes, T. B.; Case, P.; Chui, S.; Chung, D.; Haeffele, C.; Haston, K.; Lee, M.; Mai, V. P.; Marjuoa, Y.; Parker, J.; Tsui, M. Pesticide mixtures, endocrine disruption, and amphibian declines: are we underestimating the impact? *Environ. Health Perspect.* **2006**, 114 (Suppl 1), 40–50.

Herbst, A. L.; Ulfelder, H.; Poskanzer, D. C. Adenocarcinoma of the vagina—Association of maternal stilbestrol therapy with tumor appearance in young women, *N. Engl. J. Med.* **1971**, 284, 878–881.

Hunt, P. Assessing chemical risk: societies offer expertise, *Science* **2011**, 331, 1136.

Jacobs, M. Unsafe sex: how endocrine disruptors work, Pesticide Action Network UK, Briefing 4, January **2001**.

Jobling, S.; Nolan, M.; Tyler, C. R.; Sumpter, J. P. Widespread sexual disruption in wild fish, *Environ. Sci. Technol.* **1998**, 32(17), 2498–2506.

Jobling, S.; Coey, S.; Whitmore, J. G.; Kime, D. E.; Van Look, K. J. W.; McAllister, B. G., et al. Wild intersex roach (*Rutilus rutilus*) have reduced fertility, *Biol. Reprod.* **2002**, 67, 515–524.

Kavlock, R. J.; Daston, G. P.; DeRosa, C.; Fenner-Crisp, P.; Gray, L. E.; Kaattari, S.; Lucier, G.; Luster, M.; Mac M. J.; Maczka, C.; Miller, R.; Moore, J.; Rolland, R.; Scott, G.; Sheehan, D. M.; Sinks, T.; Tilson, H. A. Research needs for the risk assessment of health and environmental effect of endocrine disruptors: a report of the USEPA-sponsored workshop, *Environ. Health Perspect.* **1996**, 104(Suppl 4), 715–740.

Keith, J. A. Reproduction in a population of herring gulls (*Larus argenatatus*) contaminated by DDT, *J. Appl. Ecol.* **1966**, 3(Suppl.), 57–70.

Khanal, S. K.; Xie, B.; Thompson, M. L.; Sung, S.; Ong, S.K.; van Leeuwen, J. Fate, transport, and biodegradation of natural estrogens in the environment and engineered systems, *Environ. Sci. Technol.*, **2006**, 40(21), 6537–6546.

Kolodziej, E. P.; Harter, T.; Sedlak, D. L. Dairy wastewater, aquaculture, and spawning fish as sources of steroid hormones in the aquatic environment, *Environ. Sci. Technol.* **2004**, 38(23), 6377–6384.

Kolpin, D. W.; Furlong, E. T.; Meyer, M. T.; Thurman, E. M.; Zaugg, S. D.; Barber, L. B.; Buxton, H. T. Pharmaceuticals, hormones, and other organic wastewater contaminants in U.S. streams, 1999–2000: A national reconnaissance, *Environ. Sci. Technol.* **2002**, 36(6), 1202–1211.

Kosaka, K.; Asami, M.; Matsuoka, Y.; Kamoshita, M.; Kunikane, S. Occurrence of perchlorate in drinking water sources of metropolitan area in Japan, *Water Res.* **2007**, 41(15), 3474–3482.

Krimsky, S. *Hormone Chaos: The Scientific and Social Origins of the Environmental Endocrine Hypothesis*, Baltimore, MD: John Hopkins University Press, **2000**.

Lanphear, B. P.; Hornung, R.; Khoury, J.; Yolton, K.; Baghurst, P.; Bellinger, D. C., et al., Low-level environmental lead exposure and children's intellectual function: an international pooled analysis, *Environ. Health Perspect.* **2005**, 113, 894–899.

Legler, J.; Zeinstra, L. M.; Schuitemaker, F.; Lanser, P. H.; Bogerd, J.; Brouver, J. Comparison of in vivo and in vitro reporter gene assays for short-term screening of estrogenic activity, *Environ. Sci. Technol.* **2002**, 36(20), 4410–4415.

Li, D. K.; Zhou, Z.; Miao, M.; He, Y.; Wang, J.; Ferber, J., et al. Urine bisphenol-A (BPA) level in relation to semen quality, *Fertil. Steril.* **2011**, 95(2), 625–630.

Marty, M. S.; Carney, E. W.; Rowlands, J. C. Endocrine disruption: Historical perspectives and its impact on the future of toxicology testing, *Toxicol. Sci.* **2011**, 120(Suppl. 1), S93–S108.

McLachlan, J. A. Estrogens in the environment, *Proceedings of the Symposium on Estrogens in the Environment*, Raleigh, North Carolina, U.S.A., September 10–12, 1979, New York: Elsevier/North Holland, **1980**.

McLachlan, J. A. Estrogens in the environment II: Influences on development, *Proceedings of the Symposium*, New York: Elsevier, **1985**.

Melnick, R.; Lucier, G.; Wolfe, M.; Hall, R.; Stancel, G.; Prins, G.; Gallo, M.; Reuhl, K.; Ho, S.-M.; Brown, T., et al. Summary of the National Toxicology Program's report of the endocrine disruptors low-dose peer review, *Environ. Health Perspect.* **2002**, 110, 427–431.

Myers, J.P.; Zoeller, R.T.; vom Saal, F.S. A clash of old and new scientific concepts in toxicity, with important implications for public health, *Environ. Health Perspect.* **2009**, 117(11), 1652–1655.

Nash, J. P.; Kime, D. E.; Van der Ven, L.T.; Wester, P. W.; Brion, F.; Maack, G.; Stahlschmidt-Allner, P.; Tyler, C. R. Long-term exposure to environmental concentrations of the pharmaceutical ethynylestradiol causes reproductive failure in fish, *Environ. Health Perspect.* **2004**, 112(17), 1725–1733.

Newbold, R. R. Lessons learned from perinatal exposure to diethylstilbestrol, *Toxicol. Appl. Pharmacol.* **2004**, 199, 142–150.

Newbold, R. R. Impact of environmental endocrine disrupting chemicals on the development of obesity, *Hormones* **2010**, 9(3), 206–217.

Newbold, R. R.; Padilla-Banks, E.; Jefferson, W. N. Adverse effects of the model environmental estrogen diethylstilbestrol (DES) are transmitted to subsequent generations, *Endocrinology* **2006**, 147, S11–S17.

NRC, National Research Council, *Hormonally Active Agents in the Environment*, Washington, DC: National Academy Press, **1999**.

Orlando, E. F.; Kolok, A. S.; Binzcik, G. A.; Gates, J. L.; Horton, M. K.; Lambright, C. S.; Gray, L. E., Jr.,; Soto, A. M.; Guillette, L. J., Jr., Endocrine-disrupting effects of cattle feedlot effluent on an aquatic sentinel species, the fathead minnow, *Environ. Health Perspect.* **2004**, 112(3), 353–358.

Pardridge, W. M.; Mietus, L. J.; Frumar, A. M.; Davidson, B. J.; Judd, H. L. Effects of human serum on transport of testosterone and estradiol into rat brain, *Am. J. Physiol. Endocrinol. Metab.* **1980**, 239(1), E103–E108.

Pavuk, M.; Schecter, A.J.; Akhtar F.Z.; Michalek, J.E. Serum 2,3,7,8-tetrachlorodibenzo-p-dioxin (TCDD) levels and thyroid function in air force veterans of the Vietnam war, *Ann. Epidemiol.* **2003**, 13(5), 335–343.

Pimentel, D.; Cooperstein, S.; Randell, H.; Filiberto, D.; Sorrentio, S.; Kaye, B., et al. Ecology of increasing diseases: population growth and environmental degradation, *Hum. Ecol.* **2007**, 35, 653–668.

Purdom, C. E.; Hardiman, P. A.; Bye, V. J.; Eno, N. C.; Tyler, C. R.; Sumpter, J. P. Estrogenic effects of effluents from sewage treatment works, *Chem. Ecol.* **1994**, 8, 275–285.

Ritter, S. K. Designing away endocrine disruption, *C&E News* **2012**, 90(51), 33–34.

Roy, J. R.; Chakraborty, S.; Chakraborty, T. R. Estrogen-like endocrine disrupting chemicals affecting puberty in humans - a review, *Med. Sci. Monit.* **2009**, 15(6), RA137–RA145.

vom Saal, F. S.; Timms, B. G.; Montano, M. M.; Palanza, P.; Thayer, K. A.; Nagel, S. C.; Dahr, M. D.; Ganjam, V. K.; Parmigiani, S.; Welshons, W. V. Prostate enlargement in mice due to fetal exposure to low doses of estradiol or diethylstilbestrol and opposite effects at high doses. *Proc. Natl. Acad. Sci. U. S. A.* **1997**, 94, 2056–2061.

Sharpe, R. M.; Shakkebaek, N. F. Are oestrogens involved in falling sperm counts and disorders of the male reproductive tract? *Lancet* **1993**, 341, 1392–1395.

Smith, B. S. Tributyltin compounds induced male characteristics on female Mud Snails (*Nassarius obsoletus =Ilyanassa obsoleta*), *J. Appl. Toxicol.* **1981**, 1(3), 141–144.

Snyder, S. A.; Westerhoff, P.; Yoon, Y.; Sedlak, D. L. Pharmaceuticals, personal care products, and endocrine disruptors in water: implications for the water industry, *Environ. Eng. Sci.* **2003**, 20, 449–469.

Soto, A. M.; Justicia, H.; Wray, J. W.; Sonnenschein, C. *p*-Nonyl-phenol: an estrogenic xenobiotic released from "modified" polystyrene, *Environ. Health Perspect.* **1991**, 92, 167–173.

Soto, A. M.; Lin, T.-M.; Sakabe, K.; Olea, N.; Damassa, D.A.; Sonnenschein, C. Variants of the human prostate LNCaP cell line as a tool to study discrete components of the androgen-mediated proliferative response, *Oncol. Res.***1995**, 7, 545–558.

Soto, A. M.; Calabro, J. M.; Prechtl, N. V.; Yau, A. Y.; Orlando, E. F.; Daxenberger, A.; Kolok, A. S.; Guillette, L. J.; le Bizec, B.; Lange, I. J.; Sonnenschein, C. Androgenic and estrogenic activity in water bodies receiving cattle feedlot effluent in eastern Nebraska, USA, *Environ. Health Perspect.* **2004**, 112, 346–352.

Staples, C. A.; Dom, P. B.; Klecka, G. M.; O'Blook, S. T.; Harris, L. R. A review of the environmental fate, effects, and exposures of Bisphenol A, *Chemosphere* **1998**, 36, 2149–2173.

Sumpter, J. P. Feminized responses in fish to environmental estrogens, *Toxicol. Lett.* **1995**, 82–83, 737–742.

Swan, S. H.; Elkin, E. P.; Fenster, L. Have sperm densities declined? A re-analysis of global trend data, *Environ. Health Perspect.* **1997**, 105, 1228–1232.

Swartz, C.H.; Reddy, S.; Benotti, M. J.; Yin, H.; Barber, L. B.; Brownawell, B. J.; Rudel, R. Steroid estrogens, nonylphenol ethoxylate metabolites, and other wastewater contaminants in groundwater affected by a residential septic system on Cape Cod, MA, *Environ. Sci. Technol.* **2006**, 40(16), 4894–4902.

Thayer, K. A.; Heindel, J. J.; Bucher, J. R.; Gallo, M. A. Role of environmental chemicals in diabetes and obesity: a National Toxicology Program workshop review, *Environ. Health Perspect.* **2012**, 120, 779–789.

Toppari, J.; Larsen, J. C.; Christiansen, P., Giwercman, A.; Grandjean, P.; Guillette, L. J., Jr.,; Jejou, B.; Jensen, T. K.; Jouannet, P.; Keiding, N.; Leffers, H.; McLachlan, J. A.; Meyer, O.; Muller, J.; Rajpert-De Meyts, E.; Scheike, T.; Sharpe, R.; Sumpter, J.; Skakkebaek, N. E. Male reproductive health and environmental xenoestrogens, *Environ. Health Perspect.* **1996**, 104 (S4), 741–803.

UNEP/WHO, State of the Science of Endocrine Disrupting Chemicals–2012, Summary for decision-makers, Bergman, Å.; Heindel, J. J.; Jobling, S.; Kidd, K. A.; Zoeller, R. T., eds., Geneva, Switzerland, United Nations Environment Program and the World Health Organization, 2012. http://www.unep.org/pdf/EDCs_Summary_for_DMs%20_Jan24.pdf.

Vandenberg, L. N.; Maffini, M. V.; Sonnenschein, C.; Rubin, B. S.; Soto, A. M. Bisphenol-A and the great divide: a review of controversies in the field of endocrine disruption, *Endocr. Rev.* **2009**, 30(1) 75–95.

Vandenberg, L. N.; Colborn, T.; Hayes, T. B.; Heindel, J. J.; Jacobs, D. R., Jr.,; Lee, D. H.; Shioda, T.; Soto, A. M.; vom Saal, F. S.; Welshons, W. V.; Zoeller, R. T.; Myers, J. P. Hormones and endocrine-disrupting chemicals: low-dose effects and nonmonotonic dose responses, *Endocr. Rev.* **2012**, 33(3), 378–455.

Vos, J. G.; Dybing, E.; Greim, H. A.; Ladefoged, O.; Lambre, C.; Tarazona, J. V.; Brandt, I.; Vethaak, A. D. Health effects of endocrine-disrupting chemicals on wildlife, with special reference to the European situation, *Crit. Rev. Toxicol.* **2000**, 30, 71–133.

Welshons, W. V.; Thayer, K. A.; Judy, B. M.; Taylor, J. A.; Curran, E. M.; vom Saal, F. S. Large effects from small exposures. I. Mechanisms for endocrine-disrupting chemicals with estrogenic activity, *Environ. Health Perspect.* **2003**, 111, 994–1006.

Welshons, W. V.; Nagel, S. C.; vom Saal, F. S. Large effects from small exposures. III. Endocrine mechanisms mediating effects of bisphenol A at levels of human exposure, *Endocrinology* **2006**, 147, S56–S69.

Weybridge Workshop. European workshop on the impact of endocrine disruptors on human health and wildlife, Report of Proceedings, 2–4 December, 1996. Weybridge, UK.

WHO/UNEP, State of the Science of Endocrine Disrupting Chemicals – 2012, Report, Bergman, Å.; Heindel, J. J.; Jobling, S.; Kidd, K. A.; Zoeller, R. T., eds. World Health Organization and United Nations Environment Program, 2013. Available at: http://www.who.int/ceh/publications/endocrine/en/ (accessed 28 Jan 2014).

Ying, G.-G.; Williams, B.; Kookana, R. Environmental fate of alkylphenols and alkylphenol ethoxylates – a review, *Environ. Int* **2002**, 28, 215–226.

Zoeller, R. T.; Brown, T. R.; Doan, L. L.; Gore, A. C.; Skakkebaek, N. E.; Soto, A. M.; Woodruff, T. J.; vom Saal, F. S. Endocrine-disrupting chemicals and public health protection: a statement of principles from the Endocrine Society, *Endocrinology* **2012**, 153(9), 4097–4110.

PART I

MECHANISMS OF HORMONAL ACTION AND PUTATIVE ENDOCRINE DISRUPTORS

Endocrine Disruptors in the Environment, First Edition. Sushil K. Khetan.
© 2014 John Wiley & Sons, Inc. Published 2014 by John Wiley & Sons, Inc.

2

MECHANISMS OF ENDOCRINE SYSTEM FUNCTION

2.1 INTRODUCTION

The human endocrine system consists of glands producing and secreting hormones (such as the hypothalamus, the pituitary gland, the thyroid, the adrenals, pancreas, the ovaries, and the testes) that travel through the blood to a distant effector organ and regulate many body functions. The hormones act on receptors in the target cells of that hormone, eliciting a response in the target tissue. In general, hormones operate as chemical signals, enabling the endocrine system to regulate a variety of biological functions such as homeostasis (the body's ability to maintain a state of balance), growth, development, sexual differentiation, and reproduction (Norris and Carr, 2006). A simple archetypical endocrine system operates on the "seesaw" principle (Fig. 2.1), in which the target cells send feedback signals (usually negative feedback) to the regulating cells, with the result that secretion of the target-cell-stimulating hormone is altered (usually reduced) by one or more of the products of the target cells (Damstra et al., 2002)

2.2 HORMONAL AXES

The endocrine system is comprised of multiple pathways, or axes, each consisting of different groupings of organs and hormones with distinct regulatory functions. There are three major endocrine axes that affect reproductive development and function in the vertebrates. Axes refer to the effects of the hypothalamus, pituitary gland, and hormones operating as if these individual endocrine glands were a single

Endocrine Disruptors in the Environment, First Edition. Sushil K. Khetan.
© 2014 John Wiley & Sons, Inc. Published 2014 by John Wiley & Sons, Inc.

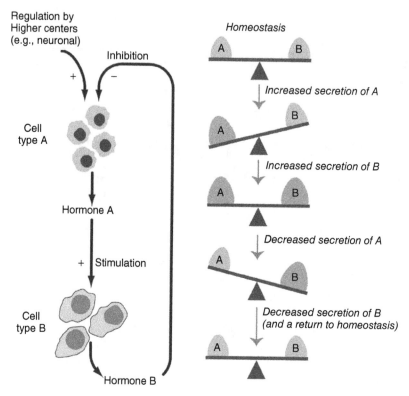

Figure 2.1 Hormonal homeostasis. In the schematic, cell type A secretes hormone A, which regulates production of hormone B by cell type B, and in turn hormone B exerts negative feedback regulation of the secretion of hormone A. In this way, swings in secretion of hormone A or B will be compensated for to maintain homeostasis (i.e., the correct levels of A and B), shown on the right. Source: Adapted from Damstra et al., 2002. Reproduced with permission of World Health Organization. Available at: http://www.who.int/ipcs/publications/new_issues/endocrine_disruptors/en/ (accessed on 28 Oct 2013).

entity as a whole. These axes are the hypothalamic–pituitary–gonadal (HPG) axis, the hypothalamic–pituitary–thyroid (HPT) axis, and the hypothalamic–pituitary–adrenal (HPA) axis, having target organs as gonads, the thyroid gland, and adrenal, respectively. Pituitary glycoproteins are used in both the HPG and HPT axes, with follicle-stimulating hormone (FSH) and luteinizing hormone (LH) in the HPG axis and thyroid-stimulating hormone (TSH) in the HPT axis. These hormones are responsible for the regulation of hormones in the pituitary. A common feature of control pathways is a feedback loop connecting the response to the initial stimulus. Negative feedback regulates many hormonal pathways involved in homeostasis. The human endocrine system is finely tuned to affect nearly all of the body's functions, and an imbalance leads to disease. Endocrine disruptors are able to disturb hormonal homeostasis of organisms by mimicking the hormonal activity of the natural hormones.

The lipophilic steroid and thyroid hormones (THs) simply diffuse across the plasma membrane and out of the cell down a concentration gradient to readily enter cells to interact with cytoplasmic or nuclear receptors.

2.2.1 Hypothalamus–Pituitary–Gonad (HPG) Axis

The primary function of the HPG axis in vertebrates is to facilitate the production of germ cells in males and to coordinate reproductive events such as ovulation, pregnancy, and lactation in females. In addition to its function in adult animals, the HPG axis regulates the differentiation of the sex-specific phenotype during early development, where sex steroids play a pivotal role.

The hypothalamus, located at the base of the brain, acts as a central processor for regulating the endocrine system by maintaining homeostasis of a variety of physiologic functions. It initiates the secretion of gonadotropin-releasing hormone (GnRH) in a pulsatile manner into the blood. At the anterior pituitary, the GnRH diffuses to its target cells, called gonadotropes. The gonadotrope cells synthesize/secrete the gonadotropins, LH, and FSH. In response to GnRH stimulation, the gonadotropes quickly release the gonadotropins from the pituitary gland into the general circulating system, and target the gonads (ovary or testis). At the gonad, gonadotropins drive the synthesis of steroid hormones via steroidogenesis and production of sperm and ova via gametogenesis. Sertoli and Leydig (testis) cells and theca and granulosa (ovary) cells have receptors for LH and FSH, and produce steroid hormones including estrogen and testosterone, as well as other factors (such as inhibin B), which induce a direct effect on hormone-responsive tissues. The steroid hormones, in turn, regulate GnRH production in the hypothalamus (and, therefore, secretion of pituitary gonadotropins). The hypothalamus and pituitary operate under negative feedback control regulated by levels of gonadotropins and steroids. This control route, hypothalamus → pituitary → gonad, is called the HPG axis (Fig. 2.2), and is one of several highly conserved hypothalamic–pituitary–hormonal axes in the vertebrates.

During puberty, the HPG axis is activated, leading to increases in LH, FSH, and sex steroids (testosterone and estradiol) levels (Grumbach and Styne, 2003). LH and FSH play important roles in the menstrual cycle. LH stimulates production of testosterone from Leydig cells and secretion by the follicle. FSH stimulates the Sertoli cells, causing the testes to produce a hormone that regulates sperm production. Sex steroids then act upon steroid hormone receptors, primarily estrogen receptors (ERs), androgen receptors (ARs), and progesterone receptors (PRs), that are widely expressed in target tissues, including the reproductive tract and genitalia, breast, and other organ systems.

Under the control of FSH, androgen is converted to estrogen by aromatizing the A ring of the steroid molecule through the actions of the enzyme aromatase

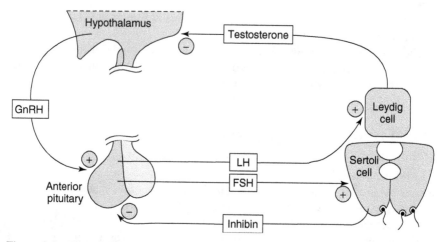

Figure 2.2 Hypothalamo–pituitary–gonadal (HPG) axis. GnRH, gonadotropin-releasing hormone; LH, luteinizing hormone; FSH, follicle-stimulating hormone. Source: Adapted from Hedge et al., 1987. Reproduced with permission of W. B. Saunders Company.

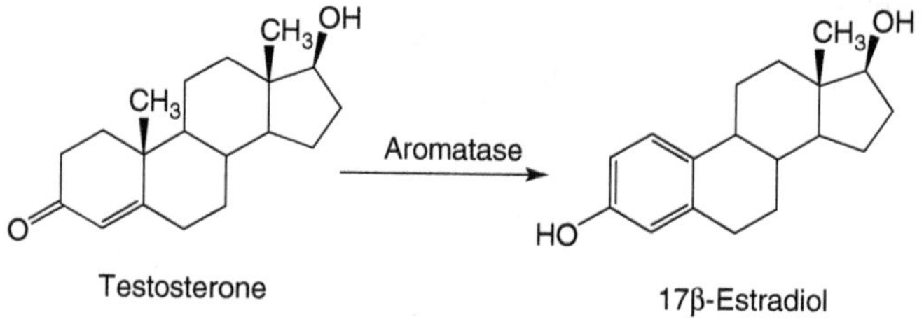

Figure 2.3 Androgen/estrogen ratio is determined by aromatase (CYP 19) activity that catalyzes, for example, aromatization of testosterone to 17β-estradiol.

(CYP19) (Fig. 2.3). The rate-limiting activity of CYP19 determines the androgen/estrogen ratio and is responsible for the irreversible estrogen biosynthesis from androgens. If aromatase production is stimulated or induced, excess estrogen will be produced, and, if it is inhibited, testosterone will remain unaltered, resulting in a shift in normal hormone concentrations.

The plasma androgen/estrogen ratio during fetal life creates a male-versus-female hormonal milieu. The balance between estrogenic and androgenic properties of EDCs (endocrine disruptor chemicals) can be biologically significant because reproduction of both sexes involves the interplay of androgens and estrogens. This delicate balance could be disrupted by xeno-hormones and lead to disorder of sexual differentiation (pseudo-hermaphroditism) (Lemaire et al., 2004).

Reproduction is coordinated with growth and development, which is tied to metabolism. At the core of metabolic and developmental regulation is the HPT axis (see later). Thus, various components of other endocrine axes are able to exert important modulatory effects on the HPG axis to alter the timing or efficiency of reproduction.

2.2.2 The Hypothalamic–Pituitary–Thyroid (HPT) Axis

Thyroid function is regulated by the dynamic interrelationships between the hypothalamus, the pituitary, and the thyroid. These dynamic relationships maintain circulating levels of THs within a narrow range under normal conditions. This functional grouping is called the HPT axis (Fig. 2.4).

To ensure stable levels of THs, the hypothalamus monitors circulating TH levels and responds to low levels by releasing the thyrotropin-releasing hormone (TRH). TRH then stimulates the pituitary to release TSH or "thyrotropin," a glycoprotein hormone from the anterior pituitary. The TSH stimulates the thyroid gland to produce the thyroid hormone thyroxine (T4) and release it from the thyroid. THs (T4 and deiodinized T3) exert a negative feedback effect on the release of pituitary TSH and on the activity of hypothalamic TRH neurons. When TH levels increase, the hypothalamus signals the pituitary to decrease the production of TSH, which in turn slows the release of new hormone from the thyroid gland. Finally, TH action is mediated through TH receptors throughout the body. THs are cleared from the blood in the liver following sulfation or sulfonation by sulfotransferases, or following glucuronidation by uridine diphosphate (UDP)-glucuronosyltransferase. These modified THs are then eliminated through the bile (Zoeller and Meeker, 2010). The

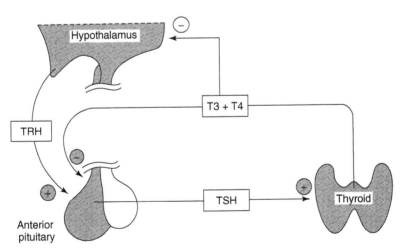

Figure 2.4 HPT Axis. The hypothalamus and anterior pituitary control the secretion of thyroid hormones through two negative feedback loops TRH, thyrotropin-releasing hormone; TSH, thyroid-stimulating hormone; T4, thyroxine; T3, deiodinized thyroxine. Source: Adapted from Hedge et al., 1987. Reproduced with permission of W. B. Saunders Company.

HPG and HPT axes function as integrated systems to produce and tightly regulate blood and tissue levels of estrogen (E), testosterone (T), and the THs.

2.2.3   The Hypothalamic–Pituitary–Adrenal (HPA) Axis

The HPA axis plays a key role in adaptation to environmental stresses. In response to physical and/or emotional stress, the hypothalamus secretes the corticotrophin-releasing hormone (CRH), which causes the release of the adrenocorticotropic hormone (ACTH) from the pituitary gland. ACTH is transported via the bloodstream to the adrenal glands, where it stimulates the secretion of the glucocorticoid hormones cortisol or corticosterone. In turn, cortisol feeds back to the brain to shut off further cortisol secretion. As in other endocrine axes, this negative feedback loop protects the organism from prolonged detrimental cortisol exposure and keeps its concentration within a wide but stable operating range (Huizenga et al., 1998) (Fig. 2.5).

The adrenal glands are a source of other important hormones, including mineralocorticoids. In humans, the glucocorticoid cortisol and the mineralocorticoid aldosterone are the physiologically most important hormones. The glucocorticoids (cortisol and corticosterone) secreted by adrenal cells have important roles in metabolism of carbohydrate, protein, and fat, with the aim to maintain blood glucose levels, regulation of blood pressure, and modulation of stress responses. Hyper-secretion of cortisol can lead to a suite of metabolic disturbances, including high blood sugar levels (hyperglycemia), redistribution of body fat, and an increased protein catabolism, and gross enlargement of the adrenal cortex. Aldosterone regulates water and electrolyte balance in the body by reducing excretion of sodium ions from the body, mainly by stimulating their reabsorption

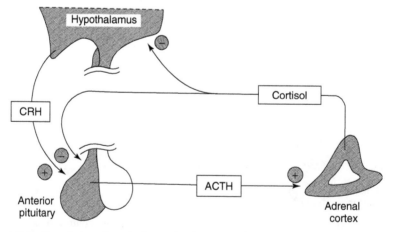

Figure 2.5   Regulation of cortisol secretion by the HPA axis. CRH, corticotropin-releasing hormone; ACTH, adreno-corticotropic hormone. Source: Adapted from Hedge et al., 1987. Reproduced with permission of W. B. Saunders Company.

in the kidney. Hyper-secretion of aldosterone causes hypertension and retention of body fluid (edema) due to excess sodium and water retention.

It is recognized that glucocorticoids have important "programing" effects during development and that alterations in the circulating levels of these hormones can affect the timing and set points of other endocrine axes. In humans, low birth weight is associated with elevated cortisol and aldosterone levels, suggesting fetal mis-programming of the HPA axis (Martinez-Aguayo et al., 2011). Urban psychosocial stress is also reported to affect plasma cortisol concentrations (Rosati et al., 2011).

EDCs may disrupt regulation of adrenal hormone secretion and function at different levels of the HPA axis. Because of its high blood supply and lipid content, a variety of persistent environmental contaminants and other chemicals are selectively taken up and retained in the adrenal cortex, both in adults and fetuses. For example, the DDT (dichlorodiphenyltrichloroethane) metabolite methylsulfonyl-DDE ($MeSO_2$-DDE), a highly potent and tissue-specific toxicant, induced degeneration and necrosis in the adrenal cortex of laboratory mice following a single dose (Lindhe et al., 2001). However, despite emerging evidence that both the HPA axis and the adrenal glands are targets for EDCs, the HPA axis has attracted relatively little attention in endocrine disruptor research (WHO/UNEP, 2013).

2.3 HORMONAL CELL SIGNALING

Steroid hormones reveal the capability to exert a variety of physiological effects in a wide range of species and target tissues to produce what are manifested as slow genomic responses, and rapid nongenomic responses. The classical genomic pathway, which involves binding of lipid-soluble steroid hormones to receptors in the cytoplasm of the target cell and subsequent modulation of gene expression, is well characterized. New evidence indicates that rapid nongenomic responses are mediated by the plasma-membrane-associated steroid receptors.

2.3.1 Receptors and Hormone Action

All hormones exert their physiological actions by binding to receptors in their target cells. The cellular hormone receptors include nuclear hormone receptors (NRs) and plasma membrane receptors of the cell. The NRs are a class of ligand-activated protein superfamily including ER, AR, the thyroid receptor (TR), peroxisome proliferator-activated receptor (PPAR), and retinoid receptors (RAR/RXR), as well as molecules with unknown function known as orphan receptors. These proteins play an important role in a wide range of physiological and toxicological processes by entering the nucleus and acting as transcription factors to transactivate or repress gene expression. The ligand-induced gene expression facilitates changes in cellular function. The steroid receptors, exemplified by the ER, are the sensors to ensure the fidelity of the steroid hormone endocrine regulation by tightly monitoring and responding to changes in circulating steroid hormone levels to maintain body homeostasis.

Plasma membrane receptors include kinase-linked receptors, which directly activate a protein kinase and G-protein coupled receptors (GPCRs), which act through the generation of a second messenger or ion channel opening.

2.3.2   Genomic Signaling Pathway

A cell is surrounded by a membrane which forms a barrier between the inside and outside of the cell. This structure consists of a double layer of phospholipid molecules interspersed with cholesterol and proteins (many of which are receptors for chemical signals) that float in or are attached to the membrane. Its lipid-rich composition provides it with the characteristic of being selectively permeable, allowing the flow of lipophilic substances across it while excluding many water-soluble ones.

In endocrine signaling, the lipophilic signaling molecules, such as steroid hormones and THs, act on target cells distant from their site of synthesis by cells of endocrine organs. Hormones are thought to simply diffuse across the plasma membrane, transported into the blood bound to low-affinity carrier proteins such as albumin, and carried from its site of release to its target (Fig. 2.6). Their cellular response depend on binding the receptor proteins usually found located in the cytosol or nucleus.

The classic model for steroid hormone action presumes that steroid hormones can freely cross the plasma membrane, enter the cytoplasm, and bind to and activate specific intracellular steroid receptor proteins. According to this model, steroid hormone binds to the hormone-binding cavity or, in some instances, to some other part of the receptor, inducing a conformational change of the receptor to activate or inhibit its ability to function as a transcription factor, often via binding of co-activator or co-repressor proteins (Fig. 2.7). The major consequence of activation is that the receptor becomes competent to directly interact with DNA response

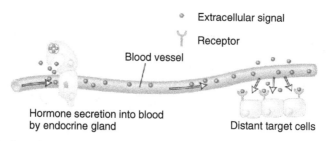

Figure 2.6   In endocrine signaling, signaling molecules, called *hormones*, are carried by the blood from its site of release to its target cells. Source: Adapted from Lodish et al., 2000. Reproduced with permission of W.H. Freeman And Company.

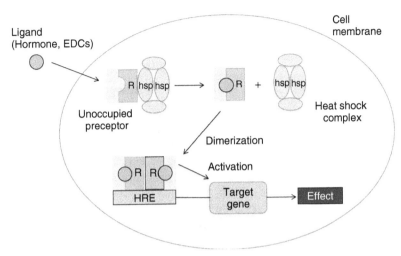

Figure 2.7   A simplified mechanism of action of steroid hormone receptors. Ligand binding to the receptor protein (R) stimulates dissociation of the heat shock proteins (hsps), causing conformational changes in the receptor and promoting dimerization of the receptor. This enables it to bind as a dimer to specific nuclear DNA sites, called *hormone response elements* (HRE). Then, DNA binding to HRE occurs to produce a complex that can trigger or suppress the transcription of a selected set of genes. Source: Adapted from Weigel, 1996. Reproduced with permission of the Biochemical Society.

elements of target genes, as well as by "cross-talking" to other signaling pathways (Fig. 2.8). It initiates a sequence of reactions regulating genes expression. Hormones of this type include the steroids (e.g., cortisol, progesterone, estradiol, and testosterone), thyroxine, and retinoic acid.

   When unbound by ligand, receptor is maintained in an inactive state in the cytosol bound to large complexes of proteins including several heat-shock proteins (hsps). Upon binding of the hormone to the receptor, dissociation of hsp results, enabling the receptor to change its conformation to the active form exposing the DNA-binding domain. Once activated, the receptor forms a homodimer complex. The dimer is then translocated to the nucleus, where it interacts with specific region of DNA known as *hormone response elements* (HREs), and modulates genes transcription, followed by production of target protein. The protein that is made from the newly synthesized messenger RNA then directs physiologic responses to maintain homeostasis, regulate growth, or control other specific processes (Fig. 2.7).

   This "classical" intracellular receptor-signaling pathway is considered as genomic, since it acts via the regulation of gene transcription. Hormone-producing signaling cells store a small supply of hormone precursor but not the mature active hormone. When stimulated, the cells convert the precursor to the active hormone. It takes a relatively long time (hours) from the translocation of the active hormone receptor into the nucleus and to the transcription, translation, and accumulation of significant amounts of newly formed protein, so the net effect appears only slowly.

2.3.3 Rapid-Response Pathway (Nongenomic Signaling)

Initially, steroid hormones were thought to act only via NRs, a class of transcription factors that regulate gene expression programs. However, the genomic action of steroid hormones cannot explain all the effects, mainly those classified as rapid effects. Some steroid effects (e.g., the opening of ion channels) detected within minutes of a change in steroid concentration are generally considered to be independent of receptors acting in the nucleus, excluding the possibility that the classical genomic pathway could mediate these hormone responses. These effects are presumed to be through the so-called nongenomic signaling pathways.

Many hormones are too large, or too polar, to pass through plasma membranes. They bind to transmembrane proteins that act as receptor sites on target cell membranes. Nongenomic mechanisms are likely to be mediated by hormones binding to receptors in the cell membrane. The binding of ligands to many cell-membrane receptors leads to a short-lived increase (or decrease) in the concentration of the intracellular signaling molecules, termed *second messengers*, and activation of various signal-transduction cascades, such as ion fluxes (often Ca^{2+}), cyclic adenosine monophosphate (cAMP) modulation, and protein kinase pathways (Lösel and Wehling, 2003). In these cases, the hormone is the first messenger, which causes activation of a second messenger in the cytoplasm (such as cAMP). Second messenger induction by nongenomic steroid action is insensitive to inhibitors of transcription and translation. These second messengers regulate numerous cellular functions from cell division to cell growth and development (within seconds or minutes). For example, in GPCR, the binding of a signal to this receptor results in activation of a G-protein, which in turn initiates a process leading to a short-lived increase (or decrease) in the concentration of a specific second messenger or modulate an ion channel (e.g., cellular Ca^{2+}), causing a change in membrane potential that will alter cellular behavior (Lodish et al., 2000). Many rapid signaling messengers, although they do not act primarily on DNA, indirectly modulate gene expression by acting on transcription factors. They might also influence genes that are targeted by the same steroid in a synergistic, immediate, and delayed manner (Lösel and Wehling, 2003).

All the members of the steroid hormones, including the gonadal hormones (estrogens, progestins, and androgens), TH, and the corticosteroids (glucocorticoids – e.g., insulin and mineralocorticoids), can exhibit nongenomic effects (Cheskis et al., 2007). Thus, transcriptional regulation of target genes by the classic genomic mechanism of steroid action mediated by intracellular receptors belonging to the nuclear steroid receptor is in addition to steroids' rapid nongenomic actions initiated at the cell surface by binding to membrane receptors frequently associated with the activation of various protein-kinase cascades (Fig. 2.8).

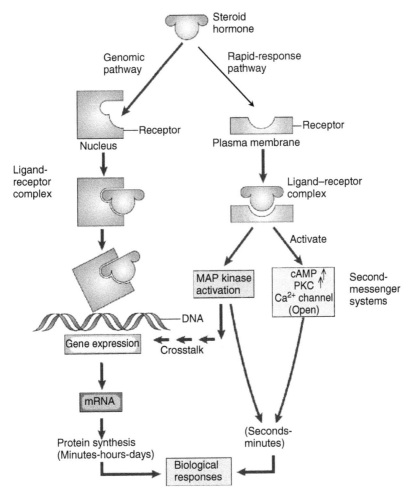

Figure 2.8 Genomic and nongenomic steroid hormone action. Genomic mechanisms initiate when the hormone binds receptors in the cytoplasm. The hormone/receptor complex migrates to the nucleus to directly alter gene expression (mRNA). This process takes hours or days to affect behavior. Nongenomic mechanisms are likely to be mediated by hormones binding to receptors in the cell membrane. These receptors then activate other cellular signaling pathways (second messengers, e.g., cAMP generation, Ca^{+2} stimulation) that can lead to rapid changes in behavior (within seconds or minutes). Source: Adapted from Norman et al., 2004. Reproduced with permission of Macmillan Publishers Ltd.

The evidence collected in the past years indicates that target cells and organs are regulated by a complex interplay of genomic and nongenomic signaling mechanisms of steroid hormones, and the integrated action of these machineries has important functional roles in a variety of pathophysiological processes. Transcriptional mechanisms are increasingly well understood, but membrane-initiated actions of these ligands remain incompletely understood.

2.3.4 Receptor Agonists, Partial Agonists, and Antagonists

Hormones and their cellular receptors have a lock-and-key relationship because of the high degree of specificity between each hormone and its receptor. The hormone molecule must fit precisely into receptor to unlock a specific biological response. A hormone is a naturally occurring ligand for its target cell receptor. A conceptual diagram of a natural hormone (A) binding to its intended receptor is shown in Fig. 2.9. Ligands that activate receptors and initiate the cellular response are termed *agonists*; so hormones are agonists to their receptors. Ligands that bind to the receptor but do not initiate the cellular response are called *antagonists*.

Many EDCs structurally resemble but are imperfect cognate ligands that bind to NRs, triggering responses that are not necessarily the same as those triggered by the endogenous hormones. These molecules are ligands that activate or inhibit the receptor function and thereby elicit a physiological response. Because of the large number of chemicals with different modes of action and different affinities to hormonal receptors, molecular locks found in cells throughout the body and their endocrine disruption potencies differ substantially. Ligands that activate a response are agonists, mimicking the action of the naturally occurring ligand, however, often with different potencies. For example, some EDCs (in Fig. 2.9b and c) can bind to

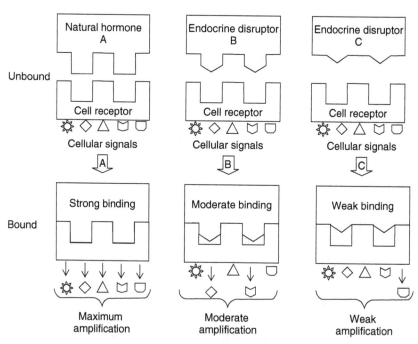

Figure 2.9 The lock-and-key relationship existing between a hormone and its receptor. Source: Adapted from Anderson, 2005. Reproduced with permission of Water Environment Research Foundation (WERF).

the receptors but far less strongly, evoking a weaker biological response, such as that triggered by the endogenous estrogens and termed as *selective ER modulators* (SERMs).

EDCs can alter the effects of the endogenous hormones by acting as receptor agonists or antagonists (or both, when acting as modulators), thereby resulting in abnormal hormonal signaling and leading to altered hormone action. EDCs can also act by affecting hormone concentrations indirectly through signaling pathways that control hormone production or elimination (Barouki et al., 2012).

2.4 SEX STEROIDS

2.4.1 Physiologic Estrogens

Estrogens are most important female sexual hormones produced in the ovary in premenopausal women, by aromatization from androgens. Steroidal estrogens are lipid-soluble compounds that are able to pass through the plasma membrane of cells by diffusion. The most abundant estrogens are 17β-estradiol (E2) and estrone (E1) extracted from ovarian tissue. E2 is the principal estrogen produced by the ovary, and two estrogens, E1 (elevated postmenopausally) and E3 (estriol – elevated during pregnancy) are largely byproducts of E2 metabolism (Fig. 2.10). E2 plays a critical role in many physiological processes in both females and males. These include normal growth, development, and cell-type-specific gene regulation in tissues of the reproductive tract, central nervous system, and skeleton (Kazeto et al., 2004). E2 is excreted in the urine of woman up to 60 μg per day, increasing to 200-400 μg during pregnancy (Ohko et al., 2002). E2 is also the ER's natural and most potent ligand among the endogenous estrogens which act solely as receptor agonists, and is found to be an important EDC in the aquatic environment (Routledge et al., 1998).

The steroid hormone estrogen regulates critical cellular signaling pathways and thus controls cell proliferation, differentiation, and homeostasis. Estrogen, the female sex hormone, is the key hormone in the initiation (puberty) and reproduction – it stimulates growth of the uterine wall in preparation for embryo implantation and the end (menopause) of reproductive life in women – and is

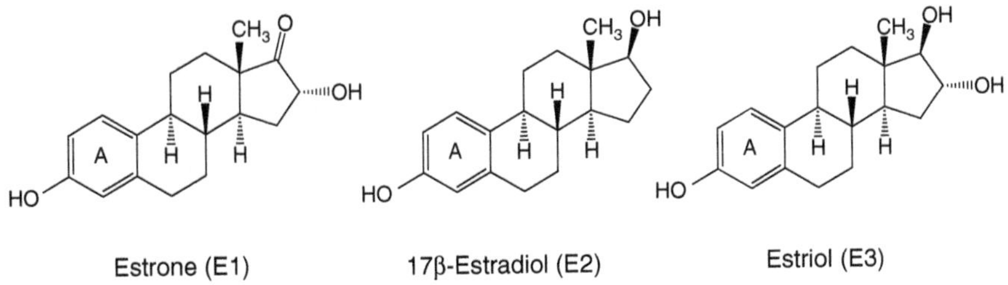

Estrone (E1)   17β-Estradiol (E2)   Estriol (E3)

Figure 2.10 Physiologic steroidal estrogens containing aromatized A ring.

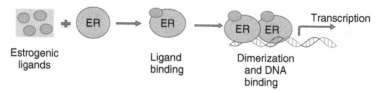

Figure 2.11 Ligand activated estrogen receptor signaling. Upon binding of estrogen to the receptor protein, accessory heat-shock proteins are dissociated from the receptors. Hormone-receptor complexes dimerize and enter the nucleus, initiating transcription of responsive genes. Adapted from Heldring et al., 2007.

thus of considerable importance in women's health. Estrogens also influence the pathological processes of hormone-dependent diseases, such as breast, endometrial, and ovarian cancers, as well as osteoporosis. Estrogens are also necessary in males for the regulation of male sexual behavior, maintenance of the skeleton and the cardiovascular system, and for normal functioning of testis and the prostate (Pettersson and Gustafsson, 2001). Estrogens are among the most potent chemicals in nature. Although environmental concentrations of these compounds are typically low, the low dose response of animals to estrogens makes their introduction into the environment a concern.

The biological actions of estrogens are mediated by ERs. ERs function as ligand-regulated transcription factors, regulating numerous important physiological processes such as the development, reproduction, behavior, metabolism, bone homeostasis, and regulation of the cardiovascular system (Heldring et al., 2007). The classical mechanism by which estrogen exerts many of its effects is by binding to its receptor in the nucleus inducing conformational changes allowing dimerization and DNA binding and activating or inhibiting the transcription of messenger RNAs, producing a new protein, which alters the function of the cell (Fig. 2.11).

Although steroid and THs were originally thought to bind only to receptors found in the cell nucleus, where effects were exerted via gene transcription, it is now known that, in addition, estrogens also elicit rapid nongenomic responses via membrane-bound receptors (Pietras & Szego 1977).

The ERs are widely distributed throughout the body, displaying distinct but overlapping expression patterns in a variety of tissues. There are two major ER isoforms (ERα or ERβ), which belong to the group of NR superfamily of ligand-activated transcription factors that also bind compounds such as steroids, THs, and retinoids (Bertrand et al., 2004). Although both ERs share similar mechanisms of action, several differences in the transcriptional abilities of each receptor have been identified, suggesting that these receptors may regulate distinct cellular pathways. While ERα is predominantly involved in the regulation of reproductive behavior and hormone secretion as well as growth and maintenance of peripheral reproductive tissues, ERβ is implicated in the control of a variety of nonreproductive functions, including the regulation of emotion and cognition (Laflamme et al., 1998; Bodo and Rissman, 2006). ERα and ERβ are encoded by separate genes on separate chromosomes and share a high degree of homology and similar affinity for 17β-estradiol (E2), the most

TABLE 2.1   Relative Molecular Volumes of Ligand-binding Cavities of Estrogen Receptors and 17β-Estradiol (Shanle and Xu, 2011)

	Molecular Volumes ($A^{\circ 3}$)
Ligand binding cavity of ERα	450
Ligand binding cavity of ERβ	390
E2	245

potent estrogen, but have opposing effects on cell growth. ERα promotes proliferation of estrogen-dependent cells, whereas ERβ is anti-proliferative and promotes differentiation, opposing functions providing a feedback loop for finite control of estrogen signaling. The opposing activities of the ER isoforms suggest that ERβ and ERα balance each other's effects and that dysregulation of one ER isoform could lead to inappropriate activity of the other (Ruegg et al., 2009). Interestingly, when ERs are coexpressed, ERβ exhibits an inhibitory action on ERα-mediated gene expression, such that ERβ has been shown to antagonize several ERα-mediated effects including cellular proliferation in breast, uterus, or prostate (Nose et al., 2009).

ERs have the unique ability to interact with a wide variety of compounds. Originally, each steroid receptor evolved to be only as specific as it had to be to bind its target ligand and exclude all others that existed at the time. The ER, which is believed to be the ancestral steroid receptor (Thornton et al., 2003), achieved this by binding substances that contain a chemical structure called an *aromatized A ring* (Fig. 2.10). Because estrogens were the only steroid hormones to have such a ring, that criterion was enough to ensure that the receptor bound only estrogens for many millions of years. Then, the chemical industry started pumping out hundreds of substances containing such aromatized rings, to which the ER unwittingly bound. It has been suggested that the promiscuity of the ERs in accepting many diverse ligands may be the result of their evolutionary history (Baker, 2004). The overall promiscuity of the ERs can be attributed to the size of the binding cavity, which has a volume almost twice that of the E2 molecular volume (Table 2.1) (Kuiper et al., 1998). The relatively large molecular volumes of the ligand-binding cavities of ERα and ERβ as compared to E2 allows access to a diverse set of small molecules to the ligand-binding cavities (Shanle and Xu, 2011).

Although the receptors ERα and ERβ bind to E2 with similar affinities, they differ by two amino acids within the ligand binding cavities, which allows selective binding to many exogenous ligands.

2.4.2   Androgens

Androgens and their receptors are crucial for the development of the male reproductive tissues and their maturation in puberty and for maintenance of male sex accessory organs, such as the prostate gland. They also play an essential role in

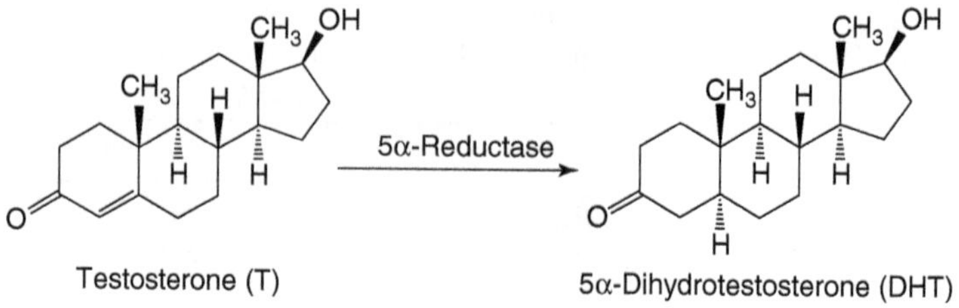

Figure 2.12   Androgen hormones.

the development and differentiation of the male embryo during the *in utero* and early postnatal development and spermatogenesis initiation and maintenance. In females, AR knock-out revealed that androgens are important for proper ovarian function and mammary development (Walters et al., 2010).

The androgen-signaling pathway shares many molecular and cellular traits with the estrogen-signaling pathway. The two physiologically active androgens that bind the human AR with the highest affinity are testosterone (T), and 5α-dihydrotestosterone (DHT) (Fig. 2.12). Free testosterone, chiefly produced by Leydig cells in the testes, is transported into the cytoplasm of target tissue cells, where it can bind to the AR, or can be reduced to DHT in prostate cells by the cytoplasmic enzyme 5α reductase. The androgen DHT is more active with a fivefold higher affinity than T for the AR (Heinlein and Chang, 2002). DHT is required for normal development of the external genitalia and prostate (Bowman et al., 2003).

In mammals, testosterone is primarily secreted in the testicles of males and the ovaries of females, although small amounts are also secreted by the adrenal glands. It is the principal male sex hormone. In men, testosterone plays a key role in the development of male reproductive tissues such as the testis and prostate, as well as promoting secondary sexual characteristics such as increased muscle, bone mass, and the growth of body hair. In addition, testosterone in the testis is responsible for supporting spermatogenesis. Testosterone is also essential for health and well-being, as well as for the prevention of osteoporosis.

In fetal life, testosterone is a key driver of the differentiation of the male reproductive tract (Wolfian duct system) into the vas deferens, epididymis, seminal vesicles, and external genitalia, and to actively remove the Mullerian duct (the precursor to the female uterine system). Conversion of T to the more potent DHT by 5α-reductase is required for differentiation of the prostate and external geni-talia. The hormone dependence of masculinization renders this process inherently susceptible to disruption by the environmental agents that interfere with hormone production, bioavailability, metabolism, or action. This susceptibility is illustrated in animal models by the high prevalence of congenital masculinization disorders, such as reduced sperm counts, increased infertility, testicular dysgenesis syndrome, and testicular and prostate cancers. Other male reproductive abnormalities associ-ated with AR disruptors in both human epidemiology studies as well as in animal models include delayed puberty (Louis et al., 2008) and reduced anogenital distance in newborn boys (Swan et al., 2005).

Testosterone is shown to act via the classical and the nonclassical pathways (Walker, 2009). In the classical pathway, testosterone diffuses through the plasma membrane and binds AR that is sequestered by *hsps* in the cytoplasm. A conformational change in AR causes the receptor to be released from the *hsps*. AR then translocates to the nucleus, where it binds to *androgen response elements* (AREs) in gene promoter regions, recruits co-regulator proteins, and regulates gene transcription (Shang et al., 2002). Rapid nongenomic action of androgens is well documented, and a membrane G-protein-coupled AR has been characterized pharmacologically in fish ovaries (Thomas et al., 2006). The most consistent nongenomic effect of androgen exposure is a rapid change in Ca^{2+}, which functions as a ubiquitous second messenger molecule, impacting a wide range of cellular processes, including cell proliferation, apoptosis, necrosis, motility, and gene expression (Foradori et al., 2008). The ability of T to induce a rapid influx of Ca^{2+} has also been reported in primary cultures of rat Sertoli cells within 4 min of testosterone treatment, which could be inhibited by the AR antagonist flutamide (Lyng et al., 2000).

Antiandrogens, narrowly defined as AR antagonists due to their ability to compete with androgens for binding to the receptor, can be broadly defined in terms of counteracting the effects of androgens in a functional sense (which would include inhibition of uptake of T precursors and of T synthesis steps) (Gray et al., 2001).

2.5 THYROID HORMONES

The THs are essential to neurologic development, skeletal growth, and normal function of the pulmonary system, metabolism, and cardiovascular system. TH levels are homeostatically controlled; that is, the body possesses compensatory mechanism to keep TH levels within a set range. The neurological development of mammals is largely dependent on normal TH homeostasis, and it is likely to be particularly sensitive to the disruption of the thyroid axis. Multiple physiologic steps, including hormone biosynthesis, transport, metabolism, and action on target cells, are required for TH homeostasis. TH biosynthesis and secretion are normally maintained within narrow limits by regulatory mechanisms that are sensitive to small changes in the circulating hormone concentrations. These regulatory mechanisms protect against both hypothyroidism (deficient TH production) and hyperthyroidism (excess TH production).

Thyroid gland releases thyroxine (T4, tetraiodo-L-thyronine), a prohormone into the blood stream, which is locally transformed in the brain into physiologically active triiodothyronine (T3) by 5'-deiodination (Fig. 2.13). T4 enters the developing brain more easily than T3, and it is necessary for normal brain development, lungs, heart, and other organs and control of metabolism, and other aspects of maintaining healthy bodies. The two THs stimulate increased expression of many cytosolic enzymes (e.g., liver hexokinase) that catalyze the catabolism of glucose,

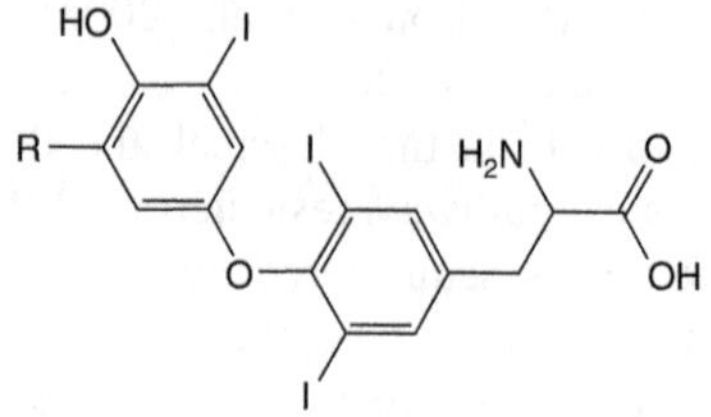

Triiodothyronine (T3): R = H
Thyroxine (T4):   R = I

Figure 2.13   The most active thyroid hormones.

fats, and proteins and of mitochondrial enzymes that catalyze oxidative phosphorylation (Miller et al., 2009).

TH exerts its effect on development and physiology perhaps primarily by interacting with specific nuclear proteins – the TRs, members of the superfamily of
ligand-regulated transcription factors. Although the THs T4 and T3 are chemically different from steroids, their classical receptors belong to the steroid-receptor
superfamily. Nuclear TR binds to a specific nucleotide sequence termed as the *TH-
responsive element* (TRE) as a homodimer or heterodimer with RXR (Chen et al.,
2010). Then, it binds to a series of proteins termed *co-activator* or *co-repressor* in a
ligand-dependent manner to regulate transcription of target genes. Similar to "true"
steroids, the THs have also been shown to have nongenomic effects (Davis et al.,
2008).

There is increasing evidence from animal and *in vitro* studies that the thyroid
is vulnerable to disruption by a variety of chemicals through changes in hormone
production, transport, and/or metabolism (Miller et al., 2009). The most commonly
used biomarker of the effect for thyroid-disrupting chemicals (TDCs) exposure is
serum total T4 concentrations (DeVito et al., 1999; Zoeller, 2007). Although serum
TSH concentration is an accepted biomarker for hypothyroidism, a number of xenobiotics alter circulating TH levels but do not change TSH (DeVito et al. 1999).
Many kinds of adverse effects are associated with either TH excess or insufficiency,
depending on the timing, severity, and duration of the perturbation. Although the
pattern of effects may differ, changes in serum TH are predictive of downstream
adverse outcomes.

2.6   CONCLUSIONS AND FUTURE PROSPECTS

Steroid and THs exert a variety of physiological effects on target tissues to produce
both slow genomic responses and rapid nongenomic responses. The hormone signaling processes are prone to disruption by EDCs because of the shared properties
of the chemicals and the similarities of the receptors and enzymes involved in the

synthesis, release, and degradation of hormones. Much progress has been made in elucidating the role of hormones in receptor activation and the mechanism by which hormone antagonists block this activity. These in turn allow better understanding of EDCs' impacts and mechanism of action.

REFERENCES

Anderson, P. D. Technical brief: Endocrine disrupting compounds and their implications for wastewater treatment, Water Environment Research Foundation (WERF), 2005. http://www.werf.org/a/ka/Search/ResearchProfile.aspx?ReportId=04-WEM-6 (accessed 25 June 2013).

Baker, M. E. Co-evolution of steroidogenic and steroid-inactivating enzymes and adrenal and sex steroid receptors, *Mol. Cell. Endocrinol.* **2004**, 215(1–2), 55–62.

Barouki, R.; Gluckman, P. D.; Grandjean, P.; Hanson, M.; Heindel, J. J. Developmental origins of non-communicable disease: implications for research and public health, *Environ. Health* **2012**, 11, 42.

Bertrand, S.; Brunet, F. G.; Escriva, H.; Parmentier, G.; Laudet, V.; Robinson-Rechavi, M. Evolutionary genomics of nuclear receptors: from twenty-five ancestral genes to derived endocrine systems, *Mol. Biol. Evolut.* **2004**, 21(10), 1923–1937.

Bodo, C.; Rissman, E.F. New roles for estrogen receptor beta in behavior and neuroendocrinology, *Front. Neuroendocrinol.* **2006**, 27, 217–232.

Bowman, C. J.; Barlow, N. J.; Turner, K. J.; Wallace, D. G.; Foster, P. M. D. Effects of in utero exposure to finasteride on androgen-dependent reproductive development in the male rat. *Toxicol. Sci.* **2003**, 74 (2), 393–406.

Chen, S. Y.; Leonard, J. L.; Davis, P. J. Molecular aspects of thyroid hormone actions, *Endocr. Rev.* **2010**, 31, 139–170.

Cheskis, B. J.; Greger, J. G.; Nagpal, S.; Freedman, L. P. Signaling by estrogens, *J. Cell. Physiol.* **2007**, 213, 610–617.

Damstra, T.; Barlow, S.; Bergman, A.; Kavlock, R.; Van Der Kraak, G. Global assessment of the state-of-the-science of endocrine disruptors, International Programme on Chemical Safety, WHO/PCS/EDC/02.2. World Health Organization, Geneva, Switzerland, 2002. Available at: http://www.who.int/ipcs/publications/new_issues/endocrine_disruptors/en/print.html (accessed 28 Oct 2013).

Davis, P. J.; Leonard, J. L.; Davis, F. B. Mechanisms of nongenomic actions of thyroid hormone, *Front. Neuroendocrinol.* **2008**, 29(2), 211–218.

DeVito, M.; Biegel, L.; Brouwer, A.; Brown, S.; Brucker-Davis, F.; Cheek, A. O., et al. Screening methods for thyroid hormone disruptors, *Environ. Health Perspect.* **1999**, 107, 407–415.

Foradori, C. D.; Weiser, M. J.; Handa, R. J. Non-genomic actions of androgens, *Front. Neuroendocrinol.* **2008**, 29, 169–181.

Gray, L. E., Jr.,; Ostby, J.; Furr, J.; Wolf, C. J.; Lambright, C.; Parks, L.; Veeramachaneni, D. N.; Wilson, V.; Price, M.; Hitchkiss, A.; Orlando, E.; Guillette, L. Effects of environmental antiandrogens on reproductive development in experimental animals, *Hum. Reprod. Update* **2001**, 7(3), 248–264.

Grumbach, M. M.; Styne, D. M. Puberty: Ontogeny, neuroendocrinology, physiology, and disorders, in *Williams Textbook of Endocrinology*, Larsen, P. R., ed., 10th ed., St. Louis: Saunders, **2003**, pp. 1115–1200.

Hedge, G. A.; Colb, H. D.; Goodman, R. L. General principles of endocrinology, in *Clinical Endocrine Physiology*, Philadelphia: WB Saunders Co., **1987**, pp. 3–33.

Heinlein, C. A.; Chang, C. The roles of androgen receptors and androgen-binding proteins in nongenomic androgen actions, *Mol. Endocrinol.* **2002**, 16(10), 2181–2187.

Heldring, N.; Pike, A.; Andersson, S.; Matthews, J.; Cheng, G.; Hartman, J., et al., Estrogen receptors: how do they signal and what are their targets, *Physiol. Rev.* **2007**, 87, 905–931.

Huizenga, N. A.; Koper, J. W.; de Lange, P.; Pols, H. A.; Stolk, R. P.; Grobbee, D. E., et al. Interperson variability but intraperson stability of baseline plasma cortisol concentrations, and its relation to feedback sensitivity of the hypothalamo–pituitary–adrenal axis to a low dose of dexamethasone in elderly individuals, *J. Clin. Endocrinol. Metab.* **1998**, 83, 47–54.

Kazeto, Y., Place, A.R., Trant, J.M. Effects of endocrine disrupting chemicals on the expression of CYP19 genes in zebrafish (Danio rerio) juveniles, *Aquat. Toxicol.* **2004**, 69, 25–34.

Kuiper, G. G. J. M.; Lemmen, J. G.; Carlsson, B.; Corton, J. C.; Safe, S. H.; van der Saag, P. T.; van der Burg, B.; Gustafsson, J. Å. Interaction of estrogenic chemicals and phytoestrogens with estrogen receptor ß, *Endocrinology* **1998**, 139(10), 4252–4263.

Laflamme, N.; Nappi, R. E.; Drolet, G., et al. Expression and neuropeptidergic characterization of estrogen receptors (ERalpha and ERbeta) throughout the rat brain: anatomical evidence of distinct roles of each subtype, *J. Neurobiol.* **1998**, 36, 357–378.

Lemaire, G.; Terouanne, B.; Mauvais, P.; Michel, S.; Rahmani, R. Effect of organochlorine pesticides on human androgen receptor activation in vitro, *Toxicol. Appl. Pharmacol.* **2004**, 196(2), 235–246.

Lindhe, Ö.; Lund, B. O.; Bergman, Å.; Brandt, I. Irreversible binding and adrenocorticolytic activity of the DDT metabolite 3-methylsulfonyl- DDE examined in tissue-slice culture. *Environ. Health Perspect.* **2001**, 109(2), 105–110.

Lodish, H.; Berk, A.; Zipursky, S. L., et al. Overview of extracellular signaling, in *Molecular Cell Biology*, 4th ed., New York: W. H. Freeman, **2000**.

Lösel, R.; Wehling, M. Nongenomic actions of steroid hormones, *Nat. Rev. Mol. Cell Biol.* **2003**, 4, 46–56.

Louis, G. M. B.; Gray, L. E., Jr.,; Marcus, M.; Ojeda, S. R.; Pescovitz, O. H.; Witchel, S. F.; Sippell, W.; Abbott, D. H.; Soto, A.; Tyl, R.W.; Bourguignon, J. P.; Skakkebaek, N. E.; Swan, S. H.; Golub, M. S.; Wabitsch, M.; Toppari, J.; Euling, S. Y. Environmental factors and puberty timing: expert panel research needs, *Pediatrics* **2008**, 121(Suppl 3), S192–S207.

Lyng, F. M.; Jones, G. R.; Rommerts, F. F. Rapid androgen actions on calcium signaling in rat sertoli cells and two human prostatic cell lines: similar biphasic responses between 1 picomolar and 100 nanomolar concentrations, *Biol. Reprod.* **2000**, 63, 736–747.

Martinez-Aguayo, A.; Aglony, M.; Bancalari, R.; Avalos, C.; Bolte, L.; Garcia, H.; Loureiro, C.; Carvajal, C.; Campino, C.; Inostroza, A.; Fardella, C. Birth weight is inversely associated with blood pressure and serum aldosterone and cortisol levels in children, *Clin. Endocrinol.* **2011**, 76, 713–718.

Miller, M. D.; Crofton, K. M.; Rice, D. C.; Zoeller, R. T. Thyroid-disrupting chemicals: interpreting upstream biomarkers of adverse outcomes, *Environ. Health Perspect.* **2009**, 117(7), 1033–1041.

Norris, D. O.; Carr, J. A., eds., *Endocrine Disruption*, New York: Oxford University Press, **2006**.

Norman, A. W.; Mizwicki, M. T.; Norman, D. P. G. Steroid-hormone rapid actions, membrane receptors and a conformational ensemble model, *Nat. Rev. Drug Discovery* **2004**, 3, 27–41.

Nose, N.; Sugio, K.; Oyama, T.; Nozoe, T.; Uramoto, H.; Iwata, T.; Onitsuka, T.; Yasumoto, K. Association between estrogen receptor-beta expression and epidermal growth factor receptor mutation in the postoperative prognosis of adenocarcinoma of the lung, *J. Clin. Oncol.*. **2009**, 27(3), 411–417.

Ohko, Y.; Iuchi, K.; Niwa, C.; Tatsuma, T.; Nakashima, T.; Iguchi, T.; Kubota, Y.; Fujishima, A. 17β-estradiol degradation by TiO_2 photocatalysis as a means of reducing estrogenic activity, *Environ. Sci. Technol.* **2002**, 36, 4175–4181.

Pettersson, K.; Gustafsson, J. A. Role of estrogen receptor β in estrogen action, *Annu. Rev. Physiol.* **2001**, 63, 165–192.

Pietras, R. J.; Szego, C. M. Specific binding sites for oestrogen at the outer surfaces of isolated endometrial cells, *Nature* **1977**, 265(5589), 69–72.

Rosati, M.V.; Sancini, A.; Tomei, F.; Andreozzi, G.; Scimitto, L.; Schifano, M. P.; Ponticiello, B. G.; Fiaschetti, M.; Tomei, G. Plasma cortisol concentrations and lifestyle in a population of outdoor workers, *Int. J. Environ. Health Res.* **2011**, 21(1), 62–71.

Routledge, E. J.; Sheahan, D.; Desbrow, C.; Brighty, G. C.; Waldock, M.; Sumpter, J. P. Identification of estrogenic chemicals in STW effluent. 2. In vivo responses in trout and roach. *Environ. Sci. Technol.* **1998**, 32, 1559.

Ruegg, J.; Penttinen-Damdimopoulou, P.; Makela, S.; Pongratz, I.; Gustafsson, J. A. Receptors mediating toxicity and their involvement in endocrine disruption, in *Molecular, Clinical and Environmental Toxicology, Vol. 1: Molecular Toxicology*, Lurch, A., ed., Switzerland: Birkhauser Verlag, **2009**, pp. 289–323.

Shang, Y.; Myers, M.; Brown, M. Formation of the androgen receptor transcription complex, *Mol. Cell* **2002**, 9, 601–610.

Shanle, E. K.; Xu, W. Endocrine disrupting chemicals targeting estrogen receptor signaling: Identification and mechanisms of action, *Chem. Res. Toxicol.* **2011**, 24(1), 6–19.

Swan, S. H.; Main, K. M.; Liu, F.; Stewart, S. L.; Kruse, R. L.; Calafat, A. M.; Mao, C. S.; Redmon, J. B.; Ternand, C. L.; Sullivan, S.; Teague, J. L. Decrease in anogenital distance among male infants with prenatal phthalate exposure, *Environ. Health Perspect.* **2005**, 113(8), 1056–1061.

Thomas, P.; Dressing, G.; Pang, Y.; Berg, H.; Tubbs, C.; Benninghoff, A.; Doughty, K. Progestin, estrogen and androgen G-protein coupled receptors in fish gonads, *Steroids* **2006**, 71(4), 310–316.

Thornton, J. W., Need, E.; Crews, D. Resurrecting the ancestral steroid receptor: ancient origin of estrogen signaling, *Science* **2003**, 301(5640), 1714–1717.

WHO/UNEP, *The State-of-the-Science of Endocrine Disrupting Chemicals – 2012*, Bergaman, A.; Heindel, J. J.; Jobling, S.; Kidd, K. A.; Zoeller, R. T., eds., Geneva: UNEP/WHO, **2013**. Available at: http://www.who.int/ceh/publications/endocrine/en/index.html (accessed 12 March 2013).

Walker, W. H. Molecular mechanisms of testosterone action in spermatogenesis, *Steroids* **2009**, 74(7), 602–607.

Walters, K. A.; Simanainen, U.; Handelsman, D. J. Molecular insights into androgen actions in male and female reproductive function from androgen receptor knockout models, *Hum. Reprod. Update* **2010**, 16(5), 543–558.

Weigel, N. L. Steroid hormone receptors and their regulation by phosphorylation, *Biochem. J.* **1996**, 319, 657–667.

Zoeller, R. T. Environmental chemicals impacting the thyroid: targets and consequences, *Thyroid* **2007**, 17(9), 811–817.

Zoeller, R.T.; Meeker, J.D. The thyroid system and its implications for reproduction, in *Environmental Impacts on Reproductive Health and Fertility*, Woodruff, T. J.; Janssen, S.; Guillette, L.; Giudice, L., eds., Cambridge University Press, **2010**.

3

ENVIRONMENTAL CHEMICALS TARGETING ESTROGEN SIGNALING PATHWAYS

3.1 INTRODUCTION

Exposures to endocrine disruptor chemicals (EDCs) can interfere with hypothalamic–pituitary–gonadal (HPG) axis signaling, leading to an interruption of the gonadotropin-releasing hormone (GnRH), luteinizing hormone (LH), and follicle-stimulating hormone (FSH) release, disrupting the homeostasis at different levels of feedback regulatory mechanisms for the regulation of steroidogenesis and spermatogenesis. The mediation of endocrine-disrupting effects on neuroendocrine reproductive function often occurs through steroid hormone receptors, particularly estrogen receptors (ERs) and androgen receptors (ARs), which are expressed abundantly in the hypothalamus. Changes in normal levels of GnRH and sex steroids in the developing fetus or newborn and their exposure to adverse environmental factors upset the normal homeostatic balance of the body, causing disturbances in their functioning throughout the subsequent life span with consequent disease susceptibility in adulthood (Langley-Evans, 2006).

Using terms like "estrogenic" may limit the scope of investigation because steroids have well-characterized function in a very small percentage of species. It is important to emphasize that, although compounds may be defined on the basis of a given outcome or mechanism of action, almost all chemicals influence multiple physiological systems and influence the way physiological systems interact with each other.

Endocrine Disruptors in the Environment, First Edition. Sushil K. Khetan.
© 2014 John Wiley & Sons, Inc. Published 2014 by John Wiley & Sons, Inc.

3.1.1   Gonadal Estrogen Function Disruptors

Environmental estrogens are the most studied EDCs. They follow the same mechanisms of action as the gonadal hormone 17β-estradiol. ERs are the major mediators of endocrine disruption by xenobiotic pollutants that mimic or block estrogen action. Numerous natural and synthetic chemicals that are quite varied in structure and potency, including pharmaceuticals, pesticides, plastics feedstocks and additives, and phytochemicals, can act as estrogen agonists or antagonists, mimicking or blocking the natural effects of estrogens on the ER (Blair et al., 2000; Gutendorf and Westendorf, 2001). Disruption of estrogen/ER signaling by such substances can have profound effects on the organism, including abnormal development of male and female reproductive tracts, feminization of males, lowered sperm counts, disrupted reproductive cycling and reduced fertility, carcinogenesis, and behavioral changes (McLachlan, 2001; Mueller, 2004; Guillette and Moore, 2006; Skakkebaek et al., 2001). Many EDCs are now ubiquitous in the global environment. Health damage by EDCs that target the ER has been documented in a variety of vertebrates, including humans (McLachlan, 2006; Sumpter and Jobling, 1995; Lauver et al., 2005; Swan, 2000).

Xenoestrogens can impact estrogen signaling through interaction with the ligand-binding domains (LBDs) of ERα and ERβ, thereby activating the receptors inappropriately. Inappropriate ER signaling can lead to disruption of normal endocrine function, resulting in multiple, diverse, and severe toxicological outcomes, such as altered pubertal development, impaired fertility, increased risk of abnormal fetal growth and development, and hormone-dependent cancer (Table 3.1) (Diamanti-Kandarakis et al., 2009). However, most phytoestrogens and xenoestrogens are partial agonists, meaning that they are unable to induce a maximal response matching that of the endogenous ligand, even at very high concentrations (Zhu, 2005).

Recent advances in endocrinology indicate that estrogens induce multiple changes in intracellular signaling cascades. Approximately 5–10% of total cellular ERs, including both ERα and ERβ, are localized to the plasma membrane in many cells. These membrane-associated receptors are capable of nongenomic steroid action in various cell types. Both physiologic estrogens and xenoestrogens can bind to ER associated with the cell membrane (membrane-associated ER

TABLE 3.1   Effects of Xenoestrogens on Development and Reproductive Action

Male fishes	Faminization
Female rodents	Altered reproductive physiology and behavior: advanced onset of puberty, premature loss of regular ovulatory cycle, abbreviated period of fertility
Male rodents	Fetal and neonatal exposure leading to increased disorder of male reproductive function termed as *testicular dysgenesis syndrome (TDS)* – Poor sperm quality (impaired spermatogenesis), cryptorchidism, hypospadias, and testicular cancer

(mER)α and mERβ) that are identical (or isoforms?) to the nuclear ER (Powell et al., 2001; Levin, 2009; Levin, 2011). Estrogens can elicit rapid nongenomic responses on gene expression via membrane-bound receptors and rapid activation of second messenger pathways, such as increases in intracellular free calcium or cyclic adenosine monophosphate (cAMP), resulting in a cellular response (Vasudevan and Pfaff, 2007). These effects are independent and distinct from the genomic, that is, ER-mediated, transcription. Additionally, one of the proteins identified in mediating estrogen action at the membrane is the orphan G-protein coupled receptor 30 (GPR30), which has been reported to act independently of classical ERs to trigger rapid signaling by estrogens (Thomas et al., 2005). In some cell types, there is evidence that GPR30 might collaborate with membrane-localized ERα as part of a large complex of proteins at the membrane, transmitting membrane ERα-generated signals to downstream kinase cascades (Levin, 2009; Levin, 2011, Shanle and Xu, 2011). For example, rapid and potent effects of many EDCs including bisphenol A (BPA), diethylstilbestrol (DES), endosulfan, dichlorodiphenyldichloroethylene (DDE), dieldrin, and nonylphenol are well documented (Ropero et al., 2006; Nadal et al., 2005).

As an estrogen-induced mechanism, only the genomic pathway to steroids acting via their nuclear receptor mediators has been examined extensively, and environmental estrogens are very weak via that mechanism. Recent findings indicate that environmental estrogens may be much more potent via the nonclassical estrogen signaling mechanisms – that is, membrane-initiated estrogen signaling or nongenomic pathway acting in nonmonotonic patters to elicit effects at concentrations far below those previously thought to be effective (Watson et al., 2011). For example, BPA and nonylphenol (NP) have shown very low potency in nuclear transcription assays for estrogen-responsive genes. In contrast, their nongenomic activities are quite robust and more effective in different responses (Kochukov et al., 2009). Therefore, inactivity in genomic assays does not predict inactivity in nongenomic mechanisms (Watson et al., 2010). Similarly, BPA was found to able to activate the membrane G-protein coupled estrogen receptor (Bouskine et al., 2009).

Thus, xenoestrogens can act directly on gene expression via the nuclear ERα and ERβ or indirectly via multiple other cellular signaling pathways, some of which can be activated quickly and at vanishingly low xenoestrogen concentrations (Watson et al., 2005; Ropero et al., 2006; Blumberg et al., 2011). It is considered likely that rapid estrogen-like signaling effects and "classic" nuclear hormone activity interact to affect physiological responses to estrogens (Levin, 2005). Xenoestrogens exerting various effects on development and reproduction are listed in Table 3.1.

Key players in the environmental estrogen story include the synthetic estrogen DES; the organochlorine pesticides (methoxychlor, dichlorodiphenyl-trichloroethane (DDT)/DDE, chlordane, dieldrin, aldrin); a host of polychlorinated biphenyls (PCBs) and the plasticizers BPA, NP, and octylphenol; and heavy metals (arsenic, cadmium). Compounds of concern were identified partially on the basis of their ability to bind to estrogen receptors (Blair et al. 2000) and the activity observed using *in vivo* biological assessments of estrogen activity such as the rat uterotropic assay (Gray et al. 2004) and production of the egg yolk protein vitellogenin (Sumpter and Jobling 1995).

It is now evident that environmental trace contaminants with estrogenic properties can impact on endocrine health of wildlife, influencing reproduction, particularly in aquatic populations. There are several reports on the feminization of male fishes in waterways due to low-level chronic exposures of EDCs. Some of the concerns about EDCs in humans also center on their interference with estrogens.

In the following, a number of putative EDCs are discussed that affect estrogen-signaling pathways. It needs to be emphasized that these chemicals do not represent their respective mode of action (MOA) in its entirety, but are cited for their capability of perturbing a particular MOA, in this case estrogen signaling.

3.2   STEROIDAL ESTROGENS

The natural and synthetic steroidal estrogens are considered compounds of concern in terms of their ability to disrupt reproductive endocrine function in resident fish populations (Sumpter and Johnson, 2008). One of the main triggers in the field of endocrine disruptors in the aquatic environment was the discovery of intersex fish in English rivers downstream of municipal wastewater discharge in 1978 (Sumpter and Johnson, 2008). The initial search for the causative agent or agents in wastewater effluents led to mainly steroid estrogens, both natural E1 and E2, and synthetic ethinylestradiol (EE2), and to a lesser extent industrial chemicals, such as alkylphenols that were recognized to be able to cause "feminization" of fishes in exposed populations (Sumpter and Johnson, 2008; Gross-Sorokin et al., 2006). Feminized responses include the formation of the egg yolk precursor vitellogenin within male and juvenile animals and histopathological changes in reproductive organs such as testes-ova and reductions in sperm count and motility.

Natural steroidal estrogens (E1, E2, and E3) and the synthetic estrogen EE2 showed affinity to ERs. EE2 exhibited greater affinity than E2 for the ERs, while E1 and E3 showed only moderate relative binding affinity (Table 3.2) (Blair et al., 2000).

TABLE 3.2   Relative Binding Affinity (RBA) of Steroidal Estrogens to Rat ERα (Blair et al., 2000)

Compounds	RBA (%)[a]
17β-Estradiol (E2)	100.00
Estriol (E3)	9.72
Estrone (E1)	7.31
17α-ethinylestradiol (EE2)	190.06

[a]RBA is the ratio of concentrations of E2 and the competitor required to reduce the binding by 50% (ratio of IC_{50} values) where RBA of E2 is set as 100.

3.2.1 Physiologic Estrogens

Physiologic estrogens E1 and E3 and metabolites such as catechol-E2, methoxy-E2, and sulfated-E2, and so on, which were considered weak estrogens because they were tested only via the genomic signaling pathway, have been found quite potent via the nongenomic signaling pathway. Their ability to act potently appears to be related to the protective action at particular life stages of women in whom these hormones are quite prominent (Watson et al., 2011). Perinatal exposure of the male fetus to potent estrogens is also known to increase the incidence of cryptochordism and hypospadias at birth, small testes, reduced sperm counts, epididymal cysts, prostatic abnormalities, and testicular cancer in adult animals. Both E2 and E1 induce vitellogenesis and feminization in fish species at dissolved concentrations as low as $1-10$ ng/L (Lintelmann et al., 2003).

3.2.2 17α-Ethinylestradiol (EE2)

17α-Ethynylestradiol (EE2) (Fig. 3.1), a synthetic steroidal estrogen used in birth control pills, enters the environment mainly through effluents from wastewater treatment facilities. It is estimated that 11.6 million women of reproductive age use birth control pills in the United States (Wise et al., 2011). In actual formulations, the EE2 takeup is about $20-35$ µg per day. The relative estrogenic activity of EE2 in estradiol equivalents is determined to be 1.81 by the yeast estrogen screen (YES) assay (Stanford and Weinberg, 2010). This strong estrogen is unmetabolized excreted through the urine and its clearance through bacteria in wastewater is incomplete. Because of the higher persistence of EE2, the concentrations of this synthetic estrogen in the environment is analogous to concentrations of the natural estrogens despite that it is excreted in a much smaller amount. EE2 was detected to be present in 16% of rivers at a median concentration of 73 ng/L as per a report on the US waterways by the U.S. Geological Survey (USGS); its biologically active concentration is as low as 1 ng/L (Kolpin et al., 2002).

EE2 is known to have a profound effect on aquatic life, adversely impacting fish populations at extremely low concentrations (low and subnanogram per liter), disrupting reproductive endocrine function and skewing sex ratios and sexual characteristics and decreased egg fertilization (Zha et al., 2008; Kidd et al., 2007). Notably, male fish can be feminized, creating egg yolk proteins that

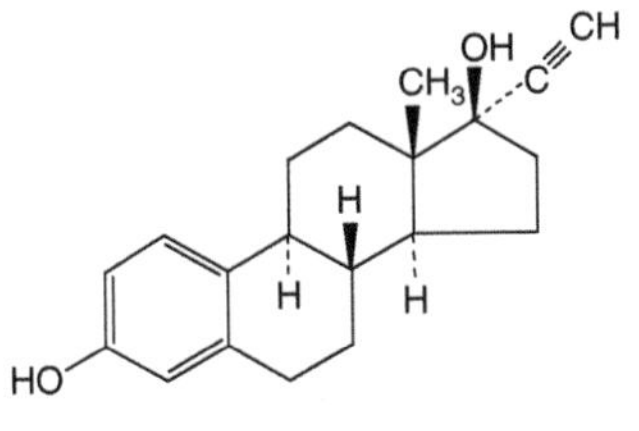

Figure 3.1   17α-Ethinylestradiol (EE2).

usually only females produce (Sumpter and Jobling, 1995; Sumpter and Johnson, 2008). Exposure of other vertebrates, such as adult male frogs, to EE2 also showed detrimental reproductive disturbances, including sex reversal, disrupted reproductive organ development, and reduced fertility, at environmentally relevant concentrations (Gyllenhammar et al. 2009). In 2004, the UK Environment Agency found that 86% of male fish sampled at 51 sites around the country were intersex, attributing feminization of male fish to EE2. Similarly, many of Europe's rivers are home to male fish that are "intersex" and so display female sexual characteristics, including female reproductive anatomy (Gilbert, 2012). It was concluded that EE2 dribbles through municipal sewage effluents and passes through wastewater treatment plants (WWTPs) and into streams and lakes.

There are a few studies that have attempted to explore the ecological relevance of the exposure to EDCs under field conditions. One example is a whole-lake study conducted over a 10-year period at the Experimental Lakes Area, an undisturbed watershed in northwestern Ontario in Canada, which is isolated from any other inputs of EDCs. The study revealed clear evidence that the potent synthetic estrogen EE2 affects reproductive failure of fish populations and their supporting food web (Kidd et al., 2007). A dose of EE2 at 5 ng/L levels was added in the natural lake three times weekly with seasonal mean concentrations of 6.1, 5.0, and 4.8 ng/L for three consecutive years, respectively. The lake contained naturally reproducing populations of lake trout, white sucker, pearl dace, and fathead minnow, along with several other smaller fish species. Subtle effects were observed in the fish in as little as 4 months, with more advanced effects on reproductive organs occurring after 12 months of dosing, followed by complete reproductive failure for the fathead minnow, a common fish species in North America, after 17 months; by the spring of 2003, only age 2 fish of this species remained (Kidd et al., 2007). As consequence of the disappearance of this food source, there was also a 30% reduction of lake trout (Halford 2008). In 3 years post addition of EE2, the fathead population recovered. The results of study demonstrated the effects of potent EE2 on fish in the natural environment at the reported concentrations in environmental waters (Kidd et al., 2007).

Concern regarding fetal and neonatal exposure to estrogenic agents also continues because of a variety of real-life circumstances, which include unintended continuation of estradiol-containing birth control pills during the first months of an undetected pregnancy (estimated at >1 million annually). The European Commission has proposed to add EE2 and E2 in the list of water pollutants that are currently monitored and controlled in EU surface waters. These additions address the potential harmful effects of their presence in the aquatic environment, where concentrations above the proposed standards can affect fish health, reducing successful reproduction and harming other living organisms (ClickGreen, 2012).

A predicted-no-effect-concentration (PNEC) for EE2 at 0.35 ng/L in surface waters has been recommended on the basis of a comprehensive review of several fish reproduction studies (Caldwell et al., 2008). This PNEC is below the no-observed-effect concentrations for vitellogenin induction previously reported in the literature and is considered to be conservative enough to protect biota in aquatic systems.

3.2.3 Phytoestrogens

Phytoestrogens are a diverse group of naturally occurring compounds produced by plants or fungi as a part of a defense system believed to provide protection against insects (Rochester and Millam, 2009) and to act as modulators of herbivore fertility (Hughes, 1988; Rochester and Millam, 2009). They bear structural resemblance to natural estrogen E2. The importance of biological activity of some phytoestrogens became clear when, some 50 years ago, the red clover flavone formononetin (Fig. 3.3b) was found to be the cause of massive infertility in sheep in Australia (Bradbury and White, 1954).

Phytoestrogens have polyphenolic structures and are classified as flavonoids, coumestanes, and lignans. Flavonoids are one of the most prevalent classes of phytoestrogens and include isoflavones such as daidzein and genistein (Fig. 3.2a and b) found in soy and fava beans. Coumestrol (Fig. 3.3a) is a coumestane present in alfalfa, soybeans, and clover.

Binding affinities for the receptors, often expressed relative to E2, have been characterized as the relative binding affinities (RBAs) of many phytoestrogenic ligands. Phytoestrogens can bind ERs with relatively low affinities but display ERβ selectivity. For example, the binding affinity of coumestrol to ERβ is sevenfold higher in comparison to ERα in a solid-phase binding assay (Table 3.3). The differential relative binding affinities to ERα and ERβ measured in solid-phase ligand binding are largely confirmed in the traditional solubilized receptor ligand-binding assay (Table 3.3). The position and number of the hydroxyl substituents in the isoflavone molecule appeared to determine the ER binding affinity. Genistein, one of the first compounds reported to have selective binding affinity for ERβ, was

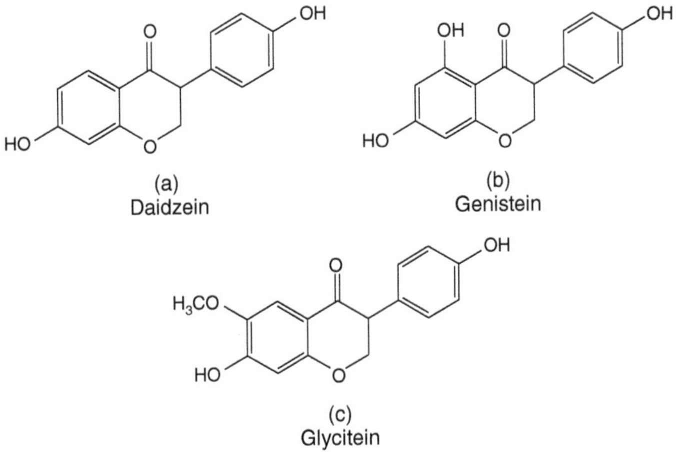

(a) Daidzein

(b) Genistein

(c) Glycitein

Figure 3.2 Naturally occurring estrogenic soy isoflavones.

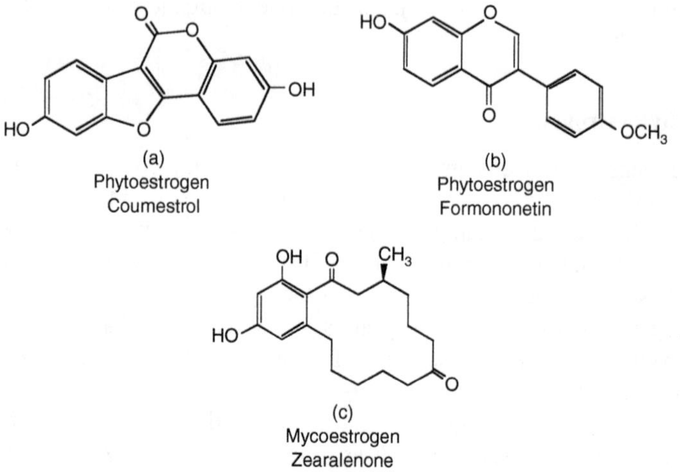

(a)
Phytoestrogen
Coumestrol

(b)
Phytoestrogen
Formononetin

(c)
Mycoestrogen
Zearalenone

Figure 3.3   Other naturally occurring estrogens.

TABLE 3.3   Differential Relative Binding Affinity (RBA) of Different Phytoestrogens for ERα and ERβ (Kuiper et al., 1998)

Compound	RBA for ERα		RBA for ERβ	
17β-Estradiol	100		100	
Coumestrol	34[a]	20[b]	100[a]	140[b]
Zearalenone	10	7	18	5
Genistein	0.7	4	13	87
Daidzein	0.2	0.1	1	0.5
Formononetin	ND	ND	<0.01	<0.01

[a]Solubilized receptor ligand-binding assay.
[b]Solid-phase binding assay.

found to have approximately 20-fold higher affinity for ERβ than for ERα (Kuiper et al., 1998). Diadzein, with the elimination of one hydroxyl group (fivefold higher than ERα), or formononetin, with elimination of two hydroxyl groups (very weak binding), showed a great loss of binding affinity (Table 3.3) (Kuiper et al., 1998).

Soy products are popular because they are a lactose-free substitute for dairy products. Recent reports of low incidence of breast cancer in Asian women and other positive effects on breast cancer risks have further spurred the use of soy products (Peeters et al., 2003). The U.S. Food and Drug Administration (FDA) has approved 25 g/day soy consumption, approximately equivalent to 75 mg of isoflavones/day (1 mg/kg/day), as being beneficial against coronary artery disease

(FDA, 1999). Individuals consuming a traditional soy-rich Asian diet (tofu and textured vegetable protein) have 7–110-fold higher plasma and 30-fold higher urinary genistein concentrations than individuals consuming a typical Western diet. The isoflavons are also the components of infant formula made using soy proteins and other components. The three main isoflavons in soy formula are genistein, daidzein, and, to a smaller extent, glycitein (Fig. 3.2c). In a study, urinary concentrations of genistein and daidzein in infants fed with soy formula were found to be about 500-fold higher than those fed on cow's milk formula (Diamanti-Kandarakis et al., 2009).

Female mice treated neonatally by subcutaneous injection of genistein (0.5–50 mg/kg) exhibited altered ovarian differentiation leading to multi-oocyte follicles. Ovarian function and estrous cyclicity were disrupted in genistein-treated mice, with increasing severity over time. Reduced fertility was observed in mice treated with genistein (0.5, 5, or 25 mg/kg), and infertility was observed at 50 mg/kg. Thus, exposure of neonatal mice to environmentally relevant concentrations of genistein led to the manifestation of reproductive abnormalities in adult life (Jefferson et al., 2007).

Maternal dietary genistein supplementation of Agouti (A^{vy}) mouse during gestation at levels comparable to humans consuming high-soy diets has been demonstrated to shift coat color distribution toward pseudoagouti and reduced incidence of obesity by hypermethylation of genome (Dolinoy et al., 2006). A similar hypermethylation was observed on nutritional exposure of A^{vy} to methyl donors, such as folic acid, shifting the offspring coat color to brown (pseudoagouti) (Cooney et al., 2002).

It is generally accepted that consumption of a diet rich in phytoestrogens is associated with beneficial effects for the organism. The consumption of genistein, the major isoflavone in soy, has been associated with decreased risk for breast and prostate cancer and decreased bone loss, and with cardio-protection. Genistein has been also associated with cancer chemoprevention and decreased DNA methyltransferases expression (Li et al., 2009). Dietary soy supplementation rich in flavonoids decreased estrogen synthesis in premenopausal women, which may explain the cancer-preventive effects of phytoestrogens. Data from *in vitro* experiments suggest that phytoestrogens competitively bind aromatase, preventing normal estrogen synthesis from androgen substrates (Moon et al., 2006). It is unclear at present what risks are involved in excessive intake of phytoestrogens (Ruegg et al., 2009). Although the expert panel convened by the National Toxicology Program has expressed minimal concern for adverse developmental effects on infants fed on soy infant formula (NIEHS, 2009), consumption of foods with high-soy content is found to be associated with lower sperm counts in men (Chavarro et al., 2008).

3.2.4   Mycoestrogen – Zearalenone (ZEN)

Mycoestrogen zearalenone (ZEN) with nonsteroidal chemical structure (Fig. 3.3c) is produced by several species of *Fusarium* fungi and it widely contaminates agricultural products, so that ZEN exists in almost all agricultural crops. ZEN is the primary toxin causing infertility, abortion, or other breeding problems, particularly in pigs. After consumption, ZEN is metabolized to provide two major stereoisomers, α- and β-zearalenol, with the α-metabolite displaying the highest estrogenic activity. In spite of its structural differences with E2, ZEN is one of the most active endocrine disruptors (le Maire et al., 2010).

3.3 NONSTEROIDAL ESTROGENIC CHEMICALS

In 1991, Soto et al. found that a chemical leaching from polystyrene laboratory tubes was causing breast cancer cells to grow *in vitro*, even though no estrogens had been added to the culture. Subsequent investigation identified the substance leached as *p*-nonylphenol, an additive commonly used in plastics, which behaves like a natural estrogen (Soto et al., 1991). This landmark discovery generated widespread interest in what we now call nonphysiologic estrogen mimetics or xenoestrogens. A wide variety of xenoestrogens, including environmental, dietary, and pharmaceutical estrogens that can mimic or antagonize the activity of physiological estrogens, involve genomic pathways by binding to nuclear estrogen receptors or nongenomic pathways by binding to cell membrane receptors (Watson et al., 2010) and activate multiple signaling pathways, leading to altered cellular functions. When superimposed, xenoestrogens can alter endogenous estrogen signaling and thereby disrupt normal signaling pathways, leading to malfunctions in many tissue types (Watson et al., 2011).

3.3.1 Diethylstilbestrol (DES)

One of the first examples of endocrine disruption in humans occurred when some 5 million pregnant women were exposed to DES (Fig. 3.4), an orally active synthetic nonsteroidal estrogen, as a therapy with the mistaken belief that it prevented miscarriage (Crews and McLachlan, 2006; McLachlan, 2006). The prenatal exposure to DES was later linked to a rare form of vaginal cancer in female offspring of mothers taking DES. Some sons of women who were given DES were also reported to have epididymal cysts, microphallus, cryptorchidism, or testicular hypoplasia (Titus-Ernstoff et al., 2008). DES is also the most potent EDC identified to date, and it continues to be one of the most well-studied examples of endocrine disruption where effects in the exposed mothers are minimal compared to effects in their offspring who were exposed during the critical windows of development (Giusti et al. 1995). It is also a powerful model estrogenic EDC for its profound effect on

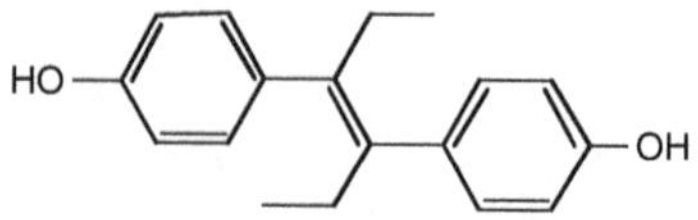

Figure 3.4   Diethylstilbestrol (DES).

the developing reproductive tract and one of the first to link a fetal exposure to a hormonally active compound with the latent development of disease years or even decades after the insult.

It has been extensively studied because of its significant adverse impacts on humans (Herbst et al., 1971; Herbst and Bern, 1981) and mice (McLachlan et al., 1980) *in utero*. Effects of developmental exposure on the female reproductive tract have been suggested to be due to alterations in genetic pathways governing uterine differentiation (Huang et al., 2005). Female offspring of mice exposed to DES during pregnancy, when mated to control males, produced a second generation of females who, although not exposed to DES themselves, expressed this same rare genital tract cancer (Newbold et al., 1998). This transgenerational transmission of a specific reproductive tract lesion in rats can be explained by invoking an epigenetic mechanism for heritable change and given the finding of altered DNA methylation patterns in a specific uterine gene in mice treated developmentally with DES (Newbold et al., 2006; Li et al., 2003). It was found that a long-term exposure of DES *in utero* resulted in hypermethylation of the *HOXA10* gene, inducing a permanent epigenetic effect on their expression (Bromer et al., 2009). However, in humans, the grandchildren of women who were given DES during pregnancy did not uncover an increased risk of disease (Titus-Ernstoff et al., 2008).

DES has been shown to induce obesity in adulthood after low-dose developmental exposure (Newbold et al., 2005; Miyawaki et al., 2007). Outbred CD-1 mice were treated with DES on days 1–5 of neonatal life using a low dose of 1 μg/kg/day. This dose did not affect body weight during treatment but was associated with a significant increase in body weight as adults (Newbold et al., 2009). Neonatal DES-treated female mice at 4–6 months of age are shown in Fig. 3.5. Male mice treated as neonates did not demonstrate this increase in body weight; on the other hand, a higher dose of 1 mg/kg/day caused a significant decrease in body weight during treatment but it was followed by a "catch-up" period around puberty and then finally resulted in an increase in body weight of the DES-treated

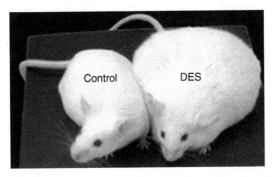

Figure 3.5 Neonatal DES-treated female mice at 4–6 months of age. Source: Newbold et al. (2009). Reproduced with permission of Elsevier.

mice compared to controls after ~2 months of age. Increased body weight in both low and high DES-treated mice compared to controls was observed throughout adulthood (Newbold, 2010).

Increased leptin has been reported with developmental exposure to DES, which is associated with increased number and size of the fat cells (adipocytes) in the DES-treated mice (Newbold et al., 2007). Leptin, an adipocyte-derived hormone associated with appetite control, directly correlates with fat mass and communicates the energy status of the organism to the body (Newbold et al., 2009). The altered hormone levels suggest that DES induces a range of changes, which set a mouse's metabolism to conserve energy as if it were living in a low-resource environment, thereby predisposing it toward obesity (Newbold et al. 2009).

3.3.2   Organochlorine Insecticides

Chemically stable and strongly lipophilic organochlorine (OC) chemicals possess estrogen-like and anti-androgenic properties at exposure levels measured in the environment. OC insecticides mimic natural hormones, inhibit the action of hormones, or alter the normal regulatory function of the endocrine system and have potential hazardous effects on male reproductive axis causing infertility. Taken together, most of these chemical compounds may act as ER agonists and/or AR antagonists in the environment, a situation leading to feminization in animals. *In vivo* and *in vitro* assays have shown the potency of OCs as estrogen agonists (Cooper and Kavlok, 1997; Gray et al., 1999), and the effects on female reproductive tracts of mammals have been reviewed (Tiemann, 2008).

3.3.2.1   *Dichlorodiphenyltrichloroethane (DDT)*   DDT is a potent and persistent xenoestrogen. It was banned in 1970s in the United States but remains an EDC of interest because of its persistence in the environment and its accumulation in adipose tissue. Technical-grade DDT is actually a mixture of three isomers: principally the p,p'-DDT (ca. 85%) (Fig. 3.6), with the o,p'-DDT and o,o'-DDT present in much lesser amounts. The estrogenicity of DDT arises primarily from o,p'-DDT, which can bind ERα or ERβ with RBAs of 0.01 and 0.02, respectively; p,p'-DDT has RBAs <0.01 for both receptors (Table 3.4) (Kuiper et al., 1998). A number of experimental studies indicate the estrogenic effect of DDT in rats: it exerted uterotropic effect (Welch et al., 1969) and inhibited *in vitro* the binding of [^{3}H]-estradiol to the cytosolic estrogen receptor in the uterus (Nelson, 1974). In mice, the uterotropic effect of DDT was manifested in a uterine weight increase and development of pseudoestrus. Statistically significant uterine weight increases (absolute and relative to body weight) were observed 24, 36, and 48 h after administration of DDT to the ovariectomized female CBA mice. Uterine weight increase was more pronounced in mice receiving DES used as a positive control, but both results (DDT and DES) were comparable. Symptoms in men working with the manufacture of DDT led to its identification as an ER agonist (Lemaire et al., 2006). Administration of DDT to young male rats led to hypomethylation of DNA (Shutoh et al., 2009). However, DDT also provides an example of a single EDC that may be both

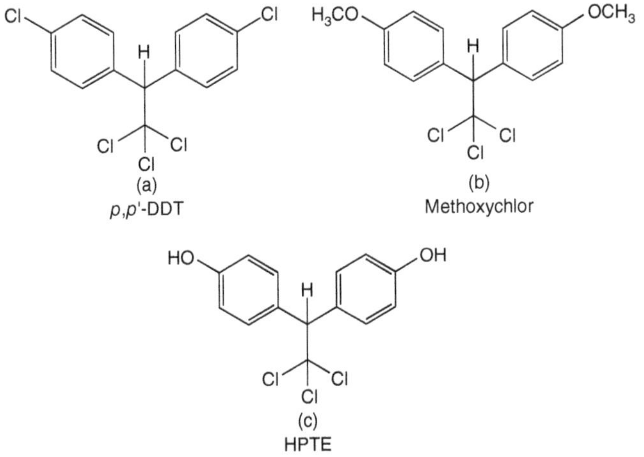

Figure 3.6 Estrogenic organochlorine insecticides.

TABLE 3.4 **Relative Binding Affinities of selected OCs to hERα (Kuiper et al., 1998) and rat ERα (Blair et al., 2000)**

Compound	RBA (%)	
	hERα	Rat ERα
17β-Estradiol	100	100
o,p'-DDT	0.01	0.001
p,p'-DDT	<0.01	
Chlordecone	0.06	0.013
Methoxychlor	<0.01	0.001
HPTE		0.253

estrogenic and antiandrogenic; the estrogen agonist DDT is metabolized into the androgen antagonist DDE (see Chapter 4) (Rasier et al., 2007).

Other examples of organochlorines that activate ER are the DDT metabolite DDE, methoxychlor, and dieldrin (Lemaire et al., 2006).

3.3.2.2 Methoxychlor Methoxychlor is a structural analog of and substitute for DDT (Fig. 3.6b), which has a relatively short half-life in the environment and in animals and appears to be less toxic in mammals. In 2003, it was banned in the United States because of its endocrine-disrupting properties (EPA, 2004). It is a weak estrogenic agonist *in vivo*. It mimics E2 action in the female rodent reproductive tract, causing adverse developmental and reproductive effects, despite its binding affinity for ERα being 10 000 times less than that for E2 (RBA of <0.01 for ERα and ERβ) (Kuiper et al., 1998). These include embryonic toxicity, precocious puberty, decreased fertility, and ovarian atrophy (Waters et al., 2001).

An investigation on the effects of methoxychlor on the pubertal development and reproductive function in the Long–Evans hooded rats by dosing from gestation through puberty showed an accelerated vaginal opening and abnormal estrus cycle in females and a suppression of testicular Leydig cell function in males (Gray et al., 1989). Exposure to methoxychlor at 1000 ppm in a long-term three-generation reproduction study found reduced fertility index, induced fetotoxicity in the form of reduced litter size, and reduced viability index (Cummings and Gray, 1989). These observations are consistent with the reports that methoxychlor mimics estrogen both *in vivo* and *in vitro*. An exposure of methoxychlor to fetal and neonatal rats resulted in transgenerational effects promoting a spermatogenic defect characterized by increased apoptosis and decreased cell number and motility in adult F1, which was carried over four generations (Zama and Uzumcu, 2009) (See Chapter 8).

Methoxychlor is metabolized *in vivo* into mono- and bisphenol demethylated derivatives which demonstrate estrogenic activity *in vivo*. The bisphenol metabolite 2,2-bis(*p*-hydroxyphenyl)-1,1,1-trichloroethane (HPTE) (Fig. 3.6c) exhibits unique estrogenic activity as an ERα-selective agonist (estrogenic) and ERβ and AR antagonist (antiestrogenic and antiandrogenic), and shows estrogenic activity which is approximately 100 times greater than that of the parent methoxychlor compound (Gaido et al., 2000). HPTE selectively antagonizes E2-mediated ERβ activation (Gaido et al., 1999). Methoxychlor has been considered to be a proestrogen because the responsibility for its *in vivo* estrogenic action is believed to be due to this metabolite. Nevertheless, an *in vitro* study in a human liver carcinoma cell line Hep G2 cells demonstrated that parent methoxychlor and its metabolites were all estrogenic through the ERs (Blum et al., 2008).

3.3.2.3 Chlordecone OC insecticide chlordecone (Fig. 3.7) activated hERα cooperatively with E2, although its activity was 10 000 times lower than that of E2 and inhibited E2-induced ERβ activation effectively. Chlordecone has been determined to be a mixed agonist for human pregnane X receptor (PXR) and ERα and an effective antagonist for liver X receptor β (LXRβ) and ERβ (Lee et al., 2008), thus increasing the risk of cancer development (le Maire et al., 2010).

The estrogenic activities of some of the OC insecticides have been evaluated for hERα in solid-phase competition binding assays (Kuiper et al., 1998) and rat (Sprague–Dawley) ERα standard binding assays (Blair et al., 2000), and are given as RBAs in Table 3.4.

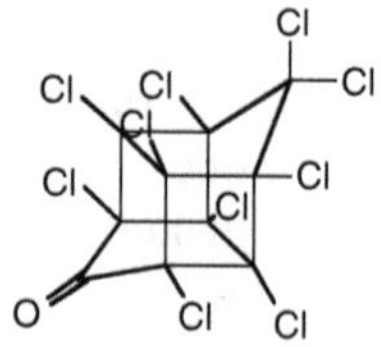

Figure 3.7 Chlordecone.

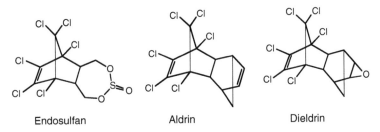

| Endosulfan | Aldrin | Dieldrin |

Figure 3.8 Estrogenic cyclopentadiene OC insecticides.

Some cyclopentadiene-based OC insecticides, such as endosulfan (Varayoud et al., 2008), aldrin (Jorgenson, 2001), and dieldrin (Soto et al., 1995) (Fig. 3.8), have also been tested as weak estrogens.

3.3.3 Polychlorinated Biphenyls (PCBs)

PCBs have been shown to have estrogenic properties, but they are weak compared to the natural hormone 17β-estradiol. It is believed that hydroxyl metabolites of PCBs may exert estrogenic effects by inhibiting the metabolism of estradiol, thus indirectly inducing estrogenic activity by increasing estradiol bioavailability in target tissues (Kester et al., 2000).

3.3.4 Alkyphenols

Alkylphenols (APs) represent a group of ubiquitous environmental estrogens that are highly related in structure. These compounds are surfactants or monomer byproducts of plastic manufacturing or product breakdown. From their use in some detergents, paints, herbicides, pesticides, and plastic polymers, APs enter the environment and bioaccumulate in algae, fish, and aquatic organisms (Nomura et al., 2008). Because of the similarity of structural features of many APs, including NPs and octylphenols, with those of the native hormone 17β-estradiol, these can target-share and thus are able to bind specifically to estrogen receptors and trigger estrogenic toxicity. NP is by far the most commercially prevalent member of the AP family, representing approximately 85% of the total AP market (Corvini et al., 2006). A directive from the European Union has prevented use of APs and their ethoxylates as coformulants in new products from 2005.

3.3.4.1 4-Nonylphenols NPs are widely used for the synthesis of nonylphenol ethoxylates (NPEs), one of the important types of nonionic surfactants, with an annual worldwide production of approximately 650 000 tons. Small quantities of NPs are also used as stabilizers or antioxidants in the manufacture of plastics such as polystyrene and polyvinyl chloride. The major source of NP contamination in the environment is the microbial degradation of NPEs, which are not estrogenically active (Lye et al., 1999; Ferrara et al., 2001). Leaching of plastic products may also

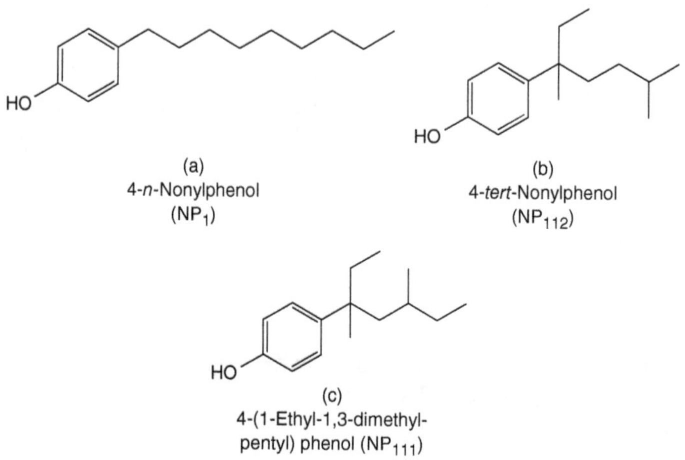

(a)
4-n-Nonylphenol
(NP$_1$)

(b)
4-$tert$-Nonylphenol
(NP$_{112}$)

(c)
4-(1-Ethyl-1,3-dimethyl-
pentyl) phenol (NP$_{111}$)

Figure 3.9   Estrogenic nonylphenols.

result in contamination by NPs (Soto et al., 1991). NPs have been detected in river water, sewage sludge, and drinking water (Ye et al., 2007). The USGS has reported that NP was one of the most frequently detected industrial chemicals in surface waters, with a median concentration of 0.8 µg/L (Kolpin et al., 2002).

4-Nonylphenols (Fig. 3.9) have been shown to be a toxic, endocrine-disrupting, and mimicking estrogen receptor agonist, and display ED activity in mammals, fishes, and other species, capable of feminizing male fish at levels as low as 50–100 ppb. These persist in aquatic environments, and are moderately bioaccumulative. In the 1990s, NPs were believed to be implicated in the feminization of fish in heavily contaminated rivers in the United Kingdom: male juveniles living downstream of WWTP effluent outlets had abnormally small testes and produced vitellogenin, an egg yolk protein normally found only in females. Among the 18 main isomers occurring in commercial NP mixtures, 4-(1-ethyl-1,3-dimethylpentyl) phenol (Fig. 3.9c) possessing a quaternary α-carbon on the branched alkyl chain was found to be a major constituent (Corvini et al., 2006).

Although NPs are weakly estrogenic (1/10 000–1/1000 of that of estradiol), they tend to accumulate in aquatic organisms because of their relatively high lipophilicity (log K_{ow} = 4.8–5.3), eventually disrupting those organism's endocrine and reproductive systems (Cionna et al., 2006). NPs are of particular concern because of their persistence, and effects on human and ecosystem health due to low concentration exposure to NPs are poorly understood and open to considerable debate and calls for better means of their degradation in the environment. In 2005 the U.S. Environmental Protection Agency (EPA) established toxicity-based 4-NP freshwater aquatic life ambient water-quality criteria of 1.7 and 6.6 µg/L for chronic and acute exposure, respectively (EPA, 2005), similar to the concentrations (10 µg/L) shown to cause endocrine disruption in fish (Schoenfuss et al., 2008). In the European Water Framework Directive, environmental quality standards for surface waters for NP have been set at 0.3 and 2.0 μg/L for annual average and maximum allowable concentrations, respectively (Giger et al., 2009).

To replace NPEs, alternative nonionic surfactant systems have been proposed, which are free of alkylphenols and are readily biodegradable. (Fernandez et al., 2005).

3.3.4.2 *4-tert-Octylphenol* It is an industrial chemical used in the manufacture of nonionic surfactants and is a chemical of widespread use in the United States. It has been detected in 57% of the US population (Calafat et al., 2008). *In vitro* tests have revealed that octylphenol is the alkylphenol that has the most powerful estrogenic effects. A concentration of 10 μg/L of octylphenol in the aquatic environment gives rise to the production of vitellogenin in male rainbow trout (Mazellier and Leverd, 2003).

3.3.4.3 *Bisphenol A* BPA (2,2-bis(4-hydroxyphenyl)propane) (Fig. 3.10), a synthetic estrogen, with the production of around 3.8 M tons in 2006, it is one of the highest volume chemicals produced worldwide (Kolvenbach et al., 2007). In the United States alone, BPA has a production volume of 800 000 tons a year (Zoeller et al., 2005) and grosses some US$6 billion a year for the five companies that produce it (Borrell, 2010). In commercial use since the 1950s, the BPA monomer is used in the production of polycarbonate plastics and epoxy and other specialty resins. Resins are used for lining of most food and beverage cans to provide a protective layer. It is found in dental sealants, eyeglasses, and compact discs as well as in cash-register receipts and American dollar bills (Vandenberg, 2011). It is also used as a stabilizer or antioxidant for many types of plastics such as polyvinylchloride (PVC). Because the ester bonds in these BPA-based polymers are subject to hydrolysis, leaching of BPA has led to widespread human exposure through ingestion of foods in contact with BPA-containing materials. Recent evidence also indicates that exposure may occur through dermal contact with the thermal paper used widely in cash-register receipts (Biedermann et al., 2010). BPA has been detected in 93% of human urine samples of the U.S. population (Calafat et al., 2008) and in 91% in Canada (Vandenberg, 2011). High urinary levels of BPA in the US adult population have lately been correlated with cardiovascular disease, liver abnormalities, and diabetes (Lang et al., 2008). A national groundwater sampling in the United States reported BPA in about 30% of groundwater samples (Barnes et al., 2008).

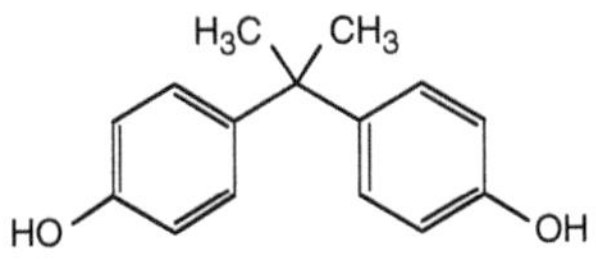

Figure 3.10 Bisphenol A.

BPA is an endocrine disruptor and can target multiple endocrine-related pathways, *in vivo*. It has been the subject of intense scientific scrutiny because of increasing evidence from animal studies that this compound poses a potential health risk, especially if exposure occurs prenatally and in early postnatal life. In animal studies, BPA has been shown to simulate the activity of the female hormone estrogen and capable of disrupting sex differentiation. BPA can impact reproductive physiology and behavior in rodents at doses even lower than the EPA-prescribed current reference or "safe" exposure limit for humans of 50 µg/kg body weight per day, set in 1988 (Vandenberg et al., 2009).

It has been observed that minute amounts of BPA were effective in causing adverse effects, whereas these effects were not exerted by larger amounts short of acutely toxic levels. It has remained unclear why minute amounts of BPA are more effective in eliciting endocrine-disrupting effects than higher doses (vom Saal and Hughes, 2005; Sekizawa, 2008). While BPA displays estrogen-like activities at nanomolar doses, the mechanism by which it exerts its biological actions remains enigmatic.

BPA was considered a weak environmental estrogen because of its relative low affinity (1000–10 000-fold lower) for the nuclear ERs ($EC_{50} = 2$–7×10^{-7} M) compared with E2 ($EC_{50} = 1$–6×10^{-13} M) (Blair et al., 2000, Oehlmann et al., 2009). Since BPA's binding to ER and its hormonal activity are extremely weak, it appeared unlikely that it interacted directly with ER to achieve its effects at low doses. However, studies have demonstrated pathways other than binding to classical nuclear ERs through which BPA can induce cellular responses at very low concentrations (Wetherill et al., 2007). Some actions of BPA are very rapid and may be explained by nongenomic actions mediated through binding to membrane ERα and to a candidate transmembrane GPR30 (Bouskine et al., 2009), or the estrogen-related receptor-γ (ERRγ) (Takayanagi et al., 2006; Okada et al., 2008).

BPA has been found to be an imperfect potent estrogen because it was found equally potent to E2 when acting via nonclassical (nongenomic) membrane versions of ER-mediated pathways (Jeng and Watson, 2011), namely the membrane-bound form of ERα and GPR30 (Vandenberg et al, 2009). BPA binds to GPR 30 with an IC_{50} of 0.630 µmol/L, a binding affinity that was 2–3% of the IC_{50} value for E2 (0.0178 µmol/L) (Thomas and Dong, 2006). There is debate as to whether this GPCR should be considered an ER because it appears to contribute to some of the early actions of estrogen, including rapid nongenomic signaling events that take place on the membrane (Olde and Leeb-Lundberg, 2009). BPA was capable of activating an estrogen-responsive luciferase reporter at levels that were 50% that of E2 activation. Thus, whereas BPA may have a significantly lower potency than endogenous estrogens *in vitro*, it is a full agonist for both ERα and ERβ.

A search among different NRs to find an actual receptor to which BPA binds led to the conclusion that it binds very strongly and activates a cellular switch known as human ERRγ, a self-activated "orphan" (without clear ligand assignment) nuclear receptor closely related to ER, for most of its estrogen-mimicking effect (Takayanagi et al., 2006; Okada et al., 2008). ERRγ shares a sequence homology with ERα and ERβ but is not activated by E2. 4-Hydroxy-tamoxifen (Fig. 3.11),

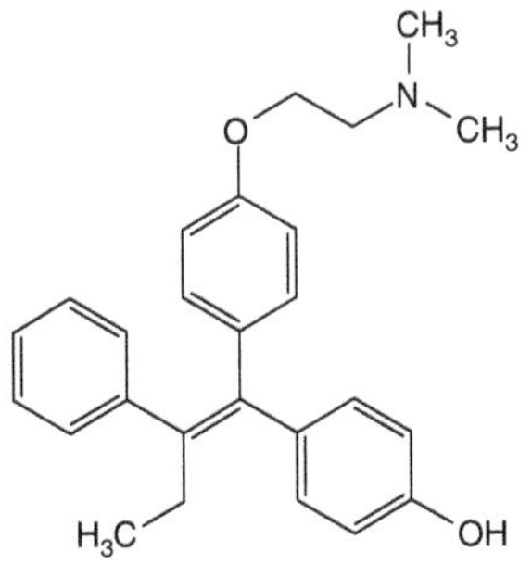

Figure 3.11   ER-antagonist 4-hydroxy-tamoxifen.

an antagonist of ERs, deactivates ERRs, characterized as the activity of an inverse agonist. BPA inhibits and reverses in a dose-dependent manner the inverse agonist activity of 4-OHT to the originally high basal activation state, and thus acts as an inverse antagonist of ERRγ. Thus, BPA is a strong binder of ERRγ, but quite silent without the inverse agonist to reveal its action.

BPA interacts with androgen and thyroid receptors as well (Moriyama et al. 2002; Wetherill et al. 2002; Zoeller et al. 2005). Recently, BPA has also been described as an agonist for the glucocorticoid receptor (GR) (Prasanth et al., 2010). During activity testing under Phase I of the USEPA's ToxCast™ (467 HTS assays), BPA had measurable activity in 101 assays involving signaling pathways for ER, AR, and TR, as well as other nuclear receptors (e.g., GR, peroxisome proliferator-activated receptor (PPAR), and PXR) that have potential relevance to endocrine signaling (CYPs, including aromatase) (Thayer and Belcher, 2011).

BPA is able to influence transcriptional regulation of genes involved in obesity and its associated metabolic complications. BPA reduces the number of fat cells but programs them to incorporate more fat so there are fewer but very large fat cells (vom Saal et al., 2012). It was found in *in vitro* studies that micromolar concentrations of BPA enhanced adipocyte differentiation and lipid accumulation in target cells in a dose-dependent manner (Masuno et al., 2005; Wada et al., 2007). It is now known that BPA may exert effects on adipogenesis *in vivo*. BPA exposure during gestation, or gestation and lactation, has been consistently reported in increase in body weight in female, but not male, rodents than controls (Somm et al., 2009; Miyawaki et al., 2007). As adipocyte differentiation in mice takes place neonatally, in all the studies in which offspring were exposed to BPA during pregnancy and lactation, weight gain occurred later in life (Vom Saal et al., 2012).

Elevated BPA levels have been linked to high body mass index and abdominal fat in humans. A positive association has been observed between higher urinary BPA levels and obesity in the U.S. National Health and Nutrition Examination Survey (Carwile and Michels, 2011). An association has also been found between urinary concentrations of BPA and body mass outcomes in children and adolescents aged 6–19 years (Trasande et al., 2012). Remarkably, obesity was not associated with exposure to other environmental phenols found in daily products such as soaps or sunscreens, which points to specificity in the association between obesity and BPA levels (Nadal, 2013).

BPA binds to estrogen receptors (ERα and ERβ), triggering nonclassical estrogenic effects that are initiated outside the nucleus, in which estrogen receptors do not act as transcription factors (Soriano, et al., 2012). Through nonclassical ER-triggered pathways, BPA alters the function of key cell types involved in metabolism, such as pancreatic β cells and adipocytes, in both mice and humans. In pancreatic β cells, whose function is the storage and release of insulin, nonclassical estrogen-triggered pathways include regulation of insulin biosynthesis and release by ERα, potentiation of glucose-induced insulin release by ERβ, and control of lipid synthesis by extranuclear ERα. Nanomolar concentrations of either E2 or BPA boost the release of insulin in mouse β cells, altering glucose metabolism on longer exposures, a key risk factor for diabetes and obesity (Alonso-Magdalena et al., 2011; Alonso-Magdalena et al., 2006). In the use of β cells from genetically modified mice that did not produce ERβ, the effect disappeared (Soriano et al., 2012).

Considering BPA's toxicity at low doses and its effects on the endocrine system, it is a public health concern and may have potential developmental and reproductive toxicity. Epidemiologic studies on BPA have linked it to several health issues, including diabetes, heart disease, and behavioral problems (Vandenberg, 2011). A study by National Toxicology Program of the National Institutes of Health (NIH) has expressed concern that BPA may affect the brain and behavioral development of fetuses, infants, and young children, and that the possibility that BPA may effect human development cannot be dismissed. Consequently, six of the largest manufacturers of baby bottles in the United States have stopped selling bottles made with BPA (Layton, 2009). BPA has been officially declared to be a "toxic substance" in Canada (Canada Gazette, 2010). Canada and Denmark have banned the chemical's use in baby bottles, toys, and other products for infants (Borrell, 2010). In March 2010, the EPA formally listed BPA as a "chemical of concern." The European Union announced that it would follow Canada's example to ban the use of BPA in baby bottles effective from 2011 (von Reppert-Bismarck and Roche, 2010). In July 2012, the FDA also placed a ban on the use of BPA in baby bottles and sippy cups (Associated Press, 2012) as well as in infant formula packaging because of the chemical's link to possible health problems (Burton, 2013).

Bisphenol S (BPS, 4,4'-dihydroxydiphenyl sulphone) (Fig. 3.12a) has been used as an alternative to BPA in plastic consumer products and thermal paper. It has enhanced thermal stability and resistance to sunlight, resulting in a less leachable compound compared to BPA (Vinas et al., 2010). However, a study has found that BPS could disrupt natural estrogen hormone actions in ways similar to BPA at very low levels (Viñas and Watson, 2013). In 2012, the new polypropylene carbonate polyols developed as a potential alternative to BPA-containing epoxy coatings to the inside of metal beverage and food containers led to a Green Chemistry Presidential Challenge Award to Geoffrey W. Coates of Cornell University for this innovation (2012 Green Chemistry Awards).

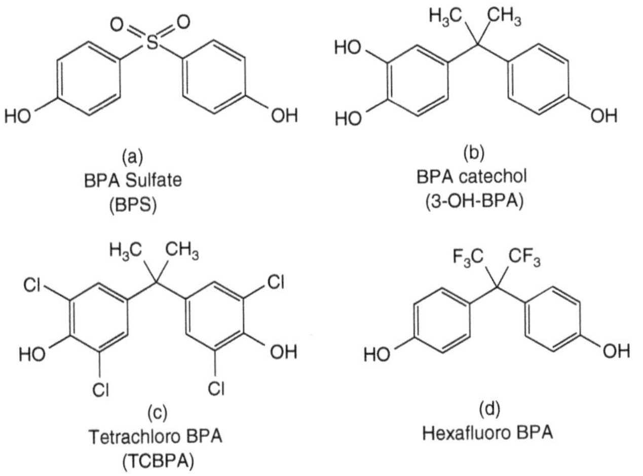

Figure 3.12 BPA and structurally similar derivatives.

3.3.4.4 BPA Derivatives A major mechanism of endocrine disruption is the action of chemicals through direct interaction with hormone receptors acting as receptor *agonists* or *antagonists*, altering endocrine function. At least one 4-hydroxyl group of BPA derivatives was found essential for the activity. The 4-hydroxyl groups of the A-phenyl ring and the B-phenyl ring of BPA derivatives are required for hormonal activities, and substituents at the 3,5-positions of the phenyl rings and the bridging alkyl moiety markedly influenced the activities.

The structure and ED activities relationships of several BPA derivatives were examined using hormone-responsive reporter assays. Estrogenic activity was examined using an ERE-luciferase reporter assay in MCF-7 cells. Tetrachloro-bisphenol A (2,2-bis-(3,5-dichloro-4-hydroxyphenyl)propane; TCBPA) (Fig. 3.12c) showed the highest activity, followed by hexafluoro-BPA (Fig. 3.12d); BPA and tetrabromo-bisphenol A (2,2-bis-(3,5-dibromo-4-hydroxyphenyl)propane; TBBPA) had lower activity (Kitamura et al., 2005). Estrogenic potencies of brominated BPAs assayed in the ER-CALUX assay with T47D Luc cells showed the highest potencies in the lowest degree of bromination (Meerts et al., 2001). A number of mono-, di-, tri- and tetrachloro derivatives of bisphenol A were also found to have more potent activity than BPA in the yeast two-hybrid assay (Fukazawa et al., 2002). A 3-hydroxyl metabolite of BPA (BPA catechol) (Fig. 3.12b) formed by human and rat liver microsomes exhibited little estrogenic activity. In contrast, the *in vivo* estrogenic activity of TCBPA by means of uterotrophic assay in ovariectomized mice was lower than that of BPA, and TBBPA showed a significant estrogenic activity in spite of having little activity in *in vitro* assay (Kitamura et al., 2005). The EC_{50} values of estrogenic activity of various BPA derivatives are shown in Table 3.5.

A halogenated derivative of BPA, such as TBBPA, is mainly used as a flame retardant to protect computer motherboards and other electronic equipment, and its presence has been reported in the environment (de Wit et al., 2009).

TABLE 3.5   *In vitro* Estrogenic Activities of Bisphenol A Derivatives in MCF-7 Estrogen Luciferase Reporter Assay (Kitamura et al., 2005)

Bisphenol compounds	EC_{50} (µM)
E2	8.6×10^{-6}
Tetrachloro-BPA	0.02
Hexafluoro-BPA	0.05
BPA	0.63, 0.3[a]
BPA catechol	1.8
3-Monobromo-BPA	0.5[a]
3,3′-Dibromo-BPA	0.4[a]
3,5,3′-Tribromo-BPA	>10[a]
Tetrabromo-BPA	19

[a]Meerts et al. (2001).

TCBPA has also been used as a flame retardant, but in much lower quantities than TBBPA. However, the origin of most chlorinated BPA in the environment is likely due to the chlorination of BPA by reaction with sodium hypochlorite, which is commonly used as a bleaching agent in paper factories and found in the effluent from waste-paper recycling plants (Fukazawa et al., 2002). Both TBBPA and TCBPA are candidate thyroid hormone disrupting chemicals (Kitamura et al., 2002; Sun et al., 2009) and potent peroxisome proliferator-activated receptor (PPARγ) agonists (Riu et al., 2011). It was observed that the bulkier brominated BPA analogs have greater capability to activate PPARγ and weaker estrogenic potential, but the halogenation degree of chlorinated bisphenols did not decrease their ERα potency (Riu et al., 2011).

A hexafluoro homolog of BPA, Bisphenol AF (BPAF), strongly binds to ERα, some 20 times more effectively than BPA, and to ERβ almost 50 times more effectively, but binds very weakly to ERRγ (Table 3.6). These differences in receptor

TABLE 3.6   Receptor Binding Characteristics of BPA, Hexafluoro-BPA, and HPTE for ERα, ERβ, and ERRγ (Matsushima et al., 2010)

Chemicals	ERα	ERβ IC_{50} (nM)[a]	ERRγ
17β-Estradiol	0.88 ± 0.04	2.17 ± 0.12	NB[b]
4-OHT	2.88 ± 0.15	3.17 ± 0.24	10.3 ± 0.8
BPA	$1,030 \pm 70$	900 ± 70	9.7 ± 0.59
BPAF	53.4 ± 3.1	18.9 ± 0.84	358 ± 3.1
HPTE	59.1 ± 1.5	18.1 ± 1.9	36.4 ± 4.4

[a]IC_{50}, the half maximal inhibitory concentration, is calculated as measure of the effectiveness in inhibiting the binding of 17β-estradiol to ERα and ERβ, and bisphenol A to ERRγ.
[b]NB means "not bound."

selectivity reflect subtle structural differences resulting from the $CH_3 \leftrightarrow CF_3$ substitution on the BPA backbone structure. BPAF is an ingredient of many plastics, electronic devices, optical fibers, and so on. It is a potent estrogen agonist for ERα, unleashing its actions just as the body's own estrogen would. However, despite BPAF's even stronger affinity for ERβ, it elicited no activity from this receptor (Matsushima et al., 2010). In doing so, it blocks the receptor's access to the body's own estrogen, preventing its triggering of the balancing function. Similar results have been reported for 2,2-bis(p-hydroxy phenyl)-1,1,1-trichloroethane (HPTE), a metabolite of methoxychlor (Table 3.6) which acts as an estrogen agonist when bound to ERα or an antagonist when bound to ERβ (Zama and Uzumcu, 2009).

3.3.5 Parabens (Hydroxy Benzoates)

Concerns have been raised that a growing number of body care formulation ingredients have been shown to be estrogenic and the potential this may have to adversely affect human health following repeated exposure (Harvey and Darbre, 2004; Gomez et al., 2005). One such group of ingredients in cosmetic formulation is the esters of p-hydroxybenzoic acid (parabens) (Fig. 3.13). Parabens have been widely used as antimicrobial preservatives – especially against molds and yeast – in cosmetics, toiletries, and pharmaceuticals. Microbial contamination of personal care products can spoil the smell and appearance of a product and spread infections to the user. Parabens, which typically include methyl-, ethyl-, propyl-, butyl-, isobutyl-, isopropyl-, and benzyl esters, are readily absorbed dermally and escape skin metabolism. Of the seven different types of parabens currently in use, benzyl-paraben appears to be most acutely toxic and methyl- and ethyl-paraben are the least acutely toxic (Terasaki et al., 2009). After dermal uptake, parabens are hydrolyzed, conjugated, and excreted through urine. Despite high dermal uptakes of parabens and their metabolites, little intact parabens were found in blood and urine (Boberg et al., 2010).

Use of parabens as preservatives in foodstuffs, including beverages, is less well known. These are identifiable on labeling as additives E214-219. Methyl-paraben (E218) and ethyl-paraben (E214) are the most commonly used parabens in food. In 2004, the European Food Safety Authority had set an acceptable daily intake (ADI) of a total of 0–10 mg/kg bodyweight per day for methyl- (E218) and ethyl-paraben (E214) (EFSA, 2004). In a study, over 90% of 267 food samples bought in the United States, comprising beverages, dairy products, fats and oils, fish and shellfish, grains, meat, fruits, and vegetables, were analyzed for measurable concentrations of methyl-, ethyl-, and propyl-parabens (Liao et al., 2013).

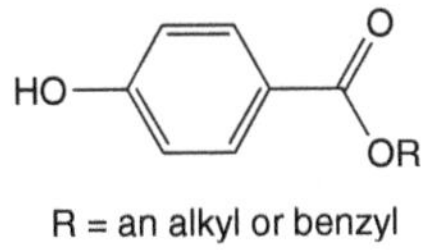

R = an alkyl or benzyl

Figure 3.13 General structure of parabens.

Parabens have displayed estrogenic activity in some *in vitro* screening tests, such as ligand binding to the estrogen receptor, regulation of CAT gene expression, and proliferation of MCF-7 human breast cancer cells. Reported *in vivo* effects include increased uterine weight (ethyl-, propyl-, butyl-, isobutyl-, and benzyl-paraben) in immature female rodents and reproductive tract effects in males (butyl-, propyl-paraben) (Lemini et al., 2003; Golden et al., 2005). In the MCF-7 cell proliferation assay, all the widely used parabens showed estrogenic activity, which increased with increased chain length and with branching of the alkyl chain (Darbre and Harvey, 2008). Additive effects were observed between different parabens and between parabens and E2. The common metabolite of paraben esters, *p*-hydroxy benzoic acid, was also found to possess estrogenic activity in both *in vitro* and *in vivo* assays (Darbre and Harvey, 2008).

Parabens significantly inhibited aromatase activity at concentrations within one order of magnitude of the effective concentration inducing cell proliferation. As aromatase is the enzyme responsible for conversion of androgens into estrogens (see Fig. 2.3), its inhibition would construe anti-estrogenic effect. Thus, in a human situation, parabens would have diminished estrogenic effects.

Many EDCs possessing estrogenic properties have also been shown to display antiandrogenic activity. In an *in vitro* study, several parabens, including methyl-, propyl-, and butyl-4-hydroxybenzoate were also found to be AR antagonists (Darbre and Harvey, 2008; Boberg et al., 2010; Chen et al., 2007). In another *in vitro* study using an AR reporter gene assay based on AR-transfected Chinese hamster ovary (CHO) cells, isobutyl-paraben antagonized the AR at concentrations of 25 µM and above (Kjærstad et al., 2010). Repeated oral dosage of propyl- and butyl-paraben in diet to juvenile rodents resulted in alterations to male reproductive functions, including spermatogenesis, testosterone secretion, and epididymal weights. While this was initially assumed to be due to estrogenic activity of parabens, the possibility that antiandrogenic activity could have contributed to the effects could not be excluded (Darbre and Harvey, 2008).

3.3.6   Sun Screens (Chemical UV Filters)

Ultraviolet (UV) filters are photostable substances used in cosmetics and other personal care products to protect human skin from UV irradiation and in plastics to prevent light-induced degradation. The majority of these are lipophilic compounds with conjugated aromatic systems that absorb UV light in the wavelength range 280–315 nm (UVB) and/or 315–400 nm (UVA). Humans are exposed to UV screens directly from cosmetics or indirectly through the food chain. These compounds can enter the aquatic environment indirectly from bathing or washing clothes, via wastewater treatment plants, and directly from recreational activities, such as swimming and sunbathing in lakes and rivers (Schlumpf et al., 2008).

Several UV filters such as 4-methylbenzylidene camphor (4-MBC), octyl-methoxycinnimate (OMC), and oxybenzone (Fig. 3.14) exhibit estrogenic activity in human breast cancer cell (MCF-7) proliferation grown *in vitro*. The induction of pS2 protein in MCF-7 cells and the blockade of the proliferative effect of 4-MBC by the estrogen antagonist fulvestrant (ICI 182,780) provided further evidence for

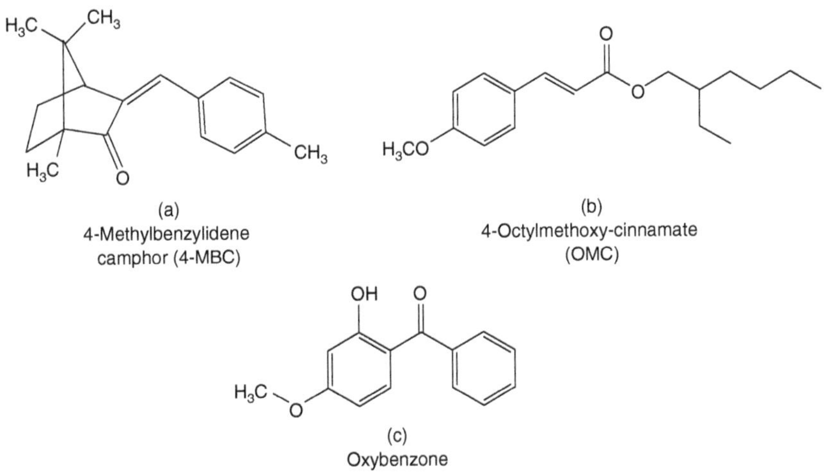

(a)
4-Methylbenzylidene
camphor (4-MBC)

(b)
4-Octylmethoxy-cinnamate
(OMC)

(c)
Oxybenzone

Figure 3.14   Estrogenic sunscreen chemicals.

estrogenic activity. In the uterotrophic assay using immature Long–Evans rats that received the chemicals for 4 days in powdered feed, uterine weight increased dose-dependently (Schlumpf et al. 2001).

Information on exposure is particularly important for the developing organism at its most sensitive early life stages. Human milk provides direct information on exposure of the suckling infant and indirect information on exposure of the mother during pregnancy. In a 3-year study during the summer and fall of 2004, 2005, and 2006, human milk was sampled from the mothers who had given birth at the University Women's Hospital in Basel, Switzerland. The chemical analytical data revealed that cosmetic UV filters such as 4-MBC were present in 85% of human milk samples, demonstrating that internal exposure of humans to cosmetic UV filters is widespread (Schlumpf et al., 2010).

The evidence from animal and *in vitro* studies indicates that some of the frequently used UV filters may also have thyroid disrupting activity. For example, OMC caused a dose-dependent decrease in serum TSH, T4, and T3 concentrations in rats (Klammer et al., 2007). In adult offspring born to 4-MBC-treated rats, thyroid weight and T3 concentration were found to increase (Schlumpf et al., 2004). Rat studies have also shown significant reduction of T4 and increase in TSH levels. 4-MBC delayed male puberty but did not affect females, and dose-dependently affected reproductive organ weights of adult offspring (Schlumpf et al., 2008).

3.4   METALLOESTROGENS

Many compounds in the environment are known to be capable of binding to cellular estrogens receptors and then mimicking the actions of physiological estrogens. The widespread origin and diversity in chemical structures of these environmental estrogens is extensive, most of these compounds being organic and in particular phenolic or carbon ring structures of varying structural complexity. Recent reports of the ability of certain metal ions to also bind to estrogen receptors and to give rise to estrogen agonist responses *in vitro* and *in vivo* have resulted in the realization that environmental estrogens can also be inorganic and these are termed as *metalloestrogens* (Darbre, 2006).

In several different estrogen-responsive *in vitro* assays, the estrogenic potencies of metal ions were 25–100% of the activity of 17β-estradiol. Thus metalloestrogens are more potent than phytoestrogens and most xenoestrogens of concern (Safe and Wormke, 2003). Metallic ions act as endocrine disruptors of reproductive tissues and fetal development in mammals, including humans. The detrimental effects occur with respect to both steroid and polypeptide hormones in the placenta. In addition to cadmium, arsenic, and lead, mercury and uranium have shown weak estrogenicity *in vitro* including proliferation of MCF-7 breast cancer cells (Dyer, 2007). Two reviews have appeared on the endocrine-disrupting activity of metals by Dyer (2007) and Iavicoli et al. (2009).

3.4.1   Cadmium (Cd)

The toxic heavy metal cadmium is a persistent environmental toxicant that enters the body through diet or cigarette smoke. Several human conditions, such as kidney dysfunction, cancer, respiratory ailments, and birth defects, are associated with Cd. It is regarded as a potential ED, since Cd exerts estrogen-like activity *in vitro* and can elicit some typical estrogenic responses in rodents upon intraperitoneal injection (Hofer et al., 2009). Low concentrations of Cd activated ERα by interacting noncompetitively with the hormone-binding domain and blocked the binding of estradiol. Cadmium treatment of MCF-7 human breast cancer cells stimulated growth, downregulated the estrogen receptor, stimulated the expression of the progesterone receptor, and stimulated estrogen response elements in transient transfection experiments – many responses elicited by estrogen (Gracia-Morales et al., 1994). Cd also possesses potent estrogen-like activity *in vivo*, where Cd treatment of Sprague–Dawley rats led to proliferations of the uterine and mammary gland tissues. These effects could be suppressed by treatment with the ER antagonist fulvestrant (ICI 182,780) (Fig. 3.15), suggesting that they are ER-mediated (Johnson et al., 2003; Kortenkamp, 2011). Similarly, female rats injected with Cd (CdCl$_2$) at a dose of 5–10 μg/kg experienced several well-characterized estrogenic responses, including earlier puberty onset, increased uterine weight, and enhanced mammary development. Both CdCl$_2$ and 17β-estradiol gave comparable responses, and these Cd-induced effects were blocked by coadministration of fulvestrant, supporting that Cd is a putative metalloestrogen (Johnson et al., 2003). It has been demonstrated that Cd at environmentally relevant concentrations also binds to the AR in human prostate cancer cells (Martin et al., 2002).

3.4.2   Lead (Pb)

Lead is a ubiquitous environmental contaminant associated with a variety of health effects. Although the Pb blood level in the US population has decreased

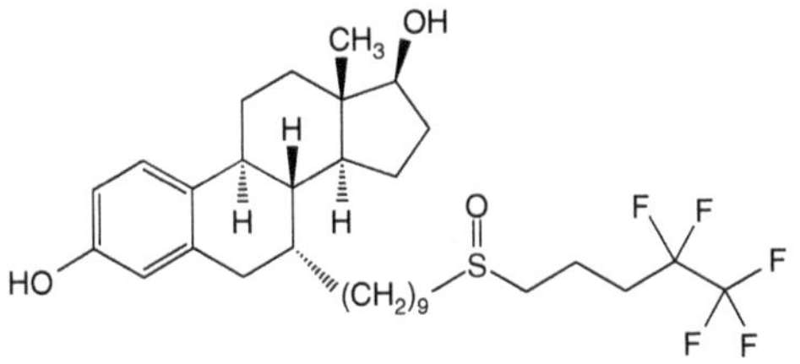

Figure 3.15   ER-antagonist fulvestrant (ICI 182,780).

considerably (from 13 μg/dL in the 1980s to <5 μg/dL now), largely due to removal of primary sources of Pb, such as leaded gasoline, lead-based paints, lead-soldered cans, and lead plumbing pipes, current levels, nonetheless, remain appreciably higher than preindustrial levels. Exposure to lead has been associated with ED effects, affecting both male and female reproductive systems, both in human populations and in experimental animals. Lead is also associated with delay in growth and pubertal development in girls (Dyer, 2007; Selevan et al., 2003).

3.4.3   Mercury (Hg)

Mercury is a metal that is widely used in foundry, mining, and manufacturing industries (chlorine-soda ash). It is a component in a number of electrical instruments and medical products (thermometers, thermostats, dental amalgams, switches, batteries, etc.). Mercuric chloride stimulated both estrogen-receptor-dependent transcription and increased proliferation of MCF-7 cells (Choe et al., 2003). In aquatic environments, sulfate-reducing bacteria mediate the transformation of inorganic divalent mercury into highly toxic bioavailable methylmercury (Zhang et al., 2011). Methylmercury stimulated MCF-7 cell foci formation in a concentration range of 0.5×10^{-7} to 1×10^{-6} M, which was blocked by the ER antagonist fulvestrant (Sukocheva et al., 2005). The estrogenic response of methylmercury did not reach the response elicited by 17β-estradiol, which is indicative of Hg being a weak estrogen mimic. Children exposed to methylmercury during pregnancy have exhibited developmental and neurological abnormalities including delayed onset of walking and/or talking, altered muscle tone, deep tendon reflexes, cerebral palsy, and reduced neurological scores (EPA, 1997).

3.4.4   Arsenic (As)

Arsenic, primarily as trivalent arsenite anion (AsO_3^{3-}), contamination of drinking water is considered a principal environmental health threat throughout the world. It is a potent endocrine disruptor, altering steroid-hormone-receptor-mediated gene regulation at very low environmentally relevant concentrations (0.01 μM) in cell culture and in whole-animal models (Kaltreider et al., 2001; Bodwell et al., 2006; Davey et al., 2007). Arsenite stimulated the growth of MCF-7 cells and inhibited by an ER antagonist. Arsenite also activated ERα at concentrations as low as 1 nM and effectively blocked estradiol binding, suggesting that it is a potent environmental estrogen (Stoica et al., 2000). Arsenic modulates transcription regulated by GR (Kaltreider et al. 2001) and other members of the hormone receptor family (androgen, progesterone, mineralcorticoid and estrogen hormones) (Bodwell et al., 2006, Davey et al., 2007), as well as the function of related nuclear receptors for thyroid hormone and retinoic acid (vitamin A) at very low environmentally relevant concentrations (0.01–2.0 μM in cell culture and at or below 10 ppb in several animal models), suggesting a common mechanism of action (Davey et al., 2008). However, the molecular mechanism by which it disrupts hormone-regulated gene expression is not yet known (Spuches and Wilcox, 2008).

Human metabolism of arsenic into methylated derivatives, once presumed to result in detoxification, may actually produce species with significantly greater pathological potential. It has been observed that formation of monomethylarsenite (MMA) within cells by intracellular methyltransferases through catalyzed oxidative addition of up to three methyl groups to arsenic is more toxic than arsenite, and that MMA, but not arsenite, competes for the binding site in GR (Spuches and Wilcox, 2008).

3.5   CONCLUSION AND FUTURE PROSPECTS

Estrogenic EDCs have received an overwhelmingly disproportionate amount of scientific attention compared to other EDCs in recent years. These naturally occurring or manmade compounds, present in the environment, are able to bind to estrogen receptors and interfere with normal cellular development in target organs and tissues. Some of the chemicals, such as EE2, have been specifically tailored to be potent estrogen receptor ligands, which are more physiologically potent and stable than endogenous natural estrogens and more persistent in the environment. The reproductive and developmental effects of estrogenic EDCs on aquatic biota are well discernable, as this tends to be the most intensively studied aspect of endocrine disruption in fishes.

REFERENCES

Alonso-Magdalena, P.; Quesada, I.; Nadal, A. Endocrine disruptors in the etiology of type 2 diabetes mellitus, *Nat. Rev. Endocrinol.* **2011**, 7(6), 346–353.

Alonso-Magdalena, P.; Morimoto, S.; Ripoll, C.; Fuentes, E.; Nadal, A. The estrogenic effect of bisphenol A disrupts pancreatic beta-cell function in vivo and induces insulin resistance, *Environ. Health Perspect.* **2006**, 114, 106–112.

Associated Press, FDA says plastic chemical BPA no longer allowed in baby bottles, sippy cups, *Washington Post*, Business, July 17, 2012.

Barnes, K. K.; Kolpin, D. W.; Furlong, E. T.; Zaugg, S. D.; Meyer, M.T.; Barber, L. B. A national reconnaissance of pharmaceuticals and other organic wastewater contaminants in the United States- I) groundwater. *Sci. Total Environ.* **2008**, 402(2–3), 192–200.

Biedermann, S.; Tschudin, P.; Grob, K. Transfer of bisphenol A from thermal printer paper to the skin, *Anal. Bioanal. Chem.* **2010**, 398, 571–576.

Blair, R. M.; Fang, H.; Branham, W. S.; Hass, B. S.; Dial, S. L.; Moland, C. L.; Tong, W.; Shi, L.; Perkins, R.; Sheehan, D. M. The estrogen receptor relative binding affinities of 100 natural and xenochemicals: structural diversity of ligands, *Toxicol. Sci.* **2000**, 54, 138–153.

Blum, J. L.; James, M. O.; Stuchal, L. D.; Denslow, N. D. Stimulation of transactivation of the largemouth bass estrogen receptors alpha, beta-a, and beta-b by methoxychlor and its mono- and bis-demethylated metabolites in HepG2 cells, *J. Steroid Biochem. Mol. Biol.* **2008**, 108(1–2), 55–63.

Blumberg, B.; Iguchi, T.; Odermatt, A. Endocrine disrupting chemicals, *J. Steroid Biochem. Mol. Biol.* **2011**, 127, 1–3.

Boberg, J.; Taxvig, C.; Christiansen, S.; Hass, U. Possible endocrine disrupting effects of parabens and their metabolites, *Reprod. Toxicol.* **2010**, 30(2), 301–312.

Bodwell JE et al., Arsenic disruption of steroid receptor gene activation: complex dose-response effects are shared by several steroid receptors, *Chem. Res. Toxicol.* **2006**, 19(12), 1619–1629.

Borrell, B. Toxicology: the big test for bisphenol A. *Nature* **2010**, 464, 1122–1124.

Bouskine, A.; Nebout, M.; Brücker-Davis, F.; Benahmed, M.; Fenichel, P. Low doses of bisphenol A promote human seminoma cell proliferation by activating PKA and PKG via a membrane G-protein–coupled estrogen receptor, *Environ. Health Perspect.* **2009**, 117, 1053–1058.

Bradbury, R. B.; White, D. Oestrogens and related substances in plants, *Vitam. Horm.* **1954**, 12, 207–233.

Bromer, J. G.; Wu, J.; Zhou, Y.; Taylor, H. S. Hypermethylation of homeobox A10 by *in utero* diethylstilbestrol exposure: an epigenetic mechanism for altered developmental programming, *Endocrinology* **2009**, 150(7), 3376–3382.

Burton, T. M. FDA bans BPA in baby-formula packaging, *The Wall Street Journal*, July 11, **2013**.

Calafat, A.M.; Ye, X.; Wong, L.Y.; Reidy, J.A.; Needham, L.L.; Exposure of the U.S. population to Bisphenol A and 4-tertiary-octylphenol: 2003–2004, *Environ. Health Perspect.* **2008**, 116910, 39–44.

Caldwell, D. J.; Mastrocco, F.; Hutchinson, T. H.; Lange, R.; Heijerick, D.; Janssen, C.; Anderson, P. D.; Sumpter, J. P. Derivation of an aquatic predicted no-effect concentration for the synthetic hormone, 17α-ethinyl estradiol, *Environ. Sci. Technol.* **2008**, 42, 7046–7054.

Canada Gazette, Order adding a toxic substance to schedule 1 to the Canadian Environmental Protection Act, 1999,Vol. 144, Number 21, October 13, 2010.

Carwile, J. L.; Michels, K. B. Urinary bisphenol A and obesity: NHANES 2003–2006, *Environ. Res.* **2011**, 111(6), 825–830.

Chavarro, J.E.; Toth, T.L.; Sadio, S.M.; Hauser, R.; Soy food and isoflavone intake in relation to semen quality parameters among men from an infertility clinic, *Hum. Reprod.* **2008**, 23(11), 2584–2590.

Chen, J.; Ahn, K. C.; Gee, N. A.; Gee, S. J.; Hammock, B. D.; Lasley, B. L. Antiandrogenic properties of parabens and other phenolic containing small molecules in personal care products, *Toxicol. Appl. Pharmacol.* **2007**, 221(3), 278–284.

Choe, S. Y.; Kim, S. J.; Kim, H. G.; Lee, J. H.; Choi, Y.; Lee, H.; Kim, Y. Evaluation of estrogenicity of major heavy metals, *Sci. Total Environ.* **2003**, 312, 15–21.

Cionna, C.; Maradonna, F.; Olivotto, I.; Pizzonia, G.; Carnevali, O. Effects of nonylphenol on juveniles and adults in the grey mullet, *Liza Aurata, Reprod. Toxicol.* **2006**, 22(3), 449–454.

ClickGreen staff, Europe to target pharmaceutical pollution with new water quality rules, January 31, 2012. Available at: www.clickgreen.org.uk/news/international-news/123110-europe-to-target-pharmaceutical-pollution-with-new-water-quality-rules.html

Corvini, P. F. X.; Schäffer, A.; Schlosser, D. The degradation of α-quaternary nonylphenol isomers by *Sphingomonas* sp. strain TTNP3 involves a type II *ipso* -substitution mechanism, *Appl. Microbiol. Biotechnol.* **2006**, 72, 223–243.

Cooney, C. A.; Dave, A. A.; Wolff, G. L. Maternal methyl supplements in mice affect epigenetic variation and DNA methylation of offspring, *J. Nutr.* **2002**, 132(8 Suppl), 2393S–2400S.

Cooper, R. L.; Kavlok, R. J. Endocrine disruptors and reproductive development, a weight-of-evidence overview, *J. Endocrinol.* **1997**, 152, 159–166.

Crews, D.; McLachlan, J. A. Epigenetics, evolution, endocrine disruption, health, and disease, *Endocrinology* **2006**, 147(6 Suppl), S4–S10.

Cummings, A. M.; Gray, L. E. Antifertility effect of methoxychlor in female rats – dose- and time-dependent blockade of pregnancy, *Toxicol. Appl. Pharmacol.* **1989**, 97(3), 454–462.

Darbre, P. D.; Harvey, P. W. Paraben esters: review of recent studies of endocrin toxicity, absorption, esterase and human exposure, and discussion of potential human health risks, *J. Appl. Toxicol.* **2008**, 28, 561–578.

Darbre, P. D. Metalloestrogens: an emerging class of inorganic estrogens with potential to add to estrogenic burden of the human breast, *J. Appl. Toxicol.*. **2006**, 26(3), 191–197.

Davey, J. C.; Nomikos, A. P.; Wungjiranirun, M.; Sherman, J. R.; Ingram, L.; Batki, C.; Lariviere, J. P.; Hamilton, J. W. Arsenic as an endocrine disruptor: arsenic disrupts retinoic acid receptor–and thyroid hormone receptor–mediated gene regulation and thyroid hormone–mediated amphibian tail metamorphosis, *Environ. Health Perspect.* **2008**, 116(2), 165–172.

Davey J. C.; Bodwell, J. E.; Gosse, J. A.; Hamilton, J. W. Arsenic as an endocrine disruptor: effects of arsenic on estrogen-mediated gene expression *in vivo* and in cell culture, *Toxicol. Sci.* **2007**, 98(1), 75–86.

de Wit, C. A.; Herzke, D.; Vorkamp, K. Brominated flame retardants in the Arctic environment - trends and new candidates, *Sci. Total Environ.* **2009**, 408, 2885–2918.

Diamanti-Kandarakis, E.; Bourguignon, J.P.; Giudice, L.C.; Hauser, R.; Prins, G.S.; Soto, A.M.; Zoeller, R.T.; Gore, A.C. Endocrine-disrupting chemicals: an Endocrine Society scientific statement. *Endocr. Rev.* **2009**, 30(4), 293–342.

Dolinoy D.C.; Weidman J.R.; Waterland R.A.; Jirtle R.L. Maternal genistein alters coat color and protects Avy mouse offspring from obesity by modifying the fetal epigenome, *Environ. Health Perspect.*. **2006**, 114(4), 567–572.

Dyer, C. A. Heavy metals as endocrine-disrupting chemicals, in *Endocrine Disrupting Chemicals*, Humana Press, **2007**, pp. 111–133.

EFSA, EFSA advises on the safety of paraben usage in food, European Food Safety Authority, 29 September, 2004. Available at: http://www.efsa.europa.eu/en/press/news/afc040929.htm?wtrl=01.

EPA, Mercury study report to Congress, Vol. 5, *Health Effects of Mercury and Mercury Compounds*, EPA-452/R-97-007, Washington, DC: U. S. Environmental Protection Agency, **1997**.

EPA, *Methoxychlor Registration Eligibility Decision (RED)*, EPA 738-R-04-010, Washington, DC: U.S. Environmental Protection Agency, June 30, **2004**.

EPA, *Aquatic Life Ambient Water Quality Criteria - Nonylphenol Final*, EPA 822-R-05-005, Washington, DC: U.S. Environmental Protection Agency, **2005**.

FDA, Federal Register 64 FR 57699, *Food Labeling: Health Claims; Soy Protein and Coronary Heart Disease*, Final Rule, U. S. Food and Drug Administration, October 26, **1999**.

Fernandez, A. M.; Held, U.; Willing, A.; Breuer, W. H. New green surfactants for emulsion polymerization, *Prog. Org. Coat.* **2005**, 53, 246−255.

Ferrara, F.; Fabietti, F.; Delise, M.; Bocca, A. P.; Funari, E. Alkylphenolic compounds in edible molluscs of the Adriatic Sea (Italy), *Environ. Sci. Technol.* **2001**, 35, 3109−3112.

Fukazawa, H.; Watanabe, M.; Shiraishi, F.; Shiraishi, H.; Shiozawa, T.; Matsushita, H.; Terao, Y. Formation of chlorinated derivatives of bisphenol A in waste paper recycling plants and their estrogenic activities, *J. Health Sci.* **2002**, 48(3), 242−249.

Gaido, K. W.; Maness, S. C.; McDonnell, D. P.; Dehal, S. S.; Kupfer, D.; Safe, S. Interaction of methoxychlor and related compounds with estrogen receptor α and β, and androgen receptor: structure-activity studies, *Mol. Pharmacol.* **2000**, 58(4), 852−858.

Gaido, K. W.; Leonard, L. S.; Maness, S. C.; Hall, J. M.; McDonnell, D. P.; Saville, B.; Safe, S. Differential Interaction of the methoxychlor metabolite 2,2-bis-(p-hydroxyphenyl)-1,1,1-trichloroethane with estrogen receptors (alpha) and (beta), *Endocrinology* **1999**, 140, 5746−5753.

Giger, W.; Gabriel, F. L. P.; Jonkers, N.; Wettstein, F. E.; Kohler, H.P. E. Environmental fate of phenolic endocrine disruptors: field and laboratory studies, *Phil. Trans. R. Soc. A* **2009**, 367, 3941−3963.

Gilbert, N. Drug-pollution law all washed up, *Nature* **2012**, 491(7425), 503.

Giusti, R. M.; Iwamoto, K.; Hatch, E. E. Diethylstilbestrol revisited: a review of the long-term health effects, *Ann. Int. Med.* **1995**, 122(10), 778−788.

Golden, R.; Gandy, J.; Vollmer, G. A review of the endocrine activity of parabens and implications for potential risks to human health, *Crit. Rev. Toxicol.* **2005**, 35 (5), 435−458.

Gomez, E.; Pillon, A.; Fenet, H.; Rosain, D.; Duchesne, M. J.; Nicolas, J. C.; Balaguer, P.; Casellas, C. Estrogenic activity of cosmetic components in reporter cell lines: parabens, UV screens, and musks, *J. Toxicol. Environ. Health A* **2005**, 68(4), 239−251.

Gracia-Morales, P.; Saceda, M.; Kenney, N.; Kim, N.; Salomon, D. S.; Gottardis, M. M.; Solomon, H. B.; Sholler, P. F.; Jordon, V. C.; Martin, M. B. Effect of cadmium on estrogen receptor levels and estrogen-induced responses in human breast cancer cells, *J. Biol. Chem.* **1994**, 269, 16896−16901.

Gray, L. E., Jr.,; Wilson, V.; Noriega, N.; Lambright, C.; Furr, J.; Stoker, T. E.; Laws, S. C.; Goldman, J.; Cooper, R. L.; Foster, P. M. D. Use of the laboratory rat as a model in endocrine disruptor screening and testing, *ILAR J.*. **2004**, 45(4), 425−437.

Gray, L. E. Jr.,; Ostby, J.; Cooper, R. L.; Kelce, W. R. The estrogenic and antiandrogenic pesticides methoxychlor alters the reproductive tract and behavior without affecting pituitarysize or LH and prolactin secretion in male rats, *Toxicol. Ind. Health* **1999**,15, 37−47.

Gray, Jr.,, L.E.; Ostby, J.; Ferrell, J. et al. A dose-response analysis of methoxychlor-induced alterations of reproductive development and function in the rat, *Fund. Appl. Toxicol.* **1989**, 12(1), 92–108.

2012 Green Chemistry Awards, *C&E News*, June 25, **2012**.

Gross-Sorokin, M. Y.; Roast, S. D.; Brighty, G. C. Assessment of feminization of male fish in english rivers by the environment agency of England and Wales, *Environ. Health Perspect.* **2006**, 114(Suppl 1), 147–151.

Guillette, Jr.,, L. J.; Moore, B. C. Environmental contaminants, fertility, and multioocytic follicles: a lesson from wildlife? *Semin. Reprod. Med.* **2006**, 24, 134–141.

Gutendorf, B.; Westendorf, J. Comparison of an array of in vitro assays for the assessment of the estrogenic potential of natural and synthetic estrogens, phytoestrogens and xenoestrogens, *Toxicology* **2001**, 166, 79–89.

Gyllenhammar, I.; Holm, L.; Eklund, R.; Berg, C. Reproductive toxicity in *Xenopus tropicalis* after developmental exposure to environmental concentrations of ethynylestradiol, *Aquat. Toxicol.* **2009**, 91, 171–178.

Halford, B. Side effects, *Chem. Eng. News* **2008**, 86, 13–17.

Harvey, P. W.; Darbre, P. Endocrine disrupters and human health: could oestrogenic chemicals in body care cosmetics affect breast cancer incidence in women? A review of evidence and call for further research, *J. Appl. Toxicol.* **2004**, 24, 167–176.

Herbst, A. L.; Ulfelder, H.; Poskanzer, D. C. Adenocarcinoma of the vagina: Association of maternal stilbestrol therapy with tumor appearance in young women, *N. Engl. J. Med.* **1971**, 284 (15), 878–881.

Herbst, A. L.; Bern, H. A. *Developmental Effects of Diethylstilbestrol in Pregnancy*, New York: Thieme-Stratton, **1981**.

Hofer, N.; Diel, P.; Wittsiepe, J.; Wihelm, M.; Gegan, G.H. Dose and route-dependent hormonal activity of the metalloestrogen cadmium in the rat uterus, *Toxicol. Lett.* **2009**, 19(2–3), 123–131.

Huang, W. W.; Yin, Y.; Bi, Q. et al., Developmental diethylstilbestrol exposure alters genetic pathways of uterine cytodifferentiation, *Mol. Endocrinol.* **2005**, 19, 669–682.

Hughes, Jr.,, C. L. Phytochemical mimicry of reproductive hormones and modulation of herbivore fertility by phytoestrogens, *Environ. Health Perspect.* **1988**, 78, 171–174.

Iavicoli, I.; Fontana, L.; Bergamaschi, A. The effects of metals as endocrine disruptors, *J. Toxicol. Environ. Health, B* **2009**, 12, 206–223.

Jefferson, W. N.; Padilla-Banks, E.; Newbold, R. R. Disruption of the female reproductive system by the phytoestrogen genistein, *Reprod. Toxicol.* **2007**, 23(3), 308–316.

Jeng, Y. J.; Watson, C. S. Combinations of physiologic estrogens with xenoestrogens alter ERK phosphorylation profiles in rat pituitary cells, *Environ. Health Perspect.* **2011**, 119(1), 104–112.

Johnson, M. D.; Kenney, N.; Stoica, A.; Hilakivi-Clarke, L.; Singh, B.; Chepko, G.; Clarke, R.; Sholler, P. F.; Lirio, A. A.; Foss, C.; Reiter, R.; Trock, B.; Paik, S.; Martin, M. B. Cadmium mimics the *in vivo* effects of estrogen in the uterus and mammary gland, *Nat. Med.* **2003**, 9, 1081–1084.

Jorgenson, J. L. Aldrin and dieldrin: a review of research on their production, environmental deposition and fate, bioaccumulation, toxicology, and epidemiology in the United States, *Environ. Health Perspect.* **2001**, 109(Suppl 1), 113–139.

Kaltreider, R.C.; Davis, A.M.; Lariviere, J.P.; Hamilton, J.W. Arsenic alters the function of the glucocorticoid receptor as a transcription factor, *Environ. Health Perspect.* **2001**,109, 245–251.

Kester, M. H. A.; Bulduk, S.; Tibboel, D.; Meinl, W.; Glatt, H.; Falany, C. N.; Coughtrie, M. W. H.; Bergman, A.; Safe, S. H.; Kuiper, G. G. J. M.; Schuur, G.; Brouwer, A.; Visser, T. J. Potent inhibition of estrogen sulfotransferase by hydroxylated PCB metabolites: A novel pathway explaining the estrogenic activity of PCBs, *Endocrinology* **2000**, 141(5), 1897–1900.

Kidd, K. A.; Blanchfield, P. J.; Mills, K. H.; Palace, V. P.; Evans, R. E.; Lazorchak, J. M.; Flick, R. W. Collapse of a fish population after exposure to a synthetic estrogen, *Proc. Natl. Acad. Sci. U. S. A.* **2007**, 104(21), 8897–8901.

Kitamura, S.; Suzuki, T.; Sanoh, S.; Kohta, R.; Jinno, N.; Sugihara, K.; Yoshihara, S.; Fujimoto, N.; Watanabe, H.; Ohta, S. Comparative study of the endocrine-disrupting activity of bisphenol A and 19 related compounds, *Toxicol. Sci.* **2005**, 84, 248–259.

Kitamura, S.; Jinno, N.; Ohta, S.; Kuroki, H.; Fujimoto, N. Thyroid hormonal activity of the flame retardants tetrabromobisphenol A and tetrachlorobisphenol A, *Biochem. Biophys. Res. Commun.* **2002**, 293, 554–559.

Kjærstad, M. B.; Taxvig, C.; Andersen, H. R.; Nellemann, C. Mixture effects of endocrine disrupting compounds in vitro, *Int. J. Androl.* **2010**, 33(2), 425–433.

Klammer, H.; Schlecht, C.; Wuttke, W.; Schmutzler, C.; Gotthardt, I.; Köhrle, J.; Jarry, H. Effects of a 5-day treatment with the UV-filter octyl-methoxycinnamate (OMC) on the function of the hypothalamo-pituitary-thyroid function in rats, *Toxicology* **2007**, 238(2–3), 192–199.

Kochukov, M. Y.; Jeng, Y.-J.; Watson, C. S. Alkylphenol xenoestrogens with varying carbon chain lengths differentially and potently activate signaling and functional responses in $GH_3/B_6/F10$ somatomammotropes. *Environ. Health Perspect.* **2009**, 117, 723–730.

Kolpin, D. W.; Furlong, E. T.; Meyer, M. T.; Thurman, E. M.; Zaugg, S. D.; Barber, L. B.; Buxton, H. T. Pharmaceuticals, hormones, and other organic wastewater contaminants in U. S. streams, 1999-2000: a national reconnaissance. *Environ. Sci. Technol.* **2002**, 36(6), 1202–1211.

Kolvenbach, B.; Schlaich, N.; Raoui, Z.; Prell, J.; Zuhlke, S.; Schaffer, A.; Guengerich, F.F.; Corvini, P.F.X. Degradation pathway of bisphenol A: Does *ipso* substitution apply to phenols containing α-carbon structure in the *para* position, *Appl. Environ. Microbiol.* **2007**, 73(15), 4776–4784.

Kortenkamp, A. Are cadmium and other heavy metal compounds acting as endocrine disrupters? *Met. Ions Life Sci.* **2011**, 8, 305–317.

Kuiper, G. G. J. M.; Lemmen, J.G.; Carlsson, B.; Corton, J.C.; Safe, S.H.; van der Saag, P.T.; van der Burg, B.; Gustafsson, J.-A.; Interaction of estrogenic chemicals and phytoestrogens with estrogen receptor β, *Endocrinology* **1998**, 139, 4252–4263.

Lang, L. A.; Galloway, T. S.; Scarlett, A.; Henley, W. E.; Depledge, M.; Wallace, R. B. et al., Association of urinary bisphenol A concentration with medical disorders and laboratory abnormalities in adults, *JAMA* **2008**, 300, 1303–1310.

Langley-Evans, S.C. Developmental programming of health and disease, *Proc. Nutr. Soc.* **2006**, 65(1), 97–105.

Lauver, D.; Nelles, K. K.; Hanson, K. The health effects of diethylstilbestrol revisited, *J. Obstet. Gynecol. Neonatal Nurs.* **2005**, 34, 494–499.

Layton, L. No BPA for baby bottles in U.S. 6 makers announce decision on chemical, *Washington Post*, March 6, **2009**, Page A06.

Lee, J.; Scheri, R. C.; Zhang, Y.; Curtis, L. R. Chlordecone, a mixed pregnane X receptor (PXR) and estrogen receptor alpha (ERα) agonist, alters cholesterol homeostasis and lipoprotein metabolism in C57BL/6 mice, *Toxicol. Appl. Pharmacol.* **2008**, 233(2), 193–202.

le Maire, A.; Bourguet, W.; Balaguer, P. A structural view of nuclear hormone receptor: endocrine disruptor interactions, *Cell. Mol. Life Sci.* **2010**, 67, 1219–1237.

Lemaire, G.; Mnif, W.; Mauvais, P.; Balaguer, P.; Rahmani, R. Activation of α- and β-estrogen receptors by persistent pesticides in reporter cell lines, *Life Sci.* **2006**, 79, 1160–1169.

Lemini, C.; Jaimez, R.; Avila, M. E.; Franco, Y.; Larrea, F.; Lemus, A. E. *In vivo* and *in vitro* estrogen bioactivities of alkyl parabens, *Toxicol. Ind. Health* **2003**, 2–6, 69–79.

Levin, E. R. Extranuclear steroid receptors: roles in modulation of cell functions, *Mol. Endocrinol.* **2011**, 25, 377–384

Levin, E. R. Plasma membrane estrogen receptors, *Trends Endocrinol. Metab.* **2009**, 20, 477– 482.

Levin, E. R. Integration of the extranuclear and nuclear actions of estrogen, *Mol. Endocrinol.* **2005**, 19(8), 1951–1959.

Li, Y.; Liu, L.; Andrews, L. G.; Tollefsbol, T. O. Genistein depletes telomerase activity through cross-talk between genetic and epigenetic mechanisms, *Int. J. Cancer* **2009**, 125, 286–296.

Li, S.; Hansman, R.; Newbold, R.; Davis, B.; McLachlan, J. A.; Barrett, J. C. Neonatal diethylstilbestrol exposure induces persistent elevation of c-fos expression and hypomethylation in its exon-4 in mouse uterus, *Mol. Carcinog.* **2003**, 38, 78–84.

Liao, C.; Liu, F.; Kannan, K. Occurrence of and dietary exposure to parabens in foodstuffs from the United States, *Environ. Sci. Technol.* **2013**, 47(8), 3918–3925.

Lintelmann, J.; Katayama, A.; Kurihara, N.; Shore, L.; Wenzel, A. Endocrine disrupters in the environment, *Pure Appl. Chem.* **2003**, 75(5), 631–681.

Lye, C. M.; Frid, C. L. J.; Gill, M. E.; Cooper, D. W.; Jones, D. M. Estrogenic alkylphenols in fish tissues, sediments, and waters from the UK Tyne and Tees estuaries, *Environ. Sci. Technol.* **1999**, 33, 1009–1014.

Martin, M. B.; Voeller, H. J.; Gelmann, E. P.; Lu, J.; Stoica, E. G.; Hebert, E. J.; Reiter, R.; Singh, B.; Danielsen, M.; Pantecost, E.; Stoica, A. Role of cadmium in the regulation of AR gene expression and activity, *Endocrinology* **2002**, 143(1), 263–275.

Masuno, H.; Iwanami, J.; Kidani, T.; Sakayama, K.; Honda, K. Bisphenol A accelerates terminal differentiation of 3T3-L1 cells into adipocytes through the phosphatidylinositol 3-kinase pathway, *Toxicol. Sci..* **2005**, 84(2), 319–327.

Matsushima, A.; Liu, X.; Okada, H.; Shimohigashi, M.; Shimohigashi, Y. Bisphenol AF is a full agonist for the estrogen receptor ERα, but a highly specific antagonist for ERβ, *Environ. Health Perspect.* **2010**, 118(9), 1267–1272.

Mazellier, P.; Leverd, J. Transformation of 4-*tert*-octylphenol by UV irradiation and by an H_2O_2/UV process in aqueous solution, *Photochem. Photobiol. Sci.* **2003**, 2, 946–953.

McLachlan, J. A. Prenatal exposure to diethylstilbestrol (DES): a continuing story, *Int. J. Epidemiol.* **2006**, 35, 868–870.

McLachlan, J. A. Environmental signaling: what embryos and evolution teach us about endocrine disrupting chemicals, *Endocr. Rev.* **2001**, 22, 319–334.

McLachlan, J. A.; Newbold, R. R.; Bullock, B. C. Long-Term Effects on the Female Mouse Genital Tract Associated with Prenatal Exposure to Diethylstilbestrol, *Cancer Res.* **1980**, 40(11), 3988–3999.

Meerts, I. A. T. M.; Letcher, R. J.; Hoving, S.; Marsh, G.; Bergman, Å.; Lemmen, J. G.; van der Burg, B.; Brouwer, A. In vitro estrogenicity of polybrominated diphenyl ethers, hydroxylated PBDEs, and polybrominated bisphenol A compounds, *Environ. Health Perspect.* **2001**, 109(4), 399–407.

Miyawaki, J.; Sakayama, K.; Kato, H.; Yamamoto, H.; Masuno, H. Perinatal and postnatal exposure to bisphenol A increases adipose tissue mass and serum cholesterol level in mice, *J. Atheroscler. Thromb.*. **2007**, 14(5), 245–252.

Moon, Y. J.; Wang, X.; Morris, M. E. Dietary flavonoids: Effects on xenobiotic and carcinogen metabolism, *Toxicol. In Vitro* **2006**, 20, 187–210.

Moriyama, K.; Tagami, T.; Akamizu, T.; Usui, T.; Saijo, M.; Kanamoto, N. et al. Thyroid hormone action is disrupted by bisphenol A as an antagonist. *J. Clin. Endocrinol. Metab.* **2002**, 87, 5185–5190.

Mueller, S. O. Xenoestrogens: mechanisms of action and detection methods, *Anal. Bioanal. Chem.* **2004**, 378, 582–587.

Nadal, A. Obesity: Fat from plastics? Linking bisphenol A exposure and obesity, *Nat. Rev. Endocrinol.* **2013**, 9, 9–10.

Nadal, A.; Alonso-Magdalena, P.; Ripoll, C.; Fuentes, E. Disentangling the molecular mechanisms of action of endogenous and environmental estrogens, *Eur. J. Physiol.* **2005**, 449, 335–343.

Nelson, J. A. Effects of dichlorodiphenyltrichloroethane (DDT) analogs and polychlorinated biphenyl (PCB) mixture on 17beta [3H] estradiol binding to rat uterine receptor, *Biochem. Pharmacol.* **1974**, 23, 447–451.

Newbold, R. R. Impact of environmental endocrine disrupting chemicals on the development of obesity, *Hormones* **2010**, 9(3), 206–217.

Newbold, R. R.; Padilla-Banks, E.; Jefferson, W. N. Environmental estrogens and obesity, *Mol. Cell. Endocrinol.* **2009**, 304(1–2), 84–89.

Newbold, R. R.; Padilla-Banks, E.; Jefferson, W. N. Adverse effects of the model environmental estrogen diethylstilbestrol are transmitted to subsequent generations, *Endocrinology* **2006**, 147, S11–S17.

Newbold, R. R., et al. Developmental exposure to estrogenic compounds and obesity, *Birth Def. Res. A Clin. Mol. Teratol.* **2005**, 73(7), 478–480.

Newbold, R.R.; Hanson, R. B.; Jefferson, W. N.; Bullock, B. C.; Haseman, J.; McLachlan, J. A. Increased tumors but uncompromised fertility in the female descendants of mice exposed developmentally to diethylstilbestrol, *Carcinogenesis* **1998**, 19, 1655–1663.

Newbold, R. R.; Padilla-Banks, E.; Snyder, R. J.; Phillips, T. M.; Jefferson, W. N. Developmental exposure to endocrine disruptors and the obesity epidemic, *Reprod. Toxicol.* **2007**, 23, 290–296.

NIEHS, Expert panel evaluation of soy infant formula, 2009. Available at: http://www.niehs.nih.gov/news/media/questions/docs/soy-infant-formula-expert-panel-summary-conclusion-12-18-09.pdf.

Nomura, S.; Daidoji, T.; Inoue, H.; Yokota, H. Differential metabolism of 4-n- and 4-*tert*-octylphenols in perfused rat liver, *Life Sci.*. **2008**, 83(5–6), 223–228.

Oehlmann, J.; Schulte-Oehlmann, U.; Kloas, W.; Jagnytsch, O.; Lutz, I.; Kusk, K. O.; Wollenberger, L.; Santos, E. M.; Paull, G. C.; Van Look, K. J.; Tyler, C. R.. A critical analysis of the biological impacts of plasticizers on wildlife, *Philos. Trans. R. Soc. Lond B Biol. Sci.* **2009**, 364(1526), 2047–2062.

Okada, H.; Tokunaga, T.; Liu, X.; Takayanagi, S.; Matsushima, A.; Shimohigashi, Y. Direct evidence revealing structural elements essential for the high binding ability of bisphenol A to human estrogen-related receptor-gamma, *Environ. Health Perspect.* **2008**, 116, 32–38.

Olde, B.; Leeb-Lundberg, L. M. GPR30/GPER1: searching for a role in estrogen physiology, *Trends Endocrinol. Metabol.* **2009**, 20(8), 409–416.

Peeters, P. H.; Keinan-Boker, L.; van der Schouw, Y. T.; Grobbee, D. E.; Phyto-estrogens and breast cancer risk. Review of the epidemiological evidence, *Breast Cancer Res. Treat.* **2003**, 77, 171–183.

Powell, C. E.; Soto, A. M.; Sonnenschein, C. Identification and characterization of membrane estrogen receptor from MCF7 estrogen-target cells, *J. Steroid Biochem. Mol. Biol.* **2001**, 77, 97–108.

Prasanth, G. K.; Divya, L. M.; Sadasivan, C. Bisphenol-A can bind to human glucocorticoid receptor as an agonist: an in silico study, *J. Appl. Toxicol.*. **2010**, 30(8), 769–774.

Rasier, G.; Parent, A. S.; Gérard, A.; Lebrethon, M. C.; Bourguignon, J. P. Early maturation of gonadotropin-releasing hormone secretion and sexual precocity after exposure of infantile female rats to estradiol or dichlorodiphenyltrichloroethane, *Biol. Reprod.* **2007**, 77, 734–742.

Riu, A.; Grimaldi, M.; le Maire, A.; Bey, G.; Phillips, K.; Boulahtouf, A.; Perdu, E.; Zalko, D.; Bourguet, W.; Balaguer, P. Peroxysome proliferator-activated receptor-γ is a target for halogenated analogues of bisphenol-A, *Environ. Health Perspect.* **2011**, 119(9), 1227–1232.

Rochester, J. R.; Millam, J. R. Phytoestrogens and avian reproduction: exploring the evolution and function of phytoestrogens and possible role of plant compounds in the breeding ecology of wild birds, *Comp. Biochem. Physiol. A, Mol. Integrat. Physiol.* **2009**, 154, 279–288.

Ropero, A. B.; Alonso-Magdalena, P.; Ripoll, C.; Fuentes, E.; Nadal, A. Rapid endocrine disruption: environmental estrogen actions triggered outside the nucleus, *J. Steroid Biochem. Mol. Biol.* **2006** 102, 163–169.

Ruegg, J.; Penttinen-Damdimopoulou, P.; Makela, S.; Pongratz, I.; Gustafsson, J. A. Receptors mediating toxicity and their involvement in endocrine disruption, in Molecular, Clinical and Environmental Toxicology, Vol. 1: Molecular toxicology, Lurch, A., ed., Switzerland: Birkhauser Verlag, **2009**, pp. 289–323.

Safe, S.; Wormke, M. Inhibitory aryl hydrocarbon receptor-estrogen receptor α cross-talk and mechanisms of action, *Chem. Res. Toxicol.* **2003**, 16, 807–816.

Schlumpf, M.; Kypke, K.; Wittassek, M.; Angerer, J.; Mascher, H.; Mascher, D.; Vökt, C.; Birchler, M.; Lichtensteiger, W. Exposure patterns of UV filters, fragrances, parabens, phthalates, organochlor pesticides, PBDEs, and PCBs in human milk: Correlation of UV filters with use of cosmetics, *Chemosphere*, **2010**, 81(10), 1171–1183.

Schlumpf, M.; Durrer, S.; Faass, O.; Ehnes, C.; Fuetsch, M.; Gaille, C.; Henseler, M.; Hofkamp, L.; Maerkel, K.; Reolon, S.; Timms, B.; Tresguerres, J. A. F.; Lichtensteiger, W. Developmental toxicity of UV filters and environmental exposure: a review, *Int. J. Androl.* **2008**, 31(2), 144–151.

Schlumpf, M.; Jarry, H.; Wuttke, W.; Ma, R.; Lichtensteiger, W. Estrogenic activity and estrogen receptor beta binding of the UV filter 3-benzylidene camphor. Comparison with 4-methylbenzyl- idene camphor, *Toxicology* **2004**, 199, 109–120.

Schlumpf, M.; Cotton, B.; Conscience, M.; Haller, V.; Steinmann, B.; Lichtensteiger, W. In vitro and in vivo estrogenicity of UV screens, *Environ. Health Perspect.* **2001**, 109(3), 239–244.

Schoenfuss, H. L.; Bartell, S. E.; Bistodeau, T. B.; Cediel, R. A.; Grove, K. J.; Zintek, L.; Lee, K. E.; Barber, L. B. Impairment of the reproductive potential of male fathead minnows by environmentally relevant exposures to 4-nonylphenol, *Aquat. Toxicol.* **2008**, 86, 91–98.

Sekizawa, J. Low-dose effects of bisphenol A: a serious threat to human health? *J. Toxicol. Sci.*. **2008**, 33(4), 389–403.

Selevan, S. G.; Rice, D. C.; Hogan, K. A.; Euling, S. Y.; Pfahles-Hutchens, A.; Bethel, J. Blood lead concentration and delayed puberty in girls, *N. Engl. J. Med.* **2003**, 348, 1527–1536.

Shanle, E. K.; Xu, W. Endocrine disrupting chemicals targeting estrogen receptor signaling: Identification and mechanisms of action, *Chem. Res. Toxicol.* **2011**, 24(1), 6–19.

Shutoh, Y.; Takeda, M.; Ohtsuka, R.; Haishima, A.; Yamaguchi, S.; Fujie, H.; Komatsu, Y.; Maita, K.; Harada, T. Low dose effects of dichlorodiphenyltrichloroethane (DDT) on gene transcription and DNA methylation in the hypothalamus of young male rats: implication of hormesis-like effects, *J. Toxicol. Sci.*. **2009**, 34(5), 469–482.

Skakkebaek N. E.; Rajpert-De Meyts, E.; Main, K. M. Testicular dysgenesis syndrome: an increasingly common developmental disorder with environmental aspects. *Hum. Reprod.* **2001**, 16, 972–978.

Somm, E.; Schwitzgebel, V. M.; Toulotte, A.; Cederroth, C. R.; Combescure, C.; Nef, S.; Aubert, M. L.; Hüppi, P. S. Perinatal exposure to bisphenol A alters early adipogenesis in the rat, *Environ. Health Perspect.* **2009**, 117, 1549–1555.

Soriano, S.; Alonso-Magdalena, P.; Marta García-Arévalo, M.; Novials, A.; Muhammed, S. J.; Salehi, A.; Gustafsson, J. A.; Ivan Quesada, I.; Nadal, A. Rapid insulinotropic action of low doses of Bisphenol-A on mouse and human islets of langerhans: role of estrogen receptor β, *PLoS ONE* **2012**, 7(2), e31109.

Soto, A. M.; Sonnenschein, C.; Chung, K. L.; Fernandez, M. F.; Olea, N.; Serrano, F. O. The E-screen assay as a tool to identify estrogens - an update on estrogenic environmental pollutants, *Environ. Health Perspect.* **1995**, 103(7), 113–122.

Soto, A. M.; Justicia, H.; Wray, J. W.; Sonnenschein, C. *p*-Nonyl-phenol: an estrogenic xenobiotic released from "modified" polystyrene, *Environ. Health Perspect.* **1991**, 92, 167–173.

Spuches, A. M.; Wilcox, D. E. Monomethylarsenite competes with Zn^{2+} for binding sites in the glucocorticoid receptor, *J. Am. Chem. Soc.* **2008**, 130(26), 8148–8149.

Stanford, B.D.; Weinberg, H. S. Evaluation of on-site wastewater treatment technology to remove estrogens, nonylphenols, and estrogenic activity from wastewater, *Environ. Sci. Technol.* **2010**, 44, 2994–3001.

Stoica, A.; Pentecost, E.; Martin, M. B. Effects of arsenite on estrogen receptor-α expression and activity in MCF-7 breast cancer cells, *Endocrinolohly* **2000**, 141(10), 3595–3602.

Sukocheva, O. A.; Yang, Y.; Gierthy, J. F.; Seegal, R. F. Methyl mercury influences growth-related signaling in MCF-7 breast cancer cells, *Environ. Toxicol.* **2005**, 20, 32–44.

Sumpter, J. P.; Johnson, A. C. 10th Anniversary perspective: Reflections on endocrine disruption in the aquatic environment: from known to unknown unknowns (and many things in between). *J. Environ. Monit.* **2008**, 10, 1476–1485.

Sumpter, J. P.; Jobling, S. Vitellogenesis as a biomarker for estrogenic contamination of the aquatic environment, *Environ. Health Perspect.* **1995**, 103 (Suppl. 7), 173–178.

Sun, H.; Shen, O. X.; Wang, X. R.; Zhou, L.; Zhen, S. Q.; Chen, X. D. Anti-thyroid hormone activity of bisphenol A, tetrabromobisphenol A and tetrachlorobisphenol A in an improved reporter gene assay, *Toxicol. In Vitro* **2009**, 23, 950–954.

Swan, S. H. Intrauterine exposure to diethylstilbestrol: long-term effects in humans, *APMIS* **2000**, 108, 793–804.

Takayanagi, S.; Tokunaga, T.; Liu, X.; Okada, H.; Matsushima, A.; Shimohigashi, Y. Endocrine disruptor bisphenol A strongly binds to human estrogen-related receptor γ (ERRγ) with high constitutive activity, *Toxicol. Lett.* **2006**, 167, 95–105.

Terasaki, M.; Makino, M.; Tatarazako, N. Acute toxicity of parabens and their chlorinated by-products with *Daphnia magna* and *Vibrio fischeri* bioassays, *J. Appl. Toxicol.* **2009**, 29, 242–247.

Thayer, K. N.; Belcher, S. Background paper on mechanisms of action of bisphenol A and other biochemical/molecular interactions, WHO/HSE/FOS/11.1, FAO/WHO Expert Meeting on Bisphenol A (BPA), Ottawa, Canada, World Health Organization, 2011. Available at: http://www.who.int/foodsafety/chem/chemicals/5_biological_activities_of_bpa.pdf.

Thomas, P.; Pang, Y.; Filardo, E. J.; Dong, J. Identity of an estrogen membrane receptor coupled to a G protein in human breast cancer cells, *Endocrinology* **2005**, 146(2), 624–632.

Thomas, P.; Dong, J. Binding and activation of the seven-transmembrane estrogen receptor GPR30 by environmental estrogens: a potential novel mechanism of endocrine disruption, *J. Steroid Biochem. Mol. Biol.* **2006**, 102, 175–179.

Tiemann, U. In vivo and in vitro effects of the organochlorine pesticides DDT, TCPM, methoxychlor, and lindane on the female reproductive tract of mammals: A review, *Reprod. Toxicol.* **2008**, 25(3), 316–326.

Titus-Ernstoff, L.; Troisi, R.; Hatch, E. E. et al. Offspring of women exposed *in utero* to diethylstilbestrol (DES): a preliminary report of benign and malignant pathology in the third generation, *Epidemiology* **2008**,19, 251–257.

Trasande, L.; Attina, T. M.; Blustein, J. Association between urinary bisphenol A concentration and obesity prevalence in children and adolescents, *JAMA* **2012**, 308, 1113–1121.

Vandenberg, L. N., Exposure to bisphenol A in Canada: invoking the precautionary principle, *CMAJ* **2011**, 183, 1265–1270.

Vandenberg, L. N.; Maffini, M. V.; Sonnenschein, C.; Rubin, B. S.; Soto, A. M. Bisphenol-A and the great divide: A review of controversies in the field of endocrine disruption, *Endocr. Rev.* **2009**, 30(1), 75–95.

Varayoud, J.; Monje, L.; Bernhardt, T.; Muñoz-de-Toro, M.; Luque, E. H.; Ramos, J. G. Endosulfan modulates estrogen-dependent genes like a non-uterotrophic dose of 17beta-estradiol, *Reprod. Toxicol.* **2008**, 26(2), 138–145.

Vasudevan, N.; Pfaff, D. W. Membrane initiated actions of estrogens in neuroendocrinology: emerging principles, *Endocr. Rev.* **2007**, 28, 1–19.

Viñas, R.; Watson, C. S. Bisphenol S disrupts estradiol-induced nongenomic signaling in a rat pituitary cell line: effects on cell functions, *Environ. Health Perspect.* **2013**. DOI: 10.1289/ehp.1205826.

Vinas, P.; Campillo, N.; Martinez-Castillo, N.; Hernandez-Cordoba, M. Comparison of two derivatization-based methods for solid-phase microextraction-gas chromatography–mass spectrometric determination of bisphenol A, bisphenol S and biphenol migrated from food cans. *Anal. Bioanal. Chem.* **2010**, 397,115–125.

vom Saal, F. S.; Nagel, S. C.; Coe, B. L.; Angle, B. M.; Taylor, J. A. The estrogenic endocrine disrupting chemical bisphenol A (BPA) and obesity, *Mol. Cell. Endocrinol.* **2012**, 354, 74–84.

vom Saal, F. S.; Hughes, C. An extensive new literature concerning low-dose effects of bisphenol A shows the need for a new risk assessment. *Environ. Health Perspect.* **2005**, 113, 926–933.

von Reppert-Bismarck, J.; Roche A. EU to ban bisphenol A in baby bottles in 2011, *Reuters* **2010**, 11, 25. Available at: www.reuters.com/article/2010/11/25/us-eu-health-plastic-idUSTRE6AO3MS20101125.

Wada, K.; Sakamoto, H.; Nishikawa, K.; Sakuma, S.; Nakajima, A.; Fujimoto, Y.; Kamisaki, Y. Life style-related diseases of the digestive system: endocrine disruptors stimulate lipid accumulation in target cells related to metabolic syndrome, *J. Pharmacol. Sci.* **2007**, 105, 133–137.

Waters, K. M.; Safe, S.; Gaido, K. W. Differential gene expression in response to methoxychlor and estradiol through ERα, ERβ, and AR in reproductive tissues of female mice, *Toxicol. Sci.* **2001**, 63(1), 47–56.

Watson, C. S.; Jeng, Y.-J.; Kochukov, M. Y. Nongenomic signaling pathways of estrogen toxicity, *Toxicol. Sci.* **2010**, 115(1), 1–11.

Watson, C. S.; Jeng, Y.-J.; Guptarak, J. Endocrine disruption via estrogen receptors that participate in nongenomic signaling pathways, *J. Steroid Biochem. Mol. Biol.* **2011**, 127(1–2), 44–50.

Watson, C. S.; Bulayeva, N. N.; Wozniak, A. L.; Finnerty, C. C. Signaling from the membrane via membrane estrogen receptor-α: estrogens, xenoestrogens, and phytoestrogens, *Steroids* **2005**, 70, 364–371.

Welch, R. M.; Levin, W.; Conney, A. H. Estrogenic action of DDT and its analogs, *Toxicol. Appl. Pharmacol.* **1969**, 14, 358–367.

Wetherill, Y. B.; Akingbemi, B. T.; Kanno, J.; McLachlan, J. A.; Nadal, A.; Sonnenschein, C.; Watson, C. S.; Zoeller, R.T.; Belcher, S. M. In vitro molecular mechanisms of bisphenol A action, *Reprod. Toxicol.* **2007**, 24(2), 178–198.

Wetherill, Y. B.; Petre, C. E.; Monk, K. R.; Puga, A.; Knudsen, K. E. The xenoestrogen bisphenol A induces inappropriate androgen receptor activation and mitogenesis in prostatic adenocarcinoma cells, *Mol. Cancer Ther.* **2002**, 1, 515–524.

Wise, A.; O'Brien, K.; Woodruff, T. Are oral contraceptives a significant contributor to the estrogenicity of drinking water? *Environ. Sci. Technol.* **2011**, 45, 51–60.

Ye, X.; Bishop, A. M.; Needham, L. L.; Calafat, A. M. Identification of metabolites of 4-nonylphenol isomer 4-(3', 6'-Dimethyl-3'-Heptyl) Phenol by rat and human liver microsomes, *Drug. Metabol. Dispos.* **2007**, 35(8), 1269–1274.

Zama, A. M.; Uzumcu, M. Fetal and neonatal exposure to the endocrine disruptor methoxychlor causes epigenetic alterations in adult ovarian genes, *Endicronology* **2009**, 150(10), 4681–4691.

Zha, J. M.; Sun, L. W.; Zhou, Y. Q. et al. Assessment of 17a ethinylestradiol effects and underlying mechanisms in a continuous, multigeneration exposure of the Chinese rare minnow (Gobiocypris rarus). *Toxicol. Appl. Pharmacol.* **2008**, 226, 298–308.

Zhang, T.; Kim, B.; Levard, C.; Reinsch, B. C.; Lowry, G. V.; Deshusses, M. A.; Hsu-Kim, H. Methylation of Mercury by Bacteria Exposed to Dissolved, Nanoparticulate, and Microparticulate Mercuric Sulfides, *Environ. Sci. Technol.* **2011**. DOI: 10.1021/es203181m.

Zhu, B. T. Mechanistic explanation for the unique pharmacologic properties of receptor partial agonists, *Biomed. Pharmacother.* **2005**, 59, 76–89.

Zoeller, R. T.; Bansal, R.; Parris, C. Bisphenol-A, an environmental contaminant that acts as a thyroid hormone receptor antagonist in vitro, increases serum thyroxine, and alters RC3/neurogranin expression in the developing rat brain, *Endocrinology* **2005**, 146, 607–612.

4

ANTI-ANDROGENIC CHEMICALS

4.1 INTRODUCTION

Male reproductive health is defined by both the proper development of the reproductive system and maintenance of function throughout adult life, including the capacity to reproduce. It has been shown that most of the anti-androgenic chemicals in the environment are able to interfere with the androgen signaling pathways by binding directly to specific intracellular androgen receptors (AR) to activate (as agonists) or repress (as antagonists) the expression of specific genes, notably those involved in the development of male primary and secondary sexual characteristics (Jolly et al., 2009). Chemicals that counteract androgen action at some stage in this period can have significant consequences for the developing animal's reproductive tract with irreversible de-masculinizing consequences and deformed sex organs. These effects can arise through antagonism of androgens at the steroid receptor level and/or via suppression of testosterone synthesis in fetal Leydig cells (testicular). Androgen deficiency during prenatal development is thought to disturb differentiation of the Wolffian duct, a process crucial to the proper development of male internal reproductive organs. Anti-androgens affect only male fetuses, whereas estrogens can harm both sexes. Many of the estrogenic effects are similar to those of anti-androgens in male fetuses (Toppari et al. 2010).

Rats (Wister, Sprague–Dawley, etc.) are often used in research studies to identify possible health concerns associated with chemical exposure. Reduced anogenital distance (AGD), retention of nipples or areolas, abnormal urinary opening (hypospadias), agenesis of sex accessory tissues, and undescended testes (cryptorchidism) have been described as consequences of disruption of

Endocrine Disruptors in the Environment, First Edition. Sushil K. Khetan.
© 2014 John Wiley & Sons, Inc. Published 2014 by John Wiley & Sons, Inc.

androgen action in the developing rat. AGD is used as a sensitive indicator of male feminization. The shorter the distance, the more female-like the animal is perceived to be. This measurement is also used in humans to predict reproductive disorders (Eisenberg et al., 2011; Mendiola et al., 2011). Human male reproductive developmental disorders such as cryptorchidism, hypospadias, testicular cancer, and decreased sperm count are also the problems associated with anti-androgen exposure.

Key anti-androgens were characterized by their antagonism of AR. Further characterization has been based on extensive batteries of examinations of the reproductive tract and secondary sex character *in vivo* in the laboratory rat. Recognized anti-androgens fell into classes including dicarboximides, such as vinclozolin (VZ) (Gray et al. 1994; Kelce & Wilson 1997) and procymidon (Gray et al., 2006; Hosokawa et al., 1993; Ostby et al., 1999), the imidazole fungicide prochloraz (Vinggaard et al. 2002; Noriega et al. 2005), the organochlorine insecticide p,p'-dichlorodiphenyldichloroethylene (DDE) (Kelce et al. 1995), the urea-based herbicide linuron (Wolf et al. 1999; Lambright et al. 2000), phthalate esters used as plasticizers (Parks et al. 2000; Howdeshell et al. 2007), and polybrominated diphenyl ethers (PBDEs) used as flame retardants (Stoker et al. 2005), in addition to flutamide used as a model anti-androgen (Noriega, 2012).

Anti-androgenic endocrine disrupting chemicals (EDCs) are primarily classified into two broad categories: (i) those that interfere with androgen biosynthesis or metabolism to indirectly modulate androgen function (non-receptor-mediated disruptors), and (ii) those that interact with the AR to interfere with the ligand-dependent transcriptional function (receptor-mediated disruptors).

4.2   TESTOSTERONE SYNTHESIS INHIBITORS

4.2.1   Phthalates

Phthalates are a group of industrial chemicals with many commercial uses, such as plasticizers and fragrance carriers used in a wide array of consumer products, especially those containing PVC. Annually, more than 3 million metric tons of phthalates are consumed globally (Bizzari et al., 2000). At least 10 different phthalates are used commercially as plasticizers, solvents, antifoam agents, or alcohol denaturants. Phthalates can be classified into two groups based on their molecular weight. Accordingly, low-molecular-weight phthalates (ester side-chain lengths, 1–4 carbons), which include dimethyl phthalate (DMP), diethyl phthalate (DEP), and di-*n*-butyl phthalate (DBP), are more commonly present in personal care products to stabilize color and scent (fragrances, shampoo, cosmetics, and nail polish). High-molecular-weight phthalates (ester side-chain lengths, five or more carbons), which include di-(2-ethylhexyl) phthalate (DEHP), di-octyl phthalate (DOP), and di-isononyl phthalate (DINP), are used in plastic tubing, in food packaging and processing materials, and in numerous PVC products. DEHP is the most commonly used phthalate plasticizer for PVC to increase its flexibility and can be found in tubing, vinyl flooring, and wall covering and some PVC medical devices (Matsumoto et al. 2002). In 2006, the National Toxicology Program (NTP) found that DEHP may pose a risk to human development, especially critically ill male infants (NTP, 2006; Barrett, 2006).

Phthalates used as plasticizers in polymers are not chemically bound to the polymers and therefore readily leach, migrate, or off-gas from the polymers to contaminate the external environment, particularly when phthalate-containing products are exposed to high temperatures, exposing humans to high concentrations of these compounds (NRC, 2008). Because phthalates are used in such a wide variety of consumer products, human exposure to them is widespread. Prenatal low-molecular-weight phthalate exposure has been associated with children clinically diagnosed with behavior or attention-deficit hyperactivity disorders. Although their biological activity may be less severe than that of other endocrine disruptors, the potential public health impact of exposure to phthalates might be greater (Engel et al., 2010). In a study investigating an association between prenatal phthalate exposure and altered genital formation in humans, it was observed that boys born to mothers with greater exposure had altered genital development (Barrett, 2005).

Phthalates represent a class of environmental endocrine-active chemicals that does not appear to act via estrogen and androgen nuclear receptors, but through a distinct mechanism of targeting the Leydig cells' testosterone biosynthesis machinery interfering with the production of androgens in the fetal testis, producing the same effect of blocking androgen action at the target tissues.

Endocrine disruption activity of biologically active phthalates DEHP and DBP is directed at early development of the fetal testis. Exposure of rats to DEHP (or MEHP) during gestation causes a significant reduction in fetal testosterone levels during the critical masculinization window between embryonic d 15 and 19. Studies have shown that male rats exposed to phthalates *in utero* during this period of sexual differentiation exhibited a number of reproductive tract abnormalities such as malformations of internal reproductive organs (epididymis, testes) (Foster, 2006). Because 5α-dihydrotestosterone (DHT) is derived from testosterone through enzymatic conversion by 5α-reductase, lower testosterone concentrations also affect the development of tissues that rely on DHT (prostate and external genitalia). DHT is further required for the regression of nipple anlagen in male rats and for the growth of the perineum to produce the normal male AGD, which is longer than in females. Because of reduced DHT levels in the wake of suppressed testosterone synthesis, retained nipples and feminized AGDs are also seen in male rats exposed to phthalates in fetal life (Christiansen et al., 2009).

Malformation of reproductive tissues in male offspring of rats is most dramatic after *in utero* and lactational exposure to phthalates, with significant postnatal developmental anomalies, including small or otherwise abnormal testes, hypospadias, cryptochidism, decreased AGD, retained nipples, and decreased sperm production, characterized as the "phthalate syndrome" (Foster, 2005; NRC, 2008). The mode of action for these effects is believed to involve an impairment of fetal Leydig and Sertoli cell function, leading to androgen deficiency in the developing reproductive tract of male rats (David, 2006). Certain similarities in humans of these malformations in rodents, described as testicular dysgenesis syndrome

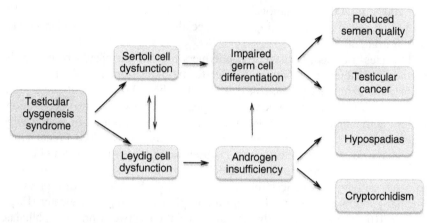

Figure 4.1 Cascade of events during the development of the testis in fetal life can be related to human reproductive disorders known as the hypothesis of testicular dysgenesis syndrome (TDS). Source: Adapted from Skakkebaek et al. (2001). Reproduced with permission of Oxford University Press.

(TDS), are speculated to be caused by exposure to anti-androgenic chemicals, which could result from reduced androgen action during fetal development (Skakkebaek et al., 2001; Wohlfahrt-Veje et al., 2009). Using the rat model, a large and convincing body of literature shows that a wide range of anti-androgenic and estrogenic EDCs can cause TDS. For example, it has been shown that exposure of rats *in utero* to DBP can induce a TDS-like syndrome in the male offspring (Mylchreest et al., 2000; Fisher et al., 2003; Foster, 2006; Dean et al., 2012; van den Driesche et al., 2012), which is manifested as dose-dependent induction of cryptorchidism, hypospadias, and impaired spermatogenesis/infertility (Fig. 4.1). In contrast, similar exposures of adult males result in none or only limited effects (Frederiksen et al., 2007). The adverse effects of phthalates observed in rodent models affecting the male reproductive system have raised concerns as to whether exposure to phthalates represents a potential health risk to humans.

DEHP, DBP, and benzyl butyl phthalate (BBP) (Fig. 4.2), which are the most investigated phthalates, have been found to produce nearly identical responses with a relative reproductive toxicity potency in the order: DEHP > DBP > BBP. With relative potency factor for DEHP assigned as 1.00, the values for DBP and BBP were calculated to be 0.64 and 0.21, respectively (Benson, 2009). DBP and BBP have been found to be AR antagonists by producing estrogenic effects in estrogen-responsive human breast cancer cells and by recombinant yeast screening (Ruegg et al., 2009). Other phthalates showing potential for reproductive toxicity include di-*n*-hexyl phthalate, di-isobutyl phthalate, and DINP (Lyche et al., 2009).

Phthalates with a certain ester side-chain length, such as DEHP, through its primary metabolite monoethylhexyl phthalate (MEHP), has been implicated as a mediator of the reproductive and developmental toxicity associated with DEHP. MEHP causes toxicity, resulting in decreased serum estradiol levels and

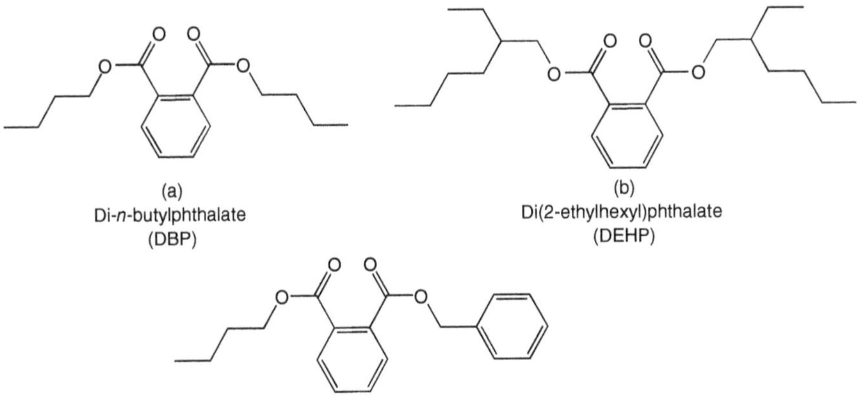

(a)
Di-*n*-butylphthalate
(DBP)

(b)
Di(2-ethylhexyl)phthalate
(DEHP)

(c)
n-Butyl benzylphthalate
(BBP)

Figure 4.2   Endocrine active phthalates.

suppression of aromatase in female rodents (Lovekamp-Swan and Davis, 2003). In male rat embryos, DEHP suppresses testosterone synthesis to those normally found in females during sexual differentiation, by interfering with the uptake of cholesterol precursors into fetal Leydig cells, where testicular androgen production takes place (Gray et al., 2000; Howdeshell et al. 2008; Parks et al., 2000). As a consequence, the development of the male reproductive tract is disrupted, leading to incomplete masculinization. MEHP is also implicated in direct activation of peroxisome proliferator-activated receptor γ (PPARγ) and promote adipogenesis, albeit to a lower extent than its full agonist rosiglitazone (Feig et al., 2007).

An expert panel of NTP found that DEHP might pose a risk to human development, especially for critically ill male infants (NTP, 2006). An association between male genital development in humans and phthalate exposure was reported, showing prenatal phthalate exposure resulting in impaired testicular function and shortened AGD among male infants (Swan et al., 2005). A study on the relationship between urinary phthalates and serum thyroid concentrations investigated in US adults and adolescents showed association of higher concentrations of metabolites of DEHP in urine among adults with decreased thyroid hormone levels in blood. This relationship was not observed among adolescents, though this group consisted of a much smaller number of participants (Meeker and Ferguson, 2011).

National monitoring studies have found one or more phthalates in over 10% of streams sampled (Kolpin et al., 2002). The only phthalate that has a drinking water standard is DEHP, which has a maximum contaminant level (MCL) based on the potential to cause mild gastrointestinal disturbances, nausea, and vertigo, but not on endocrine disrupting effects. The other phthalates have no drinking water standards as yet. In the draft risk assessment for DBP, the US EPA proposes to use changes in hormonal levels caused by DBP, which is an anti-androgen, to set the reference dose (RfD) for DBP. Specifically, it has identified reduction in fetal testosterone as the critical effect for the regulation of DBP. Despite the reduction being reversible, the EPA concluded that it could cause irreversible effects if it occurred during a critical window of development (EPA, 2006).

EPA has expressed strong concern about eight phthalates, all short-chain paraffins, that pose risks, and is considering regulations to restrict or even ban these. Under the action plan, EPA is invoking the 1976 Toxic Substances Control Act to create a list of chemicals that may present an unreasonable risk of injury to health and the environment. Once listed, the chemical producers can provide information to the EPA if they want to demonstrate that these chemicals do not pose an unreasonable risk. Also, EPA intends to add six of the phthalates to the Toxics Release Inventory. The remaining two of the eight phthalates are already listed (Hogue, 2010).

The European Union banned the use of the lower molecular weight phthalates DEHP, DBP, and BBP in cosmetic applications in 2004 and restricted their use in toys and child care articles in 2007. The US Congress took action restricting the use of phthalates in toys and other children's products by passage of the 2008 US Consumer Product Safety Improvement Act, which prohibits the sale of certain products containing phthalates (DEHP, DBP, BBP, DINP, di-iso-octyl phthalate, and di-n-octyl phthalate). Kaiser Permanente, the largest nonprofit health plan in the United States, has replaced phthalate-containing PVC in intravenous tubing, catheters, and other medical equipment. The hospital has also replaced PVC in flooring, baseboards, and wall guards – even the plastic backing on carpets (Martin, 2010). Microsoft has taken a similar action by completely ending the use of PVC in packaging material.

4.3   ANDROGEN RECEPTOR (AR) ANTAGONISTS

Pollution of surface waters with pesticides that causes endocrine disruption is of great concern. However, relatively few environmentally relevant pesticides have been tested for specific effects on endocrine end points (Orton et al., 2009).

4.3.1   Organochlorine (OC) Pesticides

There is concern that some of the OC pesticides also behave as anti-androgens, and that disruption may be mediated at the level of the AR. There is a possibility that at least some of the "estrogenic" effects observed *in vivo* may, in fact, be due to chemicals having anti-androgenic activity because a number of industrial chemicals, in particular certain pesticides, are anti-androgenic (Gray et al., 1999a). Of the several OC insecticides tested for their ability to interact with the AR *in vitro*, none reacted as agonists (Lemaire et al., 2004). The anti-androgenic activities of these compounds were compared with those of hydroxyflutamide, a known anti-androgen (Table 4.1). These results demonstrated that OCs are also weak anti-androgens, but they are capable of disrupting male hormone signaling and thus may have implications in humans and wildlife exposed to these compounds throughout their development.

TABLE 4.1 *In vitro* **Anti-androgenic Activity of Organochlorine Insecticides**

Organochlorines	Purity (%)	IC_{50} (μM)
Hydroxyflutamide		0.07 ± 0.01
DDT	Mixture	2.51 ± 0.10
o,p'-DDT	98	1.59 ± 0.28
p,p'-DDE		1.86^a
Methoxychlor	98.7	7.60 ± 0.20
Endosulfan	99.9	10.9 ± 1.75
Chlordane	Mixture of isomers	17.88 ± 0.07
Aldrin	98.5	>20
Dieldrin	98.8	7.25 ± 0.45
Endrin	99	>20

[a]Maness et al. (1998).
Adapted from Lemaire et al., 2004. Reproduced with permission of Academic Press

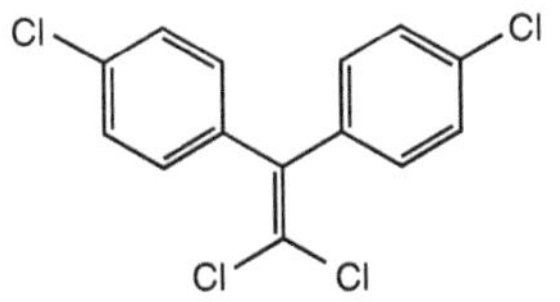

Figure 4.3 *p,p'*-DDE.

4.3.1.1 p,p'-Dichlorodiphenyldichloroethylene (DDE) *p,p'*-DDE, the major metabolite of the insecticide dichlorodiphenyltrichloroethane (DDT), has activity *in vivo* and *in vitro* as an AR antagonist. It prevented gene transcription in mammals by binding to the AR (Kelce et al., 1995). Anti-androgenic *p,p'*-DDE (Fig. 4.3) has been reported to have various effects in experimental animals, including delayed development, retarded sex accessory gland growth, cryptorchidism, and hypospadias (Orton et al., 2009). When *p,p'*-DDE (100 mg/kg daily) was administered to pregnant Long–Evans hooded rats during fetal development on days 14–18 of gestation (the period of sexual differentiation in the rat), their male pups exhibited impaired sexual development, with shortened AGD, retention of nipples, and weight reduction of androgen-dependent tissues (You et al., 1998). Sexual and reproductive abnormalities observed in male rats exposed to DDE have been attributed to endocrine disruption via binding to the AR (Kelce et al., 1995; You et al., 1998). As with rats, administration of *p,p'*-DDT or *p,p'*-DDE to rabbits during gestation resulted in reproductive abnormalities, including cryptorchidism, in the male offspring (Gray et al., 1999a, 1999b).

It has also been suggested that *p,p'*-DDE causes abnormalities in the reproductive development of wildlife. For instance, in Lake Apopka, which is heavily contaminated with *p,p'*-DDE, male alligators exhibited significantly smaller penis, testicular abnormalities, and lower plasma testosterone levels compared to alligators in a control lake, Woodruff (Guillette et al., 1996).

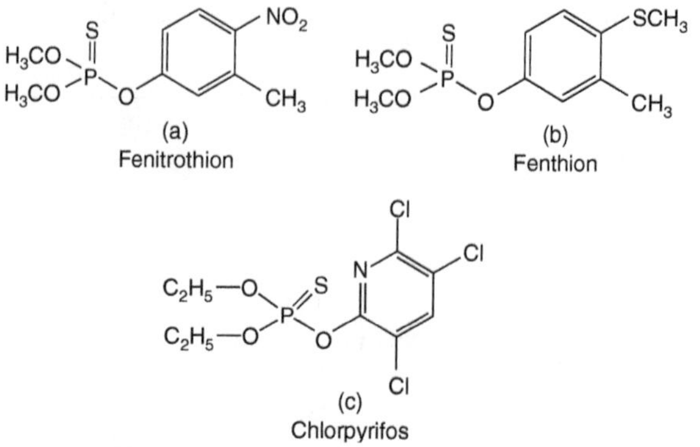

Figure 4.4 Anti-androgenic OP insecticides.

4.3.2 Organophosphorus (OP) Insecticides

Organophosphate insecticides are widely used in agriculture to control pests in the environment, and there is considerable human exposure to this class of compounds. OP insecticides are well-characterized neurotoxins; they inhibit cholinesterase activity and induce cholinergic stress.

4.3.2.1 Fenitrothion Fenitrothion (Fig. 4.4a), a widely used OP insecticide, has structural similarities with the anti-androgenic pharmaceutical flutamide used in prostate cancer treatment. Fenitrothion is reported to block the activity of human androgen receptor (hAR) *in vitro*, and antagonize the AR in a Hershberger assay *in vivo* (Tamura et al., 2001; Kitamura et al., 2003). A male three-spined sticklebacks fish, *Gasterosteus aculeatus*, was measured for kidney spiggin concentration, the glue protein that male sticklebacks use to build their nests and is directly controlled by androgens. Fenitrothion exposure significantly reduced spiggin production as well as nest-building activity, thus appearing to have anti-androgenic effects on both the physiology and behavior of the male stickleback (Sebire et al., 2009). However, in a reproductive study using rats, it was found to have no effect on the reproductive and endocrine systems of F0 and F1 generations (Okahashi et al., 2005).

The metabolic oxidative desulfuration product of fenitrothion, fenitrothion oxon, was found to have no anti-androgenic activity even in *in vitro* assay (Tamura et al., 2003). Nevertheless, a degradation product of fenitrothion, 3-methyl-4-nitrophenol, displayed anti-androgenic activity both *in vitro* recombinant yeast screen and *in vivo* Hershberger assays (Li et al., 2006).

4.3.2.2 Fenthion Structurally similar to fenitrothion, fenthion (Fig. 4.4b) is a widely used OP broad-spectrum insecticide for numerous crops. It tested positive as an antagonist of androgenic activity in the Hershberger assay using castrated male rats where it blocked androgen-dependent tissue growth (Kitamura, et al., 2003).

4.3.2.3 Chlorpyrifos Chlorpyrifos (Fig. 4.4c) has been listed as a potential EDC by the German Federal Environment Agency because of its links to male and female genital deformities. In a screen expressing hAR, chlorpyrifos was found to be anti-androgenic and, in an analysis for its effect on steriodogenesis in rat, it showed a significant decrease in testosterone biosynthesis in Leydig cells (Viswanath et al., 2010). Earlier, methyl chlorpyrifos was reported to show anti-androgenic activity by Hershberger assay (Kang et al., 2004).

4.3.3 Bisphenol A (BPA)

While the mode of action of BPA is believed to be primarily as an estrogen receptor agonist, studies have also shown that BPA can act as an AR antagonist in some cell systems (Xu et al., 2005). Once bound to AR, the AR/BPA complex may prevent endogenous androgens from regulating androgen-dependent transcription. The specificity of AR–ligand interaction may be critical in eliciting adverse effects on the male reproductive system.

Several studies using *in vitro* yeast-based assays revealed that BPA exhibits strong anti-androgenic activity (Sohoni and Sumpter, 1998; Lee et al., 2003). Using ligand competition assays, it was demonstrated that BPA could compete with DHT for binding the AR with an IC_{50} (the concentration of chemical required to reduce the specific DHT binding by 50%) value of 2.14 µM (Lee et al., 2003; Sun et al., 2006).

A study by Xu et al. has confirmed that BPA can act as an anti-androgen in a mammalian system (Xu et al., 2005). In their study, they used an hAR reporter gene assay using African monkey kidney cell line CV-1 transiently transfected with the reporter gene plasmid pMMTV-CAT. BPA showed significant inhibitory effects on the transcriptional activity induced by DHT with an IC_{50} value of ~0.8 µM, the highest anti-androgenic activity of any EDCs tested (Xu et al., 2005).

4.3.4 Polybrominated Diphenyl Ethers (PBDEs)

PBDEs are flame retardants that have been widely used in products such as foam padding, textiles, or plastics. Since PBDEs are not chemically bound to the flame-retarding material, they can enter the environment through volatilization, leaching, or degradation of PBDE-containing products (Gill et al., 2004).

Several PBDEs have been found to disrupt the endocrine system. Pregnant rats exposed to a single dose of 60 or 300 µg BDE-99 (2,2′,4.4′,5-penta BDE) per kilogram body weight on gestation day 6 resulted in decreased spermatogenesis in male offspring (Kuriyama et al., 2005). *In vitro*, DE-71 and DE-100 (2,2′,4,4′,6-penta BDE) act as a competitive inhibitors of AR binding and inhibit androgen-induced gene expression (Stoker et al., 2005). PBDE mixture DE-71 contains the predominant congeners BDE-47, -99, -100, -153, and -154. The DE-71 components BDE-47 (a tetra-BDE) and BDE-100 (but not BDE-99, -153, and -154) have shown antagonism for the AR *in vitro* (Stoker et al., 2005). Exposure of male Wistar rats to DE-71 at 60 or 120 mg/kg/day for 30 days (PND 23-53) during the peri-pubertal period caused a delay in the onset of puberty, together with decreased seminal vesicles and ventral prostate weights, indicating an anti-androgenic mechanism of action of one or more components of the mixture. In the Hershberger assay (using castrated testosterone propionate-treated rats), DE-71 caused a typical anti-androgenic profile including reduced sex accessory tissue growth and delayed puberty in male rats at all doses tested (30–240 mg/kg/day for 9 days) (Stoker et al., 2005).

4.3.5 Vinclozolin (VZ)

VZ, a nonsystemic dicarboximide fungicide, is extensively used in fruit crops, such as grapes for the wine industry. Since washing of produce is inefficient to remove the compound, humans are constantly exposed to VZ. Although it has poor affinity for the mammalian AR, VZ exhibits anti-androgenic activity after metabolism into higher affinity compounds (Kelce et al., 1994). It is rapidly metabolized in mammals into two main metabolites: 2-[[(3,5-dichlorophenyl)-carbamoyl] oxy]-2-methyl-3-butenoic acid (M1) and 3′,5′-dichloro-2-hydroxy-2-methylbut-3-enanilide (M2) (Fig. 4.5), which act as potent *in vitro* and *in vivo* AR antagonists. The antagonistic effects were in the order: M2 > VZ ≫ M1. The molecular mechanism proposed for their anti-androgenic effects is by competing with androgens (testostetrone and DHT) for binding to the AR and preventing AR binding to androgen response elements in DNA and inhibiting AR-dependent gene expression (Gray et al., 1999b; Wolf et al., 1999, 2000). The EDs affect the prostate gland through anti-androgenic pathways. Delayed puberty and reduced sperm numbers have been found in male rats exposed to VZ.

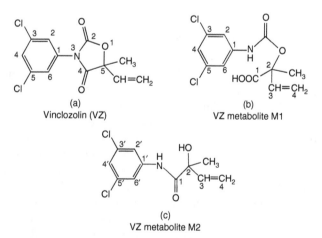

(a)
Vinclozolin (VZ)

(b)
VZ metabolite M1

(c)
VZ metabolite M2

Figure 4.5 Fungicide vinclozolin and metabolites M1 and M2.

VZ and M2 can also antagonize the activity of progesterone receptor (PR), and mineralocorticoid receptor (MR), while M2 is also a glucocorticoid receptor (GR) antagonist, *in vitro*. Furthermore, VZ and its metabolites are agonists for ERs, especially metabolite M2 via ERα (Molina-Molina et al., 2006).

Studies *in vivo* revealed that VZ-treated male offspring rats displayed demasculinizing effects including female-like reduced AGD at birth, retained nipples, undescended testes, and small sex accessory glands (Gray et al., 1994). Adult male rats were found to have reduced seminal vesicle and ventral prostate weights and lower sperm counts after embryonic or perinatal exposure to VZ (Gray et al., 1999b; Wolf et al., 1999; Hellwig et al., 2000; Uzumcu et al., 2004).

When pregnant rats were exposed to VZ at the time of mid-gestation, this transient exposure caused an adult phenotype in male mice characterized by decreased fertility, low sperm count, and sperm motility, as well as increased apoptosis in spermatogenic cells. Each generation of subsequently bred animals (up to four generations were tested) had the same disease state (Anway et al., 2006). The frequency and reproducibility of the VZ-induced transgenerational pathologies, and the finding that most of them occur in adulthood, indicate that genetic DNA-sequence mutations are not the most likely cause. The frequency of a DNA-sequence mutation, even with ionizing radiation, is normally less than 0.01%, and ranges from only 1% to 5% for hot-spot mutations. The most parsimonious explanation for these findings is that these transgenerational phenotypes result from the epigenetic reprogramming of the male germ line at the stage of gonadal sex determination (Jirtle and Skinner, 2007).

A pesticide formulation called *Switch*, which contains cyprodinil and fludioxonil, was recommended as a replacement for the VZ formulation *Ronilan* (Shah et al. 2002). However, a recent study found that both the fungicidal chemicals in this formulation were also anti-androgenic (Orton et al., 2011).

4.3.6 Procymidone

Structurally similar to the synthetic nonsteroidal anti-androgen flutamide (Fig. 4.6b) and related to the dicarboximide VZ, procymidone (Fig. 4.6a) is widely used as a fungicide. It acts solely through binding to the AR as antagonist, thus blocking the action of androgen at the cellular level, but does not affect

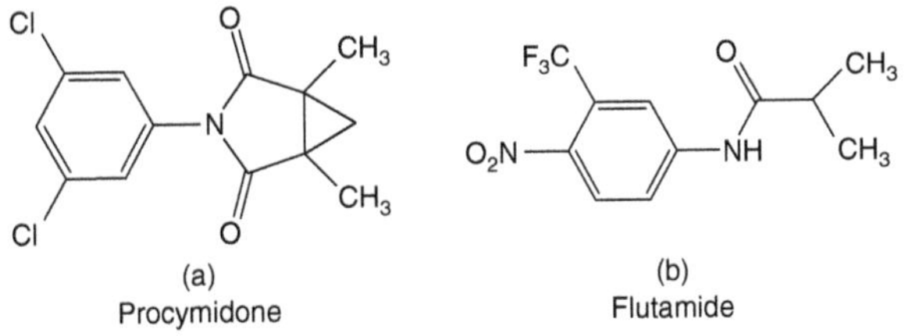

(a)
Procymidone

(b)
Flutamide

Figure 4.6 Anti-androgenic procymidone and flutamide.

fetal testosterone synthesis. It displayed effects identical to those of VZ, in rats and mice, both *in vivo* and *in vitro* (Rider et al., 2009). When procymidone was administered from day 14 of pregnancy to day 3 after birth at 0, 25, 50, 100, or 200 mg/kg/day, AGD was shortened in male pups, and the males displayed retained nipples, hypospadias, cleft phallus, a vaginal pouch, and reduced sex accessory gland size (Ostby et al., 1999). The AR-binding activity (IC_{50}) of procymidone was determined to be 80.9 ± 1.6 µM to inhibit testosterone binding to AR by 50% (Okubo et al., 2004).

4.4 AR ANTAGONISTS AND FETAL TESTOSTERONE SYNTHESIS INHIBITORS

4.4.1 Prochloraz

Prochloraz (Fig. 4.7a), an imidazole fungicide, disrupts androgen activity by dual mechanisms of action, namely, by antagonizing the AR and by inhibiting the conversion of progesterone to testosterone formed in testis by Leydig cells (Christiansen et al., 2009). *In vivo*, prochloraz acted as an anti-androgen in the Hershberger assay by reducing weights of reproductive organs, affecting androgen-regulated gene expressions in the prostate, and increasing luteinizing hormone levels. Pregnant Wistar dams dosed perinatally with 30 mg/kg prochloraz significantly reduced plasma and testicular testosterone levels in gestational day 21 male fetuses, whereas testicular progesterone was increased, indicating inhibition of testosterone production. It led to malformations in male offspring, closely resembling those seen with VZ, in the production of hypospadias (NRC, 2008; Blystone et al., 2007). In male pups, a significant increase in nipple retention was found. Abnormalities such as vaginal morphology in males, initially classified as feminization of the male offspring after perinatal exposure and later more accurately described as extreme cases of de-masculinization towards a default female morphology, are due in part to diminished fetal steroidogenesis (Vinggaard et al., 2006; Noriega et al., 2005).

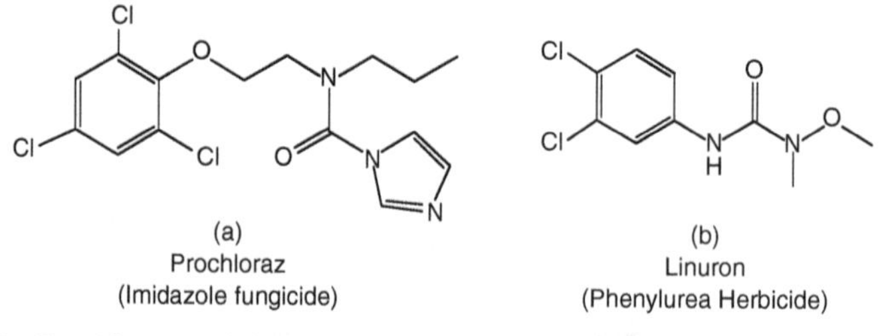

(a)
Prochloraz
(Imidazole fungicide)

(b)
Linuron
(Phenylurea Herbicide)

Figure 4.7 Prochloraz and linuron disrupt androgen action by two mechanisms as AR antagonists and inhibitors of fetal testosterone synthesis.

4.4.2 Linuron

Linuron (3-(3,4-dichlorophenyl)-1-methoxy-1-methylurea), a phenylurea herbicide (Fig. 4.7b), applied to suppress broadleaf and grassy weeds, is a weak competitive AR antagonist *in vitro* and is demonstrated to exhibit anti-androgenic effect on reproductive parameters *in vivo* in mice (Lambright et al., 2000). Prenatal exposure to linuron (75 mg/kg/day) during gestational days 14–18 in rats reduced fetal testosterone production and resulted in epididymis predominantly, a phenotype similar to that noted after fetal testicular testosterone inhibition of phthalates (Hotchkiss et al., 2004). These findings suggest that linuron disrupts the development of androgen-dependent tissues primarily by acting as an AR antagonist and by inhibiting testosterone synthesis by the fetal testis. Additionally, linuron was found to be a potent anti-estrogenic than anti-androgenic in the yeast estrogen screen (YES) test and inhibited ovulation in *Xenopus* oocyte, while building up progesterone levels (Orton et al, 2009).

4.5 COMPARATIVE ANTI-ANDROGENIC EFFECTS OF PESTICIDES TO ANDROGEN AGONIST DHT

Three pesticides, the OP insecticide fenitrothion, the thiourea herbicide linuron, and the fungicide VZ, were tested for anti-androgenic activity *in vivo* and *in vitro* assays in the three-spined stickleback (*G. aculeatus*) using the magnitude of inhibition of DHT-induced spiggin (an androgen-induced protein) production as an endpoint. In *in vitro* assay, employing cultures of primed female stickleback kidney cells exposed to a range of concentrations of the test compounds together with DHT at 10^{-8} M, fenitrothion, and flutamide significantly inhibited DHT-induced spiggin production at 10^{-12} M, while linuron and VZ induced a significant decrease at 10^{-10} M, respectively. Thus, the *in vitro* anti-androgenic potency of the compounds followed the order: fenitrothion ≥ flutamide ≥ linuron > VZ. In an *in vivo* study carried out in parallel, female sticklebacks were exposed to a range of concentrations of the same chemicals with DHT (5 µg/L) for 21 days. Here again, fenitrothion and flutamide were found to be the most potent compounds significantly reducing DHT-induced spiggin production at 10 and 25 µg/L, respectively; both linuron and VZ decreased spiggin production at 100 µg/L. The order of anti-androgenic potency in *in vivo* testing was: fenitrothion > ftuamide ≥ VZ > linuron (Jolly et al., 2009). Earlier, in human cell line transfected with the human AR and in the Hershberger assay, the potency of fenitrothion as a competitive AR antagonist was found comparable to that of flutamide (Tamura et al., 2001).

4.6 CONCLUSIONS AND FUTURE PROSPECTS

Environmental chemicals with a potential to alter the androgen signaling pathway *in utero* with distinct modes of action have been identified. These include chemicals that interfere with the biosynthesis, metabolism, or action of endogenous andro-gens resulting in a deflection from normal male developmental programming and reproductive tract growth and function. Since male sexual differentiation is entirely androgen-dependent, it is highly susceptible to androgen disruptors. Androgen disruption also occurs when a ligand binds the AR ligand-binding domain without inducing activation. In this case, the ligand serves as a functional antagonist and competes for receptor binding sites with endogenous androgens. Consequently, normal transcription induced by the endogenous ligand is lessened or ablated by the competing disruptor as a result of reduced receptor availability. Several classes of chemicals have been shown in laboratory studies to disrupt reproductive development by acting as AR antagonists and/or inhibitors of fetal Leydig cell testosterone production. Dysfunction of fetal Leydig cells induced by EDCs may cause incomplete masculinization and development of various malformations in the male reproductive tract of humans and animals. Animal models and epidemiological evidence link exposure to androgen disrupting chemicals with reduced sperm counts, increased infertility, testicular dysgenesis syndrome, and testicular and prostate cancers. Their widespread use and ubiquitous presence in the environment has raised concern about possible adverse effects in humans and wildlife. Some studies have pointed such effects in population level studies.

The presence of androgens in the environment has also come into light. For example, effluents from pulp and paper mills display androgenic activity of sufficient potency to masculinize and/or sex-reverse female fish. Effluent from beef-cattle-concentrated animal feedlot operations from the United States also displays androgenic activity *in vitro*, due, in part, to the presence of a steroid used to promote growth in beef cattle.

REFERENCES

Anway M. D.; Memon M. A.; Uzumcu M.; Skinner M.K. Transgenerational effect of the endocrine disruptor vinclozolin on male spermatogenesis, *J. Androl.* **2006**, 27, 868–879.

Barrett, J. R. NTP draft brief on DEHP, *Environ. Health Perspect.* **2006**, 114(10), A580–A581.

Barrett, J. R. Phthalates and baby boys: potential disruption of human genital development, *Environ. Health Perspect.* **2005**, 113(8), A542.

Benson, R. Hazard to the developing male reproductive system from cumulative exposure to phthalate esters–dibutyl phthalate, diisobutyl phthalate, butylbenzyl phthalate, diethylhexyl phthalate, dipentyl phthalate, and diisononyl phthalate, *Regul. Toxicol. Pharmacol.* **2009**, 53(2), 90–101.

Bizzari, S.; Oppenberg, B.; Iskikawa, Y. Plasticizers, *Chemical Economics Handbook*, Palo Alto, CA: SRI International, **2000**.

Blystone, C. R.; Lambright, C. S.; Howdeshell, K. L.; Furr, J.; Sternberg, R. M.; Butterworth, B.C.; Durhan, E. J.; Makynen, E. A.; Ankley, G. T.; Wilson, V. S.; Leblanc, G. A.; Gray, L. E., Jr., Sensitivity of fetal rat testicular steroidogenesis to maternal prochloraz exposure and the underlying mechanism of inhibition, *Toxicol. Sci.* **2007**, 97(2), 512–519.

Christiansen, S.; Scholze, M.; Dalgaard, M.; Vinggaard, A. M.; Axelstad, M.; Kortenkamp, A.; Hass, U. Synergistic disruption of external male sex organ development by a mixture of four antiandrogens, *Environ. Health Perspect.* **2009**, 117(12), 1839–1846.

David, R. M. Proposed mode of action for in utero effects of some phthalate esters on the developing male reproductive tract, *Toxicol. Pathol.* **2006**, 34, 209–219.

Dean, A.; Smith, L. B.; Macpherson, S.; Sharpe, R. M. The effect of dihydrotestosterone exposure during or prior to the masculinization programming window on reproductive development in male and female rats, *Int. J. Androl.* **2012**, 35, 330–339.

Eisenberg, M. L.; Hsieh, M. H.; Walters, R. C.; Krasnow, R.; Lipshultz, L. I. The relationship between anogenital distance, fatherhood, and fertility in adult men, *PLos ONE* **2011**, 6(5), e18973.

Engel, S. M.; Miodovnik, A.; Canfield, R. L.; Zhu, C.; Silva, M. J.; Calafat, A. M.; Wolff, M. S. Prenatal phthalate exposure is associated with childhood behavior and executive functioning, *Environ. Health Perspect.* **2010**, 118(4), 565–571.

EPA, *Toxicological Review of Dibutyl Phthalate (CAS No. 84-74-2)*, Washington, DC, US Environmental Protection Agency, June **2006**.

EPA, *Phthalates Action Plan Summary*, Washington, DC, US Environmental Protection Agency, **2010**. Available at: http://www.epa.gov/oppt/existingchemicals/pubs/actionplans/phthalates.html (accessed 18 Jan 2014).

Feig, J. N.; Gelman, L.; Rossi, D.; Zoete, V.; Metivier, R.; Tudor, C.; Anghel, S. I.; Grosdidier, A.; Lathion, C.; Engelborghs, Y.; Michielin, O.; Wahli, W.; Desvergne, B. The endocrine disruptor monoethyl-hexyl-phthalate is a selective peroxisome proliferator-activated receptor modulator that promotes adipogenesis, *J. Biol. Chem.* **2007**, 282(26), 19152–19166.

Fisher, J. S.; Macpherson, S.; Marchetti, N.; Sharpe, R. M. Human "testicular dysgenesis syndrome": a possible model using in-utero exposure of the rat to dibutyl phthalate, *Hum. Reprod.* **2003**, 18, 1383–1394.

Foster, P. M. Disruption of reproductive development in male rat offspring following in utero exposure to phthalate esters, *Int. J. Androl.* **2006**, 29(1), 140–147.

Foster, P. M. Mode of action: impaired fetal Leydig cell function-effects on male reproductive development produced by certain phthalate esters, *Crit. Rev. Toxicol.* **2005**, 35(8–9), 713–719.

Gill, U.; Chu, I.; Ryan, J. J.; Feeley, M. Polybrominated diphenyl ethers: human tissue levels and toxicology, *Rev. Environ. Contam. Toxicol.* **2004**, 183, 55–97.

Frederiksen, H.; Skakkebaek, N. E.; Andersson, A. M. Metabolism of phthalates in humans, *Mol. Nutr. Food Res.* **2007**, 51(7), 899–911.

Gray, L. E.; Wilson, V. S.; Stoker, T.; Lambright, C.; Furr, J.; Noriega, N.; Howdeshell, K.; Ankley, G. T.; Guillette, L. Adverse effects of environmental antiandrogens and androgens on reproductive development in mammals, *Int. J. Androl.* **2006**, 29, 96–104.

Gray, L. E.; Ostby, J.; Furr, J.; Price, M.; Veeramachaneni, D. N.; Parks, L. Perinatal exposure to the phthalates DEHP, BBP, and DINP, but not DEP, DMP, or DOTP, alters sexual differentiation of the male Rat, *Toxicol. Sci.* **2000**, 58, 350–365.

Gray, L. E., Jr.; Ostby, J.; Cooper, R. L.; Kelce, W. R. The estrogenic and antiandrogenic pesticides methoxychlor alters the reproductive tract and behavior without affecting pituitary size or LH and prolactin secretion in male rats, *Toxicol. Ind. Health* **1999a**, 15, 37–47.

Gray, L.; Ostby, J.; Monosson, E.; Kelce, W. R. Environmental antiandrogens: low doses of the fungicide vinclozolin alter sexual differentiation of the male rat, *Toxicol. Ind. Health* **1999b**, 15(1–2), 48–64.

Gray, L. E., Jr., Ostby, J. S., and Kelce, W. R. Developmental effects of an environmental antiandrogen: the fungicide vinclozolin alters sex differentiation of the male rat, *Toxicol. Appl. Pharmacol.* **1994**, 129, 46–52.

Guillette, L. J., Jr.; Pickford, D. B.; Crain, D. A.; Rooney, A. A.; Percival, H. F. Reduction in penis size and plasma testosterone concentrations in juvenile alligators living in a contaminated environment, *Gen. Comp. Endocrinol.* **1996**, 102, 32–42.

Hellwig, J.; van Ravenzwaay, B.; Mayer, M.; Gembardt, C. Pre- and postnatal oral toxicity of vinclozolin in Wistar and Long-Evans rats, *Regul. Toxicol. Pharmacol.* **2000**, 32, 42–50.

Hogue, C. Targeted for regulation–Toxic Substances: EPA names four categories of chemicals for action, including restrictions and bans, *C&E News* **2010**, 88(2), 9.

Hosokawa, S.; Murakami, M.; Ineyama, M.; Yamada, T.; Yoshitake, A.; Yamada, H.; Miyamoto, J. The affinity of procymidone to androgen receptor in rats and mice, *J. Toxicol. Sci.* **1993**, 18, 83–93.

Hotchkiss, A. K., Parks-Saldutti, L. G.; Ostby, J. S.; Lambright, C.; Furr, J.; Vandenbergh, J. G.; Gray, L. E., Jr., A mixture of the "antiandrogens" linuron and butyl benzyl phthalate alters sexual differentiation of the male rat in a cumulative fashion, *Biol. Reprod.* **2004**, 71(6), 1852–1861.

Howdeshell, K. L.; Wilson, V. S.; Furr, J.; Lambright, C. R.; Rider, C. V.; Blystone, C. R. et al. A mixture of five phthalate esters inhibits fetal testicular testosterone production in the Sprague-Dawley rat in a cumulative, dose-additive manner, *Toxicol. Sci.* **2008**, 105, 153–165.

Howdeshell, K. L.; Furr, J.; Lambright, C. R.; Rider, C. V.; Wilson, V. S.; Gray, L. E., Jr., Cumulative effects of dibutyl phthalate and diethylhexyl phthalate on male rat reproductive tract development: altered fetal steroid hormones and genes, *Toxicol. Sci.* **2007**, 99(1), 190–202.

Jirtle, R. L.; Skinner, M. K. Environmental epigenomics and disease susceptibility, *Nat. Rev. Genet.* **2007**, 8, 253–262.

Jolly, C.; Katsiadaki, I.; Morris, S.; Le Belle, N.; Dufour, S.; Mayer, I.; Pottinger, T. G.; Scott, A. P. Detection of the anti-androgenic effect of endocrine disrupting environmental contaminants using *in vivo* and *in vitro* assays in the three-spined stickleback, *Aquat. Toxicol.* **2009**, 92(4), 228–239.

Kang, H. G.; Jeong, S. H.; Cho, J. H.; Kim, D. G.; Park, J. M.; Cho, M. H. Chlorpyrifos-methyl shows anti-androgenic activity without estrogenic activity in rats, *Toxicology* **2004**, 199, 219–230.

Kelce, W. R.; Wilson, E. M. Environmental antiandrogens: Developmental effects, molecular mechanisms, and clinical implications, *J. Mol. Med.* **1997**, 75, 198–207.

Kelce, W. R.; Stone, C. R.; Laws, S. C.; Gray, L. E.; Kemppainen, J. A.; Wilson, E. M. Persistent DDT metabolite p,p′-DDE is a potent androgen receptor antagonist, *Nature* **1995**, 375(6532), 581–585.

Kelce, W. R.; Monosson, E.; Gamcsik, M. P.; Laws, S. C.; Gray, L. E., Jr., Environmental hormone disruptors: evidence that vinclozolin developmental toxicity is mediated by antiandrogenic metabolites, *Toxicol. Appl. Pharmacol.* **1994**, 126, 276–285.

Kitamura, S.; Suzuki, T.; Ohta, S.; Fujimoto, N. Antiandrogenic activity and metabolism of the organophosphorus pesticide fenthion and related compounds, *Environ. Health Perspect.* **2003**, 111, 503–508.

Kolpin, D. W.; Furlong, E. T.; Meyer, M. T.; Thurman, E. M.; Zaugg, S. D.; Barber, L. B.; Buxton, H. T. Pharmaceuticals, hormones, and other organic wastewater contaminants in U.S. streams, 1999-2000: a national reconnaissance, *Environ. Sci. Technol.* **2002**, 36(6), 1202–1211.

Kuriyama, S. N.; Talsness, C. E.; Grote, K.; Chahoud, I. Developmental exposure to low dose PBDE 99: effects on male fertility and neurobehavior in rat offspring, *Environ. Health Perspect.* **2005**, 113(2), 149–154.

Lambright, C.; Ostby, J.; Bobseine, K. et al. Cellular and molecular mechanisms of action of linuron: An antiandrogenic herbicide that produces reproductive malformations in male rats, *Toxicol. Sci.* **2000**, 56, 389–399.

Lee, H. J.; Chattopadhyay, S.; Gong, E. Y.; Ahn, R. S.; Lee, K. Antiandrogenic effects of bisphenol A and nonylphenol on the function of androgen receptor, *Toxicol. Sci.* **2003**, 75(1), 40–46.

Lemaire, G.; Terouanne, B.; Mauvais, P.; Michel, S.; Rahmani, R. Effect of organochlorine pesticides on human androgen receptor activation in vitro, *Toxicol. Appl. Pharmacol.* **2004**, 196(2), 235–246.

Li, C.; Taneda, S.; Suzuki, A. K.; Furuta, C.; Watanabe, G.; Taya, K. Anti-androgenic activity of 3-methyl-4-nitrophenol in diesel exhaust particles, *Eur. J. Pharmacol.* **2006**, 543(1–3), 194–199.

Lovekamp-Swan, T.; Davis, B. J. Mechanisms of phthalate ester toxicity in the female reproductive system, *Environ. Health Perspect.* **2003**, 111, 139–45.

Lyche, J. L.; Gutleb, A. C.; Bergman, Å.; Eriksen, G. S.; Murk, A. T. J.; Ropstad, E.; Saunders, M.; Skaare, J. U. Reproductive and developmental toxicity of phthalates, *J. Toxicol. Environ. Health, B., Crit. Rev.* **2009**, 12(4), 225–249.

Maness, S. C.; McDonnell, D. P.; Gaido, K. W. Inhibition of androgen receptor-dependent transcriptional activity by DDT isomers and methoxychlor in HepG2 human hepatoma cells, *Toxicol. Appl. Pharmacol.* **1998**, 151(1), 135–142.

Martin, D. S. Companies, hospitals move away from toxic material, CNN Health, May, 26, 2010. Available at: http://articles.cnn.com/2010-05-26/health/abandoning.pvc_1_pvc-dioxin-polyvinyl-chloride/2?_s=PM:HEALTH (accessed 14 Jan 2014).

Matsumoto, J.; Yokota, H.; Yuasa, A. Developmental increases in rat hepatic microsomal UDP-glucuronosyl-transferase activities toward xenoestrogens and decreases during pregnancy, *Environ. Health Perspect.* **2002**, 110, 193–196.

Meeker, J. D.; Ferguson, K. K. Relationship between urinary phthalate and bisphenol A concentrations and serum thyroid measures in U.S. adults and adolescents from the National Health and Nutrition Examination Survey (NHANES) 2007–2008, *Environ. Health Perspect.* **2011**, 119, 1396–1402.

Mendiola, J.; Stahlhut, R. W.; Jørgensen, N.; Liu, F.; Swan, S. H. Shorter Anogenital distance predicts poorer semen quality in young men in Rochester, New York, *Environ. Health Perspect.* **2011**, 119(7), 958–963.

Molina-Molina, J. M.; Hillenweck, A.; Jouanin, I.; Zalko, D.; Cravedi, J. P.; Fernandez, M. F.; Pillon, A.; Nicolas, J. C.; Olea, N.; Balaguer, P. Steroid receptor profiling of vinclozolin and its primary metabolites, *Toxicol. Appl. Pharmacol.* **2006**, 216, 44–54.

Mylchreest, E.; Wallace, D. G.; Cattley, R. C.; Foster, P. M. Dose-dependent alterations in androgen-regulated male reproductive development in rats exposed to di(n-butyl) phthalate during late gestation. *Toxicol. Sci.* **2000**, 55, 143–151.

Noriega, N. C. Evolutionary perspectives on sex steroids in the vertebrates, in *Sex Steroids*, Kahn, S. M., ed., InTech, **2012**, pp. 1–33. Available at: http://www.intechopen.com/ books/sex-steroids/evolutionary-perspectives-on-sex-steroids-in-the-vertbrates (accessed 18 Jan 2014).

Noriega, N. C.; Ostby, J.; Lambright, C.; Wilson, V. S.; Gray, L. E., Jr., Late gestational exposure to the fungicide prochloraz delays the onset of parturition and causes reproductive malformations in male but not female rat offspring, *Biol. Reprod.* **2005**, 72(6), 1324–1335.

NRC, *Phthalates Cumulative Risk Assessment – The Tasks Ahead*. Committee on Phthalates Health Risks, National Research Council, National Academy of Sciences, Board on Environmental Science and Technology, National Academy Press, Washington, DC, 2008.

NTP-CERHR *Monograph on the Potential Human Reproductive and Developmental Effects of Di(2-Ethylhexyl) Phthalate (DEHP)*, National Toxicology Program (NTP) -NIH Publication No. 06-4476, November **2006**.

Okahashi, N.; Sano, M.; Miyata, K.; Tamano, S.; Higuchi, H.; Kamita, Y. et al. **2005**. Lack of evidence for endocrine disrupting effects in rats exposed to fenitrothion *in utero* and from weaning to maturation, *Toxicology* **2005**, 206(1), 17–31.

Okubo, T.; Yokoyama, Y.; Kano, K.; Soya, Y.; Kano, I. Estimation of estrogenic and antiestrogenic activities of selected pesticides by MCF-7 cell proliferation assay, *Arch. Environ. Contam. Toxicol.* **2004**, 46(4), 445–453.

Orton, F.; Rosivatz, E.; Scholze, M.; Kortenkamp, A. Widely used pesticides with previously unknown endocrine activity revealed as *in vitro* antiandrogens, *Environ. Health Perspect.* **2011**, 119, 794–800.

Orton, F.; Lutz, I.; Kloas, W.; Routledge, E. J. Endocrine disrupting effects of herbicides and pentachlorophenol: *in vitro* and *in vivo* evidence, *Environ. Sci. Technol.* **2009**, 43(9), 2144–2150.

Ostby, J.; Kelce, W. R.; Lambright, C.; Wolf, C. J.; Mann, P.; Gray, L. E. The fungicide procymidone alters sexual differentiation in the male rat by acting as an androgen-receptor antagonist *in vivo* and *in vitro*, *Toxicol. Ind. Health* **1999**, 15, 80–93.

Parks, L. G.; Ostby, J. S.; Lambright, C. R.; Abbott, B. D.; Klinefelter, G. R.; Barlow, N. J.; Gray, L. E., Jr., The plasticizer diethylhexyl phthalate induces malformations by decreasing fetal testosterone synthesis during sexual differentiation in the male rat, *Toxicol. Sci.* **2000**, 58(2), 339–349.

Rider, C. V.; Wilson, V. S.; Howdeshell, K. L.; Hotchkiss, A. K.; Furr, J. R.; Lambright, C. R.; Gray, L. E., Jr., Cumulative effects of *In utero* administration of mixtures of "antiandrogens" on male rat reproductive development, *Toxicol. Pathol.* **2009**, 37(1), 100–113.

Ruegg, J.; Penttinen-Damdimopoulou, P.; Makela, S.; Pongratz, I.; Gustafsson, J. A. Receptors mediating toxicity and their involvement in endocrine disruption, in *Molecular, Clinical and Environmental Toxicology, Vol. 1: Molecular toxicology*, Lurch, A., ed., Switzerland: Birkhauser Verlag, **2009**, pp. 289–323.

Sebire, M.; Scott, A. P.; Tyler, C. R.; Cresswell, J.; Hodgson, D. J.; Morris, S.; Sanders, M. B.; Stebbing, P. D.; Katsiadaki, I. The organophosphorus pesticide, fenitrothion, acts as an anti-androgen and alters reproductive behavior of the male three-spined stickleback, *Gasterosteus aculeatus*, *Ecotoxicology* **2009**, 18(1), 122–133.

Shah, D. A.; Dillard, H. R.; Cobb, A. C. Alternatives to vinclozolin (Ronilan) for controlling gray and white mold on snap bean pods in New York, *Plant Health Prog.* **2002**. Available at: http://www.plantmanagementnetwork.org/pub/php/research/snapbean/ (accessed 18 Jan 2014).

Skakkebaek, N. E.; Rajpert-De Meyts, E.; Main, K. M. Testicular dysgenesis syndrome: an increasingly common developmental disorder with environmental aspects, *Hum. Reprod.* **2001**, 16, 972–978.

Sohoni, P.; Sumpter, J. P. Several environmental oestrogens are also anti-androgens, *J. Endocrinol.* **1998**, 158(3), 327–339.

Stoker, T. E.; Cooper, R. L.; Lambright, C.S.; Wilson, V. S.; Furr, J.; Gray, L. E. In vivo and in vitro anti-androgenic effects of DE-71, a commercial polybrominated diphenyl ether (PBDE) mixture, *Toxicol. Appl. Pharmacol.* **2005**, 207, 78–88.

Sun, H.; Xu, L. C.; Chen, J. F.; Song, L.; Wang, X. R. Effect of bisphenol A, tetrachlorobisphenol A and pentachlorophenol on the transcriptional activities of androgen receptor-mediated reporter gene, *Food Chem. Toxicol.* **2006**, 44(11), 1916–1921.

Swan, S. H.; Main, K. M.; Liu, F.; Stewart, S. L.; Kruse, R. L.; Calafat, A. M.; Mao, C. S.; Redmon, J. B.; Ternand, C. L.; Sullivan, S.; Teague, J. J. Decrease in anogenital distance among male infants with prenatal phthalate exposure, *Environ. Health Perspect.* **2005**, 113(8), 1056–1061.

Tamura, H.; Yoshikawa, H.; Gaido, K. W.; Ross, S. M.; DeLisle, R. K.; Welsh, W. J.; Richard, A. M. Interaction of organophosphate pesticides and related compounds with androgen receptor, *Environ. Health Perspect.* **2003**, 111(4), 545–552.

Tamura, H.; Maness, S. C.; Reischmann, K.; Dorman, D. C.; Gray, L. E.; Gaido, K. W. Androgen receptor antagonism by the organophosphate insecticide fenitrothion, *Toxicol. Sci.* **2001**, 60, 52–56.

Toppari, J.; Virtanen, H. E.; Skakkebaek, N. E. Environmental contaminants and reproductive and fertility effects in the male, in *Environmental Impacts on Reproductive Health and Fertility*, Woodruff, T. J.; Janssen, S. J.; Guillette, L. J., Jr.; Giudice, L. C., eds.; Cambridge, UK: Cambridge University Press, **2010**, pp.147–153.

Uzumcu M.; Suzuki H.; Skinner M. K. Effect of the anti-androgenic endocrine disruptor vinclozolin on embryonic testis cord formation and postnatal testis development and function, *Reprod. Toxicol.* **2004**, 18, 765–774.

van den Driesche, S.; Kolovos, P.; Platts, S.; Drake, A. J.; Sharpe, R. M. Inter-relationship between testicular dysgenesis and Leydig cell function in the masculinization programming window in the rat, *PLoS One.* **2012**, 7, 11; doi: 10.1371/journal.pone.0030111.

Vinggaard, A. M.; Hass, U.; Dalgaard, M.; Andersen, H. R.; Bonefeld-Jorgensen, E.; Christiansen, S.; Laier, P.; Poulsen, M. E. Prochloraz: an imidazole fungicide with multiple mechanisms of action, *Int. J. Androl.* **2006**, 29(1), 186–192.

Vinggaard, A. M.; Nellemann, C.; Dalgaard, M.; Jorgensen, E. B.; Andersen, H. R. Antiandrogenic effects in vitro and in vivo of the fungicide prochloraz, *Toxicol. Sci.* **2002**, 69, 344–353.

Viswanath, G.; Chatterjee, S.; Dabral, S.; Nanguneri, S. R.; Divya, G.; Roy, P. Anti-androgenic endocrine disrupting activities of chlorpyrifos and piperophos, *J. Steroid Biochem. Mol. Biol.* **2010**, 120(1), 22–29.

Wohlfahrt-Veje, C.; Main, K. M.; Skakkebaek, N. E. Testicular dysgenesis syndrome: foetal origin of adult reproductive problems, *Clin. Endocrinol.* (Oxf) **2009**, 71, 459–465.

Wolf, C., Jr.; Lambright, C.; Mann, P.; Price, M.; Cooper, R. L.; Ostby, J.; Gray, L. E., Jr., Administration of potentially antiandrogenic pesticides (procymidone, linuron, iprodione, chlozolinate, p,p'-DDE, and ketoconazole) and toxic substances (dibutyl- and diethylhexyl phthalate, PCB 169, and ethane dimethane sulphonate) during sexual differentiation produces diverse profiles of reproductive malformations in the male rat, *Toxicol. Ind. Health* **1999**, 15(1–2), 94–118.

Wolf, C. J.; LeBlanc, G. A.; Ostby, J. S.; Gray, L. E., Jr., Characterization of the period of sensitivity of fetal male sexual development to vinclozolin. *Toxicol. Sci.* **2000**, 55, 152–161.

Xu, L. C.; Sun, H.; Chen, J. F.; Bian, Q.; Qian, J.; Song, L., et al. Evaluation of androgen receptor transcriptional activities of bisphenol A, octylphenol and nonylphenol in vitro, *Toxicology* **2005**, 216(2/3), 197–203.

You, L.; Casanova, M.; Archibeque-Engle, S.; Sar, M.; Fan, L. Q.; Heck, H. A. Impaired male sexual development in perinatal Sprague-Dawley and Long-Evans hooded rats exposed in utero and lactationally to p,p'-DDE, *Toxicol. Sci.* **1998**, 45, 162–173.

5

THYROID-DISRUPTING CHEMICALS

5.1 INTRODUCTION

Thyroid-disrupting chemicals (TDCs) are broadly defined as xenobiotics that interfere with thyroid hormone (TH) signaling. The neurological development of mammals is largely dependent on normal TH homeostasis, and it is likely to be particularly sensitive to the disruption of the thyroid axis. For THs, homeostasis is defined as the normal range of THs and thyroid-stimulating hormone (TSH) in circulation and tissues. A wide range of structurally diverse TDCs interfere with the hypothalamic–pituitary–thyroid (HPT) axis by different mechanisms to alter TH homeostasis, at the receptor level, in binding to transport proteins, in cellular uptake mechanisms, or in modifying the metabolism of THs (Boas et al., 2006). TH homeostasis involves a complex interplay of homeostatic regulatory processes. Regulation of THs includes control of iodine uptake, synthesis and storage of THs in the thyroid gland, release into and transport of THs within an out-of-circulation-tissue-specific deiodination, and degradation by catabolic hepatic enzymes (Fig. 5.1).

Concern about TDCs has increased because of the critical role that THs play in brain development (Crofton, 2008). Even transient disruption of normal thyroid homeostasis will lead to disastrous outcomes, especially in the developing nervous system (Crofton, 2008). The changes of normal TH levels can adversely affect pregnancy outcome, fertility, and postnatal development in humans and animals. Especially, when changes occur in a critical developmental phase, such as deficiency of TH during pre- and early postnatal period, it may cause profound and irreversible damage to the newborn, resulting in abnormal brain development

Endocrine Disruptors in the Environment, First Edition. Sushil K. Khetan.
© 2014 John Wiley & Sons, Inc. Published 2014 by John Wiley & Sons, Inc.

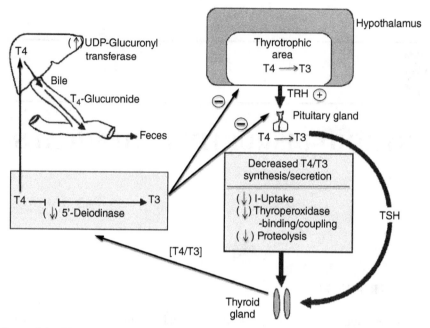

Figure 5.1 TH control pathways and sites of disruption by xenobiotic chemicals. TRH, thyrotropin-releasing hormone; TSH, thyroid-stimulating hormone. Modified from Capen (2008). Reproduced with permission of The McGraw-Hill Companies.

known as *cretinism* in humans. Screening for neonatal hypothyroidism is actively conducted in most industrialized countries to prevent sporadic cretinism induced by congenital abnormalities (Kolbuchi, 2009).

The chemically identical THs in mammals are also present in amphibians and fish, where they play different, but still important, roles. THs play a central role in amphibian metamorphosis, guiding the complex process of differentiation and growth, and also morphological changes, including tail resorption, emergence of limbs, and development of the digestive system (Diamanti-Kandarakis et al., 2009). This process is exploited in short-term endocrine disruptor screening assays, such as the amphibian metamorphosis assay which is part of the EPA's Endocrine Disruptor Screening Program (see Chapter 12). The assay is highly sensitive and is thought to provide insight into potential for interactions with the thyroid system in mammals (including humans) and also in amphibians and fish.

Multiple chemicals have been identified that interfere with thyroid function by each of the identified mechanisms discussed below. Several environmental chemicals have a high degree of structural resemblance to the THs T4 and T3 and therefore interfere with binding of THs to receptors or transport proteins leading to hypothyroidism.

5.2   THYROID SYNTHESIS INHIBITION BY INTERFERENCE IN IODIDE UPTAKE

5.2.1   Perchlorate

Perchlorate is a powerful oxidant that has emerged as an important threat to drinking water sources in the United States, with over 400 public water systems reporting perchlorate in their water (Kolpin et al., 2002). Perchlorate is a contaminant that comes from rocket fuel, fireworks, road flares, fertilizer, and other sources. Perchlorate is an anion that is very water soluble and environmentally stable and is not removed by conventional water treatment processes. It is known to interfere with the normal function of the thyroid gland. Iodine is needed by the thyroid in order to create THs. Normally, iodine is transported into the thyroid gland through an energy-requiring mechanism called the *sodium–iodide symporter* (NIS). Perchlorate blocks this transport and prevents uptake of iodine into the gland, with subsequent decrease in iodine-based TH synthesis. Interference with the production of these vital hormones, which are essential in fetal and postnatal neurodevelopment, affects normal metabolism, growth, and development (Solomon, 2010). Interestingly, perchlorate does not appear to be transported by the NIS, indicating that it is a blocker of NIS function, not a competitive inhibitor (Fig. 5.2).

A decrease in circulating TH during gestation or the first year of life can result in neurodevelopmental abnormalities leading to permanent brain dysfunction. Many studies have shown subtle but lasting deficits in cognitive function, language, hearing, behavior, attention span, and vestibular function (balance) in those that had early life or prenatal thyroid suppression. According to the Centers for Disease

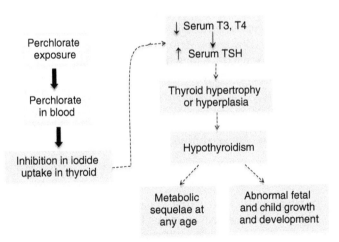

Figure 5.2   Proposed mode of action for perchlorate toxicity in humans. Solid arrows represent outcomes observed in humans during perchlorate exposure, while dashed arrows represent biologically plausible outcomes. Modified from Capen (2008). Reproduced with permission of The McGraw-Hill Companies.

Control and Prevention (CDC), about 30% of women of reproductive age in the United States have suboptimal dietary iodine, making them particularly susceptible to compounds (such as perchlorate) that block iodine uptake into the thyroid gland.

Although there is no federal regulation for perchlorate in drinking water in the United States, several states have promulgated enforceable regulations, with Massachusetts having the most stringent standard at 2 µg/L (Pisarenko et al., 2010).

5.3 TH TRANSPORT DISRUPTORS AND ESTROGEN SULFOTRANSFERASES INHIBITORS

TH disruptors also target enzymes involved in conjugating sulfotransferases (SULT) and UDP-gucuronosyltransferases (UGTs). The SULT family comprises important phase II conjugation enzymes for the detoxification of xenobiotics and modulation of the activity of physiologically important endobiotics such as THs, steroids, and neurotransmitters. SULT enzymes catalyze the transfer of a sulfuryl group, donated by 3′-phosphoadenosine-5′- phosphosulfate (PAPS), to an acceptor substrate that may be a hydroxy group or an amine group in a sulfonation process (Glatt, 2000). For example, sulfation by the specific estrogen sulfotransferase (SULT1E1) is an important pathway for the inactivation of E2 (Fig. 5.3) (Glatt, 2000). The estrogen sulfates formed by SULT1E1, which possess a considerably longer half-life than their parent compounds, are unable to bind to the ER and therefore do not elicit genomic action (Pasqualini, 2009).

Human exposure to certain environmental chemicals, such as hydroxylated polychlorinated biphenyls (OH-PCBs), hydroxylated polyhalogenated aromatic hydrocarbons, and pentachlorophenol, may lead to the inhibition of SULT activity. Inhibition of the SULT-mediated biotransformation of biologically active estrogens by endocrine disruptor chemicals (EDCs) can lead to an increased *in situ* availability of these endogenous steroids, which has been related to various estrogen-dependant unwanted features (Fig. 5.4). Inhibition of individual human SULT isoforms may cause adverse effects on human health (Wang and James, 2006).

Polyhalgenated phenolic compounds may exhibit ED activity by increasing the bioavailability of endogenous THs through inhibition of hormone-conjugating enzymes in target tissues (adapted from Kester et al., 2002).

5.3.1 Polychlorinated Biphenyls (PCBs)

Polychlorinated biphenyls (PCBs) (Fig. 5.5a) comprise a family of ubiquitous, persistent, and bioaccumulated environmental contaminants that include 209 congeners used for products ranging from fluorescent light fixtures to coolant fluids inside parts of consumer electronics. PCB exposure has been linked to adverse effects in animals and wildlife, which ultimately led to their ban in the United States since 1977 and are out of use or highly restricted throughout much of the world. However, PCBs made and used for nearly 50 years before the ban remain in the

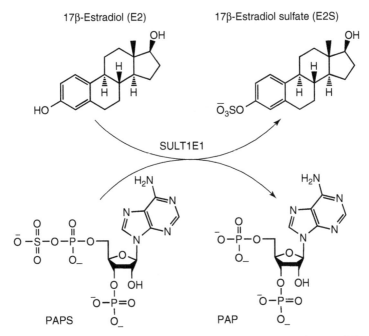

Figure 5.3 SULT1E1-catalyzed 3-sulfonation of the prototype substrate 17β-estradiol (E2) into 17β-estradiol-3-sulfate (E2S).

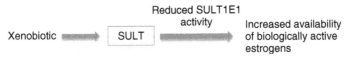

Figure 5.4 The xenobiotic can act as an SULT1E1 inhibitor and thereby disrupt its involvement in the sulfonation of endogenous steroids and prevent the associated protection of peripheral tissues from estrogenic effects.

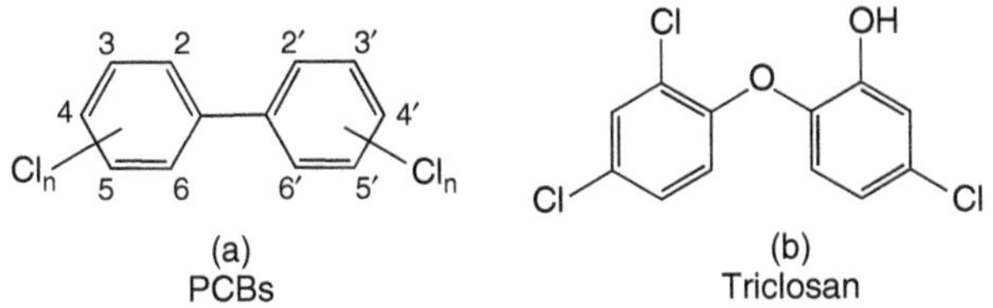

Figure 5.5 TH transport disruptors and sulfotransferase inhibitor compounds.

environment and are found throughout the food chain, including in human tissues and breast milk.

PCBs have been demonstrated to exert effects on TH levels in animals and humans. Depending on the chemical structure of the PCB congener, these compounds may disturb estrogen, androgen, or TH receptor pathways, and their effects have been reported on the immune system, development, and reproduction (Carpenter, 2006). One of the most consistent findings is that PCB exposure decreases the levels of circulating THs (total T4 and T3) and an increase in TSH level in the animals and that these effects are dose-dependent (Boas et al., 2009), resulting in developmental deficits, including deficits in hearing. PCBs are able to bind with TH transport proteins and compete with THs, thus modifying ratios of the free to bound hormone. Additionally, PCBs may be transported to normally inaccessible sites of action, including fetal development and fetal brain, with a resultant decrease in fetal brain T4 levels (Boas et al., 2006). Monkeys exposed orally to PCB for 18–23 weeks showed a significant dose-dependent reduction of T4, free T4 (FT4), and T3, and an increase in TSH (van den Berg et al., 1988).

Both *in vivo* and *in vitro* studies suggest that PCBs activate the pregnane X receptor (PXR) in rodents, which leads to upregulation of hepatic catabolic enzymes and subsequent declines in circulating concentrations of T4. The PXR is involved in activating the expression of several P450 detoxifying enzymes, including CYP3A4 in the adult and CYP3A7 in the fetus, in response to xenobiotics and steroids. CYP3A4 is the major human hepatic P450, and has been suggested as being involved in the metabolism of over 60% of drugs in clinical use (Marel, 1996). The steroid X receptor (SXR) is the human equivalent for rodent PXR. It appears unlikely the PCB congeners or their metabolites competitively bind to the TR, but it may well be that they produce allosteric effects on TRs that alter their ability to mediate TH action (Miller et al., 2009).

PCBs are metabolized to OH-PCBs, which are also biologically active, and have a high degree of structural resemblance to thyroxin (T4) (Boas et al., 2009). The OH-PCBs are known to interfere with TH transport in laboratory animals due to their strong binding affinity for the transport protein transthyretin (TTR), which can be even higher than that of the indigenous ligand T4, thus altering plasma levels of TH (Meerts et al., 2002).

In vitro studies have shown that the OH-PCBs inhibit SULT1E1, which is partially responsible for their ED effects. OH-PCBs inhibit E2 sulfonation, which may prolong the bioavailability of endogenous E2 (Kester et al., 2000) and inhibit TH sulfonation, thereby potentially disrupting the TH system and thus contributing to the known toxic effects of these compounds (Wang and James, 2006). Different OH-PCBs, for example, altered the sexual differentiation of the turtle (Kester et al., 2000).

5.3.2 Triclosan

Triclosan (5-chloro-2-(2,4-dichloro-phenoxy)-phenol), a chlorinated phenolic compound (Fig. 5.5b), has broad-spectrum antimicrobial activity against most Gram-negative and Gram-positive bacteria. It is widely used in personal care products, including soaps, toothpastes, and chopping boards. It acts by interrupting the fatty acid synthesis in bacteria. It has become distributed ubiquitously across the ecosystem, and recent reports that it can cause endocrine disruption in aquatic species have increased concern. A high pK_{ow} of 4.8 indicates that triclosan is hydrophobic and suggests the possibility for bioaccumulation.

Triclosan has been reported to disrupt TH signaling and decrease serum T4 in male juvenile rats (Zorrilla et al., 2009). Oral exposure of rats to triclosan produced hypothyroxinemia with dose-responsive T4 decreases without compensatory TSH increase, similar to PCBs. Triclosan upregulated phase II glucuronidation and sulfation, and this increased catabolism of T4 may be partially responsible for the triclosan-induced hypothyroxinemia adversely effecting TH homeostasis (Paul et al., 2010; Zorrilla et al., 2009).

Triclosan was shown to possess intrinsic estrogenic and androgenic activity in a range of assays *in vitro*; it displaced estradiol from ERs of MCF-7 human breast cancer cells and displaced testosterone from binding to the ligand-binding domain of the rat AR (Gee et al., 2008). In the uterotrophic assay, the uterine weight of the female Wistar rats treated with oral doses of triclosan was not affected. However, a dose-dependent increase was observed when cotreated with E2 and triclosan as compared with E2 alone, indicating a potentiation of the estrogenic effect of E2 (Stoker et al., 2010).

Male mosquito fish from relatively clean water exposed to triclosan for a month at about 100 times concentrations of what is usually found in water induced to produce notable amounts of egg yolk protein, something only females are supposed to do. Sperm production in these fish also took a big hit, falling by a third when compared to untreated males. These data indicate that triclosan is weakly estrogenic and has the potential to act as an endocrine-disrupting agent in aquatic organisms (Raut and Angus, 2010).

Triclosan is also reported to be a potent inhibitor of SULT1E1 activity in human liver fractions (Wang et al., 2004). Studies of the effect of triclosan on sheep placental cytosolic SULT1E1 activity showed that it was a very potent inhibitor of both estradiol and estrone sulfonation (James et al., 2010). The high potency of triclosan as an inhibitor of SULT1E1 activity raises concern about its possible effects on the ability of the placenta to supply estrogen to the fetus and, in turn, on fetal growth and development (James et al., 2010). Estrogen is vital for the growth and development of major organs, such as the lungs and liver, in a growing fetus. Miscarriage can occur when estrogen is unable to cross the placenta.

There has been evidence for microbial degradation of triclosan, but the compound is still readily detected in the environment. It was one of 30 compounds most frequently detected in a survey of 85 urban rivers in the United States. It was detected in 58% of the samples and found at a maximum concentration of 2.3 µg/L (Kolpin et al., 2002).

5.4 THYROID HORMONE LEVEL DISRUPTORS

5.4.1 Polybrominated Diphenyl Ethers (PBDEs)

Polybrominated diphenyl ethers (PBDEs) are a group of brominated aromatic compounds that have been widely used as flame retardants in numerous industrial and

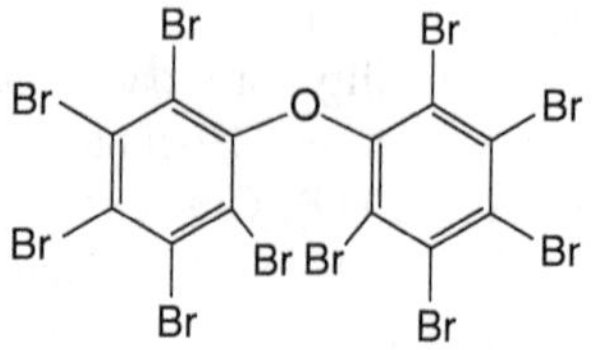

Figure 5.6   Deca BDE structure.

consumer products such as textiles, electronics, building insulation, polyurethane foam, and wires and cables. These brominated flame retardants work by releasing bromine free radicals when heated, which scavenge other free radicals that are part of the flame propagation process. There is a growing concern about their persistence in the environment, as PBDEs have tendency to bioaccumulate in the food chain. Their structure, persistence, and bioaccumulative properties are similar to those of the PCBs. Because they are additives rather than chemically bound to consumer products, they are more likely to leach out of the product into the environment. Industrial and urban effluents are significant sources of PBDEs to surface waters and sediments. Human exposure is primarily through diet and house dust in the home, with toddlers particularly highly exposed because of their low body weight and their hand-to-mouth behaviors.

Three PBDE technical mixtures were commercially available, but Deca is the only one currently produced in large quantities worldwide (Fig. 5.6). The major component of Deca is decabromodiphenyl ether (BDE-209), the fully brominated congener (Laguardia et al., 2006). It is the most widely used PBDE globally, primarily in high-impact polystyrene (HIPS) plastic that is frequently used to make the back part of television sets and in other electronic devices. *In vivo* and *in vitro* studies have evidenced effects of BDE-209 on TH homeostasis and direct effects on nervous cells. The major US importers and manufacturers of Deca BDE have announced that this mixture will be phased out by the end of 2013 for all but essential uses for which no alternative is available (Hogue, 2012).

Several studies have demonstrated that exposure to PBDEs may have endocrine-disrupting effects. Most of these studies have focused on TH disruption and a smaller number on the disruption of the estrogen/androgen hormone system (Darnerud, 2008). In studies with rats and mice, *in vivo* PBDE exposure has been found to affect thyroid function, which is observed as induction of thyroid hyperplasia and disrupt TH balance with decreased levels of total and free T4 and increased serum TSH (Hallgren et al., 2001). These observations are dependent to some extent upon the specific PBDE mixture employed in the study, with the lower brominated compounds appearing more potent in reducing serum TH levels. For example, Administration of a common flame retardant, 2,2′,4,4′-tetrabromodiphenyl ether (BDE-47), at doses relevant to human exposure affected the reproductive system and thyroid gland of female Wistar rats (Talsness et al., 2008). Most PBDEs have also anti-androgenic activity *in vitro* and *in vivo* (Stoker et al., 2005).

PBDEs have structural similarities to PCBs and can bind to the Ah receptor, but unlike PCBs they do not appear to activate the Ah receptor–AhR nuclear translocator protein–XRE complex. Investigations for the potential mechanisms by which PBDE exposure may lead to reduction in circulating levels of TH include metabolism and excretion of serum T4 or to an interaction of PBDEs with the TH transport system by interacting with TTR, a TH binding protein in plasma, displacing T4 and lowering the level of T4. A possible role of OH-PDBEs metabolites, which are more potent in displacing T4 from TTR, is implied here (Stoker et al., 2005; Costa et al., 2008; Szabo et al., 2009). It is reported that the TTR-binding potencies of OH-PBDEs are orders of magnitude higher than that of BDE-47, which also supports this contention (Hamers et al., 2008). Several OH-PBDEs were found to inhibit CYP19 (aromatase), a key enzyme in steroidogenesis, in human pacental microsomes.

In vitro and animal studies have been associated with various PBDEs with a variety of neurological and developmental deficits, including low intelligence and learning disabilities (Kodavanti et al., 2010; Dingemans et al., 2011). Endocrine disruption during critical developmental periods may result in irreversible effects on differentiating tissue, including the brain. Causal relationships between prenatal exposure to PBDEs and indices of developmental neurotoxicity have been observed in experimental animal models (Costa et al., 2008).

For the endocrine disrupting effects of PBDEs, readers are referred to two recent reviews (Costa et al., 2008; Darnerud, 2008). As PBDEs are phased out in the United States, chemicals of uncharacterized toxicity are replacing these (Dodson et al., 2012). These replacement chemicals include tris(2,3-dibromopropyl) phosphate (banned in children's sleepwear), Firemaster 550 (a mixture of 2-ethylhexyl-2,3,4,5-tetrabromobenzoate, bis(2-ethylhexyl)-3,4,5,6-tetrabromo phthalate, triphenyl phosphate, and a yet-to-be-fully characterized isopropylated triaryl phosphate mixture). In an animal study, Firemaster 550 components exposed to rats (100 and 100 µg/d across gestation and lactation) were found accumulated in tissues of exposed dams and their offspring and exhibited advanced female puberty, weight gain, male cardiac hypertrophy, and altered exploratory behaviors (Patisaul et al., 2013).

A line of halogen gree polyphosphonate plastics are being offered by the US based FRX polymers as less toxic flame retardants. These include Nofia HM1100 for blending, Nofia copolymer as stand-alone and oligomer FR materials as additives (Lebel, 2013).

5.5 SELECTIVE THYROID HORMONE ANTAGONISTS

5.5.1 Bisphenols

Several studies have shown that chemicals such as bisphenol A (BPA) and halogenated BPA can bind to the TR with relatively high affinity (Kitamura et al., 2002; Moriyama et al., 2002). BPA, a weak estrogen, binds to rat TR and antagonizes T3 activation *in vitro*, inhibiting TR-mediated gene activation (Moriyama et al., 2002). Sprague–Dawley rats exposed to BPA during pregnancy and lactation caused increased serum T4 in pups postnatally without affecting serum TSH. In humans, estrogen elevates serum T4, but in rats it decreases. The result was indicative that BPA exerts a selective TH antagonism independent of estrogenic effect *in vivo* (Zoeller, 2005). In another *in vivo* study, BPA was reported to block TH-induced tail resorption during Xenopus metamorphosis (Iwamuro et al., 2003).

In a study investigating relationships between maternal BPA exposure and thyroid function in pregnant women and neonates, BPA was found to have effects on both the mother's and her baby's thyroid function. A linkage with urinary BPA concentrations in third trimester of pregnancy was found to reduce total T4 in pregnant women and significantly decrease TSH in male, but not female newborns (Chevrier et al., 2013). BPA circulates in pregnant women's blood, and it passes through the placenta to the fetus in the womb. The idea that "many lifelong chronic diseases start in the womb" has gained wide support in recent years.

Halogenated BPA, such as tetrabromobisphenol A and tetrachlorobisphenol A, show closer structural relationship to T4 than PCBs: both these tetrahalogenated bisphenols induce thyroid-dependent growth in pituitary GH3 cell line at concentrations 4–6 orders of magnitude higher than T3 (Kitamura et al., 2002).

5.5.2 Perfluoroalkyl Acids (PFAAs)

PFAAs' actions on the thyroid system are multiple and complex, showing impairment in thyroid homeostasis in animal studies. A study with perfluorodecanoic acid showed that it could reduce serum TH levels by displacing circulating THs from their plasma protein-binding sites (Gutshall et al., 1989).

Rats exposed to perfluorooctane sulfonate (PFOS) have been reported to result in reduced serum T4 and T3 without the concomitant increase in TSH (Lau et al., 2003; Luebker et al., 2005; Seacat et al., 2003).PFOS was the key ingredient in Scotchgard®, a fabric protector made by 3M, and numerous stain repellents, and has been used to make aqueous film-forming foam (AFFF), a component of firefighting foams. PFOS has been shown to significantly reduce circulating TH levels in mammals (Yu et al., 2009a) and cross-over studies of rats exposed *in utero* and/or in lactation document that both prenatal and postnatal exposure to PFOS may reduce TH levels in the offspring (Yu et al., 2009a, 2009b). PFOS-induced hypothyroxinemia in rats indicated that increased conjugation of T4 in the liver and increased thyroidal conversion of T4 to T3 by type 1 deiodinase may be partly responsible for the effects (Yu et al., 2009b). However, no differences in free TH levels have been observed in PFOS-dosed animals or in the HPT axis (Chang et al., 2008). Thus, although PFOS exerted significant effects on the total levels of circulating hormones, it did not affect the free hormone concentrations.

5.5.3 Phthalates

To date, few studies have investigated the effects of phthalates on the action of TH. Rodent exposure to DEHP, di-*n*-octyl phthalate (DOP), and di-*n*-hexyl phthalate

(DHP) found histopathological changes in the rat thyroid glands, corresponding to thyroid hyperactivity (Hinton et al., 1986; Howarth et al., 2001). Oral rat exposure to DEHP did not affect the levels of circulating THs (Bernal et al., 2002), whereas intravenous exposure in doses corresponding to levels of DEHP solubilized in blood bags for human transfusions resulted in significant increase in the serum T3 and T4, which returned to normal after 7 days (Gayathri et al., 2004). In contrast, di-*n*-butyl phthalate (DBP) decreased T3 and T4 in rats in a dose-dependent manner (O'Connor et al., 2002).

5.6   CONCLUSIONS AND FUTURE PROSPECTS

THs are strongly involved in vertebrate brain development, from early embryogenesis to subsequent prenatal and perinatal development in mammals. A large variety of ubiquitous chemicals have been shown to have thyroid-disrupting properties. However, only the effects of environmental levels of PCBs have been extensively investigated in humans, wildlife, animal experiments, and *in vitro* (Boas et al., 2012). Serum levels of TSH, T3, and T4 are tightly regulated within a given individual, maintaining an individual set point. Up to a (yet unknown) threshold of exposure, the human body may be able to compensate for adverse effects, that is, decrease in peripheral T4 and T3, by negative feedback mechanisms, namely, increase in TSH. Nevertheless, minor alterations in thyroid homeostasis in the individual may have adverse health effects, especially during sensitive developmental windows such as the development of the central nervous system in fetal life and infancy. The combination of mechanistic, epidemiological, and exposure studies indicates that the environmental exposure to industrial chemicals may impose a serious threat to human and wildlife thyroid homeostasis (Boas et al., 2009). Thus, thyroid toxicants are of great concern for human health.

REFERENCES

Bernal, C. A.; Martinelli, M. I.; Mocchiutti, N. O. Effect of the dietary exposure of rat to di(2-ethyl hexyl) phthalate on their metabolic efficiency, *Food Addit. Contam.* **2002**, 19(11), 1091–1096.

Boas, M.; Feldt-Rasmussen, U.; Skakkebaek, N. E.; Main, K. M. Environmental chemicals and thyroid function, *Eur. J. Endocrinol.* **2006**, 154(5), 599–611.

Boas, M.; Feldt-Rasmussen, U.; Main, K. M. Thyroid effects of endocrine disrupting chemicals, *Mol. Cell. Endocrinol.* **2012**, 355(2), 240–248.

Boas, M.; Main, K. M.; Feldt-Rasmussen, U. Environmental chemicals and thyroid function: an update, *Curr. Opin. Endocrinol. Diabetes Obes.* **2009**, 16, 385–391.

Capen, C. C. Toxic responses of the endocrine system, in *Casarett and Doull's Toxicology, The Basic Science of Poisons*, 7th Ed., Klaassen, C. D., ed., New York: McGraw Hill Medical, **2008**, pp. 807–879.

Carpenter, D. O. Polychlorinated biphenyls (PCBs): routes of exposure and effects on human health, *Rev. Environ. Health* **2006**, 21(1), 1–23.

Chang, S. C.; Thibodeaux, J. R.; Eastvold, M. L., et al. Thyroid hormone status and pituitary function in adult rats given oral doses of perfluorooctane sulfonate (PFOS), *Toxicology* **2008**, 243(3), 330–339.

Chevrier, J.; Gunier, R. B.; Bradman, A.; Holland, N. T.; Calafat, A. M.; Eskenazi, B.; Harley, K. G. Maternal urinary bisphenol A during pregnancy and maternal and neonatal thyroid function in the CHAMACOS study, *Environ. Health Perspect.* **2013**, 121(1), 138–144.

Costa, L. G.; Giordano, G.; Tagliaferri, S.; Caglieri, A.; Mutti, A. Polybrominated diphenyl ether (PBDE) flame retardants: environmental contamination, human body burden and potential adverse health effects, *Acta Biomed.* **2008**, 79, 172–183.

Crofton, K. M. Thyroid disrupting chemicals: mechanisms and mixtures, *Int. J. Androl.* **2008**, 31(2), 209–223.

Darnerud, P. O. Brominated flame retardants as possible endocrine disruptors. *Int. J. Androl.* **2008**, 31(2), 152–160.

Diamanti-Kandarakis, E.; Bourguignon, J.P.; Giudice, L.C.; Hauser, R.; Prins, G.S.; Soto, A.M.; Zoeller, R.T.; Gore, A.C. Endocrine-disrupting chemicals: an Endocrine Society scientific statement. *Endocr. Rev.* **2009**, 30(4), 293–342.

Dingemans, M. M. L., et al. Neurotoxicity of brominated flame retardants: (in) direct effects of parent and hydroxylated polybrominated diphenyl ethers on the (developing) nervous system, *Environ. Health Perspect.* **2011**, 119(7), 900–907.

Dodson, R. E.; Perovich, L. J.; Covaci, A.; Van den Eede, N.; Ionas, A. C.; Dirtu, A. C.; Brody, J. G.; Rudel, R. A. After the PBDE phase-out: a broad suite of flame retardants in repeat house dust samples from California, *Environ. Sci. Technol.* **2012**, 46(24), 13056–13066.

Gayathri, N. S.; Dhanya, C. R.; Indu, A. R.; Kurup, P. A. Changes in some hormones by low doses of di (2-ethyl hexyl) phthalate (DEHP), a commonly used plasticizer in PVC blood storage bags and medical tubing, *Indian J. Med. Res.* **2004**, 119(4), 139–144.

Gee, R. H.; Charles, A.; Taylor, N.; Darbre, P. D. Oestrogenic and androgenic activity of triclosan in breast cancer cells, *J. Appl. Toxicol.* **2008**, 28(1), 78–91.

Glatt, H. Sulfotransferases in the bioactivation of xenobiotics, *Chem. Bio. Interact.* **2000**, 129(1–2), 141–170.

Gutshall, D. M.; Pilcher, G. D.; Langley, A. E. Mechanism of the serum thyroid hormone lowering effect of perfluoro-n-decanoic acid (PFDA) in rats, *J. Toxicol. Environ. Health* **1989**, 28(1), 53–65.

Hallgren, S.; Sinjari, T.; Hakansson, H.; Darnerud, P. O. Effects of polybrominated diphenyl ethers (PBDEs) and polychlorinated biphenyls (PCBs) on thyroid hormone and vitamin A levels in rats and mice. *Arch. Toxicol.* **2001**, 75, 200–208.

Hamers, T.; Kamstra, J. H.; Sonneveld, E.; Murk, A. J.; Visser, T. J.; Van Velzen, M. J.; Brouwer, A.; Bergman, A. Biotransformation of brominated flame retardants into potentially endocrine-disrupting metabolites, with special attention to 2,2',4,4'-tetrabromodiphenyl ether (BDE-47), *Mol. Nutr. Food Res.* **2008**, 52(2), 284–298.

Hinton, R. H.; Mitchell, F. E.; Mann, A.; Chescoe, D.; Price, S. C.; Nunn, A.; Grasso, P.; Bridges, J. W. Effects of phthalic acid esters on the liver and thyroid, *Environ. Health Perspect.* **1986**, 70, 195–210.

Hogue, C. EPA targets flame retardants, *C&E News* **2012**, 90(44), 34–37.

Howarth, J. A.; Price, S. C.; Dobrota, M.; Kentish, P. A.; Hinton, R. H. Effects on male rats of di(2-ethylhexyl) phthalate and di-n-hexylphthalate administered alone or in combination, *Toxicol. Lett.* **2001**, 121(1), 35–43.

Iwamuro, S.; Sakakibara, M.; Terao, M., et al, Teratogenic and anti-metamorphic effects of bisphenol-A on embryonic and larval Xenopus laevis, *Gen. Comp. Endocrinol.* **2003**,133, 189–198.

James, M. O., Li, W.; Summerlot, D. P.; Rowland-Faux, L.; Wood, C. E. Triclosan is a potent inhibitor of estradiol and estrone sulfonation in sheep placenta, *Environ. Int.* **2010**, 36(8): 942–949.

Kester, M. H.; Bulduk, S.; Tibboel, D.; Meinl, W.; Glatt, H.; Falany, C. N.; Coughtrie, M. W.; Bergman, A.; Safe, S. H.; Kuiper, G. G.; Schuur, A. G.; Brouwer, A.; Visser, T. J. Potent inhibition of estrogen sulfotransferase by hydroxylated PCB metabolites: a novel pathway explaining the estrogenic activity of PCBs, *Endocrinology* **2000**, 141(5), 1897–900.

Kester, M. H.; Bulduk, S.; van Toor, H.; Tibboel, D.; Meini, W.; Glatt, H., et al. Potent inhibition of estrogen sulfotransferase by hydroxylated metabolites of polyhalogenated aromatic hydrocarbons reveals alternative mechanism for estrogenic activity of endocrine disruptors, *J. Clin. Endocrinol. Metab.* **2002**, 87(3), 1142–1150.

Kitamura, S.; Jinno, N.; Ohta, S.; Kuroki, H.; Fujimoto, N. Thyroid hormonal activity of the flame retardants tetrabromobisphenol A and tetrachlorobisphenol A. *Biochem. Biophys. Res. Commun.* **2002**, 293(1), 554–559.

Kodavanti PRS, et al. Developmental exposure to a commercial PBDE mixture, DE-71: neurobehavioral, hormonal, and reproductive effects, *Toxicol. Sci.* **2010**, 116(1), 297–312.

Kolbuchi, N. Mechanism of chemical disruptors of thyroid function, *Hot Thyroidol.* **2009**. Available at: www.hotthyroidology.com/editorial_220.html (accessed 19 Jan 2014).

Kolpin, D. W.; Furlong, E. T.; Meyer, M. T.; Thurman, E. M.; Zaugg, S. D.; Barber, L. B.; Buxton, H. T. Pharmaceuticals, hormones, and other organic wastewater contaminants in U. S. streams, 1999-2000: a national reconnaissance. *Environ. Sci. Technol.* **2002**, 36(6), 1202–1211.

Laguardia, M. J.; Hale, R. C.; Harvey, E. Detailed polybrominated diphenyl ether (PBDE) congener composition of the widely used penta-, octa-, and deca-PBDE technical flame-retardant mixtures, *Environ. Sci. Technol.* **2006**, 40, 6247–6254.

Lau, C.; Thibodeaux, J. R.; Hanson, R. G.; Rogers, J. M.; Grey, B. E.; Stanton, M. E.; Butenhoff, J. L.; Stevenson, L. A. Exposure to perfluorooctane sulfonate during pregnancy in rat and mouse. II: Postnatal evaluation, *Toxicol. Sci.* **2003**, 74(2), 382–392.

Lebel, M. A. Green chemistry to replace bromine-based flame retardants, *EcoChem conference, Basel, Switzerland*, November 19–21, **2013**.

Luebker, D. J.; Case, M. T.; York, R. G.; Moore, J. A.; Hansen, K. J.; Butenhoff, J. L. Two-generation reproduction and cross-foster studies of perfluorooctanesulfonate (PFOS) in rats, *Toxicology* **2005**, 215(1–2), 126–148.

Marel, P. The CYP 3 family, in *Cytochromes P450: Metabolic and Toxicological Aspects*, Ionnides, C., ed., Boca Raton, FL: CRC Press, Inc., **1996**, pp. 241–270.

Meerts, I. A. T. M.; Assink, Y.; Cenijn, P. H.; van den Berg, J. H. J.; Weijers, B. M.; Bergman, Å.; Koeman, J. H.; Brouwer, Å. Placental transfer of a hydroxylated polychlorinated biphenyl and effectsn on fetal and maternal thyroid hormone homeostasis in the rat. *Toxicol. Sci.* **2002**, 68, 361–371.

Miller, M. D.; Crofton, K. M.; Rice, D. C.; Zoeller, R. T. Thyroid-disrupting chemicals: interpreting upstream biomarkers of adverse outcomes, *Environ. Health Perspect.* **2009**, 117, 1033–1041.

Moriyama, K.; Tagami, T.; Akamizu, T.; Usui, T.; Saijo, M.; Kanamoto, N.; Hataya, Y.; Shimatsu, A.; Juzuya, H.; Nakao, K. Thyroid hormone action is disrupted by bisphenol A as an antagonist, *J. Clin. Endocrinol. Metab.* **2002**, 87(11), 5185–5190.

O'Connor, J. C.; Frame, S. R.; Ladics, G. S. Evaluation of a 15-day screening assay using intact male rats for identifying antiandrogens, *Toxicol. Sci.*, **2002**, 69(1), 92–108.

Pasqualini, J. R. Estrogen sulfotransferases in breast and endometrial cancers, *Ann. N. Y. Acad. Sci.* **2009**, 1155, 88–98.

Patisaul, H. B.; Roberts, S. C.; Mabrey, N.; Mccaffrey, K. A.; Gear, R. B.; Braun, J.; Belcher, S. M.; Stapleton, H. M. Accumulation and endocrine disrupting effects of the flame retardant mixture Firemaster® 550 in rats: an exploratory assessment, *J. Biochem. Mol. Toxicol.* **2013**, 27(2), 124–136.

Paul, K. B.; Hedge, J. M.; DeVito, M.J.; Crofton, K. M. Short-term exposure to triclosan decreases thyroxine *In vivo* via upregulation of hepatic catabolism in Young Long-Evans rats, *Toxicol. Sci.* **2010**, 113(2), 367–379.

Pisarenko, A. N.; Stanford, B. D.; Quinones, O.; Pacey, G. E.; Gordon, G.; Snyder, S. A. Rapid analysis of perchlorate, chlorate and bromate ionsin concentrated sodium hypochlorite solutions, *Anal. Chim. Acta*, **2010**, 659(1–2), 216–223.

Raut, S. A.; Angus, R. A. Triclosan has endocrine-disrupting effects in male western mosquitofish, *Gambusia affinis*, *Environ. Toxicol. Chem.* **2010**, 29(6), 1287–1291.

Seacat, A. M.; Thomford, P. J.; Hansen, K. J.; Clemen, L. A.; Eldridge, S. R.; Elcombe, C. R.; Butenhoff, J. L. Sub-chronic dietary toxicity of potassium perfluorooctanesulfonate in rats, *Toxicology* **2003**, 183(1–3), 117–131.

Solomon, G. M. Endocrine disrupting chemicals in drinking water: risks to human health and the environment, *Testimony before the U.S. Congress*, Committee on energy and commerce, subcommittee on energy and the environment, Natural Resources Defense Council, February 25, 2010.

Stoker, T. E.; Cooper, R. L.; Lambright, C.S.; Wilson, V. S.; Furr, J.; Gray, L. E. In vivo and in vitro anti-androgenic effects of DE-71, a commercial polybrominated diphenyl ether (PBDE) mixture, *Toxicol. Appl. Pharmacol.* **2005**, 207, 78–88.

Stoker, T. E.; Gibson, E. K.; Zorrilla, L. M. Triclosan exposure modulates estrogen-dependent responses in the female wistar rat, *Toxicol. Sci.* **2010**, 117(1), 45–53.

Szabo, D. T.; Richardson, V. M.; Ross, D. G.; Diliberto, J. J.; Kodavanti, P. R.; Birnbaum, L. S. Effects of perinatal PBDE exposure on hepatic phase I, phase II, phase iII, and deiodinase 1 gene expression involved in thyroid hormone metabolism in male rat pups, *Toxicol. Sci.* **2009**, 107, 27–39.

Talsness, C. E.; Kuriyama, S. N.; Sterner-Kock, A.; Schnitker, P.; Grande, S. W.; Shakibaei, M., et al. *In utero* and lactational exposures to low doses of polybrominated diphenyl ether-47 alter the reproductive system and thyroid gland of female rat offspring, *Environ. Health Perspect.* **2008**, 116, 308–314.

Van den Berg, K. J.; Zurcher, C.; Brouwer, A.; Effects of 3,4, 3',4'-tetrachlorobiphenyl on thyroid function and histology in marmoset monkeys, *Toxicol. Lett.* **1988**, 41, 77–86.

Wang, L.-Q.; James, M. O. Inhibition of sulfotransferases by xenobiotics, *Curr. Drug Metabol.* **2006**, 7(1), 83–104.

Wang, L.-Q.; Falany, C. N.; James, M. O. Triclosan as a substrate and inhibitor of 3'-phosphoadenosine 5'phosphosulfate-sulfotransferase and UDP-glucuronosyl transferase in human liver fractions, *Drug Metab. Dispos.* **2004**, 32, 1162.

Yu, W. G.; Liu, W.; Jin, Y. H., et al. Prenatal and postnatal impact of perfluorooctane sulfonate (PFOS) on rat development: a cross-foster study on chemical burden and thyroid hormone system, *Environ. Sci. Technol.* **2009a**, 43(21), 8416–8422.

Yu, W. G.; Liu, W.; Jin, Y. H. Effects of perfluorooctane sulfonate on rat thyroid hormone biosynthesis and metabolism, *Environ. Toxicol. Chem.* **2009b**, 28(5), 990–996.

Zoeller, R. T. Environmental chemicals as thyroid hormone analogues: new studies indicate that thyroid hormone receptors are targets of industrial chemicals? *Mol. Cell. Endocrinol.* **2005**, 242(1–2), 10–15.

Zorrilla, L. M.; Gibson, E. K.; Jeffay, S. C.; Crofton, K. M.; Setzer, W. R.; Cooper, R. L.; Stoker, T. E. The effects of triclosan on puberty and thyroid hormones in male Wistar rats, *Toxicol. Sci.* **2009**, 107(1), 56–64.

6

ACTIVATORS OF PPAR, RXR, AhR, AND STEROIDOGENIC FACTOR 1

6.1   INTRODUCTION

Most studies on endocrine disrupting chemicals (EDCs) have focused on their effects on hormonal signaling mediated by nuclear hormone receptor (NR) family of proteins the estrogen receptors (ERs), the androgen receptor (AR), and thyroid hormone receptors (TRs), even though every possible cellular hormonal pathway can be their target. More recently, retinoid X receptor (RXR), and peroxisome proliferator-activated receptors (PPARs) are shown to be targets for EDC action and possible involvement in the development of obesity and impaired glucose tolerance, where normal insulin levels are insufficient to reduce circulating levels of glucose or triglycerides leading to increased risk for diabetes and cardiovascular disease. Perfluorooctanoic acid and sulfonate and monophthalate esters activate PPAR, while organotin compounds, such as tributyltin (TBT) and triphenyltin (TPT), activate both PPAR and RXR.

Some biological effects of EDCs are mediated by binding to receptors that are characterized for involving in xenobiotic recognition and responses. Most important among these is the aryl hydrocarbon receptor (AhR), a ligand-activated transcription factor and a xenosensor that mediates the biological response to a wide spectrum of xenobiotics, in particular, the toxic effects of the dioxin TCDD (2,3,7,8-tetrachlorodibenzo-p-dioxin).

Steroidogenic factor-1 (SF-1), which is an orphan member of the NR family, encoded by the *NR5A1* gene and a key regulator of steroidogenesis, regulating the transcription of key genes involved in sexual development and reproduction, is activated by the herbicide atrazine. Its targets include genes at every level of the

Endocrine Disruptors in the Environment, First Edition. Sushil K. Khetan.
© 2014 John Wiley & Sons, Inc. Published 2014 by John Wiley & Sons, Inc.

hypothalamic–pituitary–gonadal (HPA) axis, as well as many genes involved in gonadal and adrenal steroidogenesis.

6.2 PEROXISOME PROLIFERATOR-ACTIVATED RECEPTOR (PPAR) AGONISTS

PPARs are lipid-sensing and liporegulatory receptors. The PPARs got their name because they cause proliferation of peroxisomes, that is, organelles that catabolize long-chain fatty acids. Given PPARs' large ligand-binding pocket, it is not surprising that PPARs are activated by their main natural ligands – large fatty acids of approximately 14–18 carbons (Desvergne and Wahli, 1999; Xu et al., 1999), as well as synthetic compounds, such as fibrates (hypolipidemic drugs) and thiazolidinedions (antidiabetic drugs). In response to ligand activation, PPARs heterodimerize with the retinoid-X-receptor-α (RXRα), interact with co-activators and peroxisome proliferator-response elements (PPREs) found in the promoter region of target genes, and modulate expression of target genes (Shearer and Hoekstra, 2003).

This subfamily of nuclear receptors can be activated by both dietary fatty acids and their metabolic derivatives in the body, and thus serve as lipid sensors which when activated can markedly redirect metabolism. PPARs have important roles in reproduction and development, and their expression may influence the responses of an embryo exposed to PPAR agonists. PPARs consist of three isoforms, namely PPARα, PPARβ, and PPARγ (Shearer and Hoekstra, 2003). PPARα regulates target genes that modulate fatty acid degradation; PPARγ regulates target genes that modulate glucose homeostasis; and PPARβ may regulate fatty acid metabolism in skeletal muscle (Berger and Moller, 2002).

PPARγ is a key regulator in the formation of fat cells and is crucial in adipose tissue differentiation and adipocyte function, such as fat storage and energy dissipation, and is pivotal in glucose metabolism (Tontonoz and Spiegelman, 2008). PPARγ may be particularly susceptible to chemical "imposters" because it has a large ligand-binding pocket that can accommodate many chemical structures. When a molecule capable of activating the receptor enters the pocket, it turns on the adipogenic program. If PPARγ is activated in a preadipocyte, it becomes a fat cell; if it already is a fat cell, it puts more fat in the cell. However, not all chemicals that activate PPARγ are adipogenic or correlated with obesity in humans (Janesick and Blumberg, 2011a, 2011b).

Both PPARs and estrogen receptors (ERs) are involved in regulating adiposity. Interestingly, PPAR/RXR heterodimers have been shown to bind to estrogen response elements, and PPARs and ERs share certain cofactors, suggesting that signal crosstalk between these two nuclear receptors may participate in the control of obesity (Lau et al., 2010). Since 1990, when the PPAR family members were cloned and characterized, a number of environmental contaminants have been shown to activate PPARs. These include di-(2-ethylhexyl)phthalate (DEHP) (Feige et al., 2010), diisobutyl phthalate (Boberg et al., 2008), bisphenol

A (Kwintkiewicz et al., 2010), perfluoroalkyl acids (PFAAs) (Wolf et al., 2008), and organotins (Hiromori et al., 2009).

The PPAR isoforms PPARγ and PPARα are known to influence lipogenesis/weight gain, and environmental compounds such as TBT, phthalates, and PFOA are shown to be regulated by these receptors (Grün et al., 2006).

6.2.1 Organotin Antifoulant Biocides

Organotin compounds, such as TBT (Fig. 6.1a) and TPT (Fig. 6.1b), have been widely utilized as antifouling paints for ships and fishing nets, wood preservatives, and rodent repellents. Because of its widespread use as an antifoulant in boat paints since the 1960s, organotins are a common contaminant of marine and freshwater ecosystems. Exposure of aquatic invertebrates, particularly marine snails (gastropods), to very low concentrations of these compounds induces an irreversible sexual abnormality in females termed *imposex* (simultaneous presence of both male and female reproductive organs) (Smith, 1981). The consequence has been impaired reproductive fitness and possibly sterility, resulting in population decline or mass extinction (Grün et al., 2006). Imposex induced by TBT has been reported in over 150 species of snails as a very specific response to organotin compounds. Even in very weak doses, such as 0.1 ng/l (Oehlmann et al., 2007), an imposex phenomenon can be observed where females develop penises and, a sperm canal. However, there are no reports of TBT inducing an intersex condition in other groups of invertebrates. Human exposure to organotins occurs through fish and shellfish consumption.

There are different hypotheses postulated to explain the mechanism of organotin compounds' action on imposex induction, which is thought to be one of the mechanisms of endocrine disruption in wildlife (Nishikawa, 2006). In female gastropods, the growth of the male sex organs can be stimulated by testosterone, and studies have illustrated that TBT increases testosterone levels by inhibiting the enzyme aromatase, which converts testosterone to estradiol (Oberdörster and McClellan-Green, 2002).

Chemically induced PPARγ activity causes obesity. RXR is a key regulatory receptor during development and reproduction. Organotin compounds including TBT and TPT were identified as nanomolar agonists for both PPARγ and retinoid X

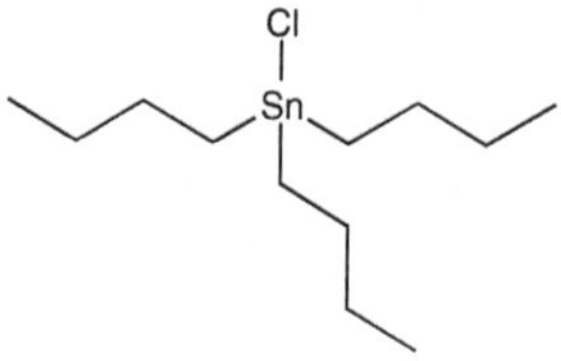

(a)
Tributyltin

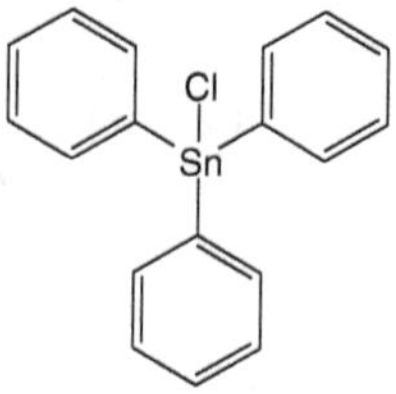

(b)
Triphenyltin

Figure 6.1 Organotin antifoulants.

receptor (RXR). These compounds act as high-affinity ligands at levels comparable to that of the known natural ligand of RXR, 9-*cis*-retinoic acid (9-*cis*-RA) or the well-known PPARγ ligand rosiglitazone, a thiazolidinedione linked to weight gain in humans (Blumberg, 2011) and used to treat type II diabetes (Nishikawa et al., 2004; Kanayama et al., 2005). The ability of TBT to activate PPARγ and induce adipogenesis in mouse models is well documented (Grün et al., 2006; Grün and Blumberg, 2009; Janesick and Blumberg, 2011a, 2011b).

The organotin compounds, by binding to RXRs, are able to efficiently activate these receptors inducing various toxicities ranging from weight gain, adipogenesis, and obesity in mammals to the development of male reproductive organs in female snails (le Maire et al., 2010; Nishikawa et al., 2004). In an experiment, 9-*cis*-RA-induced imposex in *Nucella lapillus* with the same severity as the positive control TBTCl, suggesting that both compounds may be acting through the same signaling pathway (Sousa et al., 2010). These results suggested that RXR plays an important role in the induction, differentiation, and growth of male genital organs in female gastropods (Nishikawa, 2006; Sternberg et al., 2010).

TBT has been shown to cause permanent physiological changes in both male and female mice exposed during prenatal development, resulting in a predisposition for weight gain. *In utero* TBT exposure induced body weight gain in adulthood, particularly through a rise in adipocyte proliferation, resulting in an increase of adipose mass, not only at the level of the adipose tissue but also by augmenting adiposity of diverse organs such as muscles (Grün and Blumberg, 2006). A 45-day chronic TBT exposure study demonstrated a dose-dependent increase in body weight of young male mice, which was significant at 5 μg/kg body weight; at this dose mice gained 9% in total body weight compared to control group (Zuo et al., 2011). Transgenerational effects on increased fat depot, fat cell size, and number through at least the F3 generation were observed when C57BL/6J female mice (F0) were exposed to TBT prenatally throughout pregnancy via the drinking water (Chamorro-García et al., 2013). In this study, F1 animals were exposed *in utero* and F2 mice were potentially exposed as germ cells in the F1, but F3 animals were never exposed to the chemicals (Chamorro-Gracia et al., 2013). In cellular assays, TBT exhibited exceptionally low EC_{50} values for activation of RXRα and PPARγ with values of 5 and 20 nM, respectively; *in vitro* binding affinities were comparable (Grün et al., 2006). The effect of TBT was blocked by the addition of a PPARγ antagonist.

In 2003, the International Marine Organization and the European Union (EU) banned the use of TBT in boat paints. Although this action led to a significant reduction in TBT release into the environment, it still persists in seas/oceans owing to its long half-life (>365 days) (Sousa et al., 2009). A new antifoulant, Sea-Nine®, 4,5-dichloro-2-*n*-octyl-4-isothiazolin-3-one (Fig. 6.2) was developed by Rohm and Haas as an environmentally acceptable alternative to TBT. Its metabolic breakdown products were found to be ring-opened compounds with greatly reduced toxicity that did not bioaccumulate in fish (Jacobson and Willingham, 2000). For this development, Rohm and Haas were awarded the 1996 Presidential Green Chemistry Award.

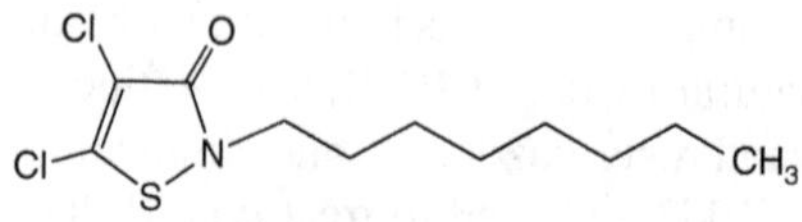

Figure 6.2 Isothiazolone antifoulant Sea-Nine developed as an alternative to TBT.

6.2.2   Perfluoroalkyl Compounds (PFCs)

PFCs are a family of synthetic, highly stable perfluorinated compounds (PFCs) with a wide range of uses in industrial and consumer products, including carpets, textiles, personal care products, and leveling and wetting agents, and in food-contact materials (D'eon and Mabury, 2011). Among these, perfluorooctanoate (PFOA) (Fig. 6.3a) and perfluorooctane sulfonate (PFOS) (Fig. 6.3b) are used as surfactants in the production of fluoro-polymers, grease and stain repellents, friction reducers (wiring, computers), and water-proofing and insulating agents and in fire-extinguishing foam, which has resulted in their widespread presence in the environment, and in human tissues, and are known to be toxic in animals and humans (White et al., 2011). PFCs are unusual chemically, in that they are both hydrophobic (repel water) and lipophobic (repel lipids/grease). They contain one of the strongest chemical bonds (C–F) known, which is resistant to hydrolysis, photolysis, and metabolism. Because of these properties, they are highly stable in the environment and are classified as persistent organic pollutants. Estimated half-lives of PFOS and PFOA in humans are 5.4 and 3.8 years, respectively (Olsen et al., 2007). Their persistence and accumulation properties, as well as toxicity in animal models, have raised concern over low-level chronic exposure effects on human health. PFOA was found in the serum of >99% of the general US population in the 2003–2004 National Health and Nutrition Examination Survey (NHANES), with a median concentration of 4.0 µg/l (Calafat et al., 2007). The US Environmental Protection Agency (EPA) has now listed PFOA and PFOS on the new CCL-3 (EPA, 2009).

Perfluorinated alkyl acids, including PFOA and PFOS, activate PPARα which has a critical role in modulating gene expression to maintain lipid homeostasis. It also plays important roles in regulating inflammatory responses, cell proliferation, and differentiation (Abbott, 2009), and enhances the catabolism and elimination of cholesterol (Pyper et al., 2010). PPARα is highly expressed in rodent liver but weakly expressed in humans. Laboratory rodents exposed to PFOA or PFOS

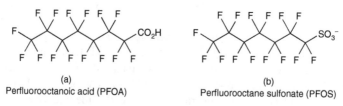

(a)
Perfluorooctanoic acid (PFOA)

(b)
Perfluorooctane sulfonate (PFOS)

Figure 6.3   PPARα agonists perfluoroalkyl compounds.

during gestation exhibited developmental effects such as reduced birth weight and increased neonatal mortality (Luebker et al., 2005). PFOA treatment during various critical developmental stages in mice has revealed general development toxicity and stimulatory to postnatal mammary gland development which may include long-lasting effects in reproductive tissues and metabolic reprogramming (Abbott, 2009; Abbott et al., 2007; White et al., 2011). Since PFOA is a known PPARα agonist, effects on the mammary gland may involve this pathway. However, the stimulatory effect of PFOA on mammary gland development observed in wild-type mice was also observed in PPARα knockout mice (C57Bl/6) at low dose (5 mg/kg) (Zhao et al., 2010; Yang et al., 2009), suggesting that this effect is independent of the expression of PPARα. PFOA, which is known to alter sexual maturation in animals, is also found to cause delayed puberty in children with high blood levels of PFOA (C&E News May 16, 2011).

A low-dose developmental exposure of PFOA (0.01, 0.1 mg PFOA per kilogram) on CD-1 female mouse led to significantly increased mean weight and rate of weight gain in mid-life (up to and including 37 weeks of age) than controls (Fig. 6.4) (Hines et al., 2009). These were found to be in agreement with low-dose hormone data that indicate important metabolic changes supporting the findings of increased weight. *In utero* exposure to PFOA in the mouse led to an extended developmental exposure period via lactational exposure (all of gestation and nearly 3 months postnatally). Once the offspring reached adulthood, they became obese, reaching significantly higher weight levels than controls.

In utero exposure to PFOS has been shown to adversely affect postnatal growth of surviving rat pups. PFOS-exposed pups lagged significantly behind controls in a dose-dependent manner (10–20%), and this effect persisted past weaning and body weight gain, although the onset of sexual maturation was not delayed (Lau et al., 2003; Luebker et al., 2005).

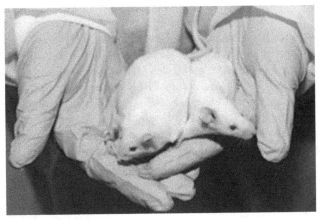

Figure 6.4   Mice exposed prenatally to PFOA were more likely than controls to become obese when they reached adulthood. Source: Adapted from Hines et al. (2009). Reproduced with permission from Elsevier.

In 2002, the 3M Company–a leading manufacturer of PFOS and PFOA–voluntarily stopped manufacturing both PFOS and the chemicals that degrade to form PFOS because they were accumulating in humans globally and in animals–such as polar bears–that live in remote areas (Butt et al., 2010). PFOS has a half-life in people of 4–5 years (Olsen et al., 2009). In May 2009, PFOS was included in Annex B of the Stockholm Convention on persistent organic pollutants by the Fourth Conference of Parties. In early 2006, the EPA, Teflon manufacturer DuPont, and seven other companies announced an agreement to reduce PFOA in emissions from manufacturing plants and in consumer products by 95% by the year 2010.

As opposed to the obesogen hypothesis, exposure to PFCs in rodents and monkeys has been demonstrated to have potent anorexigenic effects. PFCs, acting via PPARα, inhibit feeding behavior and weight gain (Asakawa et al., 2008).

6.2.3   Phthalates

Phthalates are widely used industrial chemicals that primarily serve as plasticizers to soften poly(vinyl chloride) (PVC) but are also found in cosmetics, perfumes, and certain drugs as well as in industrial paints and solvents. Contamination of phthalates occurs through environmental and food-chain sources. These are well-characterized inducers of hepatic peroxisome proliferation, and the phthalate monoesters appear to be the active metabolites that function as ligands of PPARs (Zoete et al., 2007; Bility et al., 2004). Several phthalate monoesters (MEHP, MBenP, and MButP) activate PPARα and PPARγ, and lower concentrations are required for activation of mouse PPARα than human PPARα (Hurst and Waxman, 2003). Various phthalates and their metabolites have documented biochemical activity as PPARγ activators, as thyroid hormone axis antagonists, or as anti-androgens.

Phthalates represent a class of candidate obesogens ingested from food sources with several metabolites present in more than 80% of the population and fetal exposure levels readily detectable. In mouse liver, DEHP activates PPARα and regulates the expression of its target genes (Eveillard et al., 2009). The DEHP metabolite mono-(2-ethylhexyl) phthalate (MEHP), in particular, is an agonist for PPARγ and selectively activates different PPARγ target genes and promotes adipogenesis (Feige et al., 2007; Desvergne et al., 2009). Prenatal exposure of mice to DEHP doses higher than 5 mg/kg body weight induces an anti-adipogenic effect, acting through activation of PPARα. By contrast, chronic exposure to this same dose induces adipogenesis through activation of PPARγ (Hurst and Waxman, 2003). An epidemiological study in male human subjects reported a positive and significant correlation between urinary phthalate levels (mono-benzyl phthalate and MEHP metabolites) in urine with increased waist diameter (Stahlhut et al., 2007). A positive correlation between urinary phthalate metabolites and body mass index (BMI) and measures of insulin resistance was also reported in women (Hatch et al., 2008).

Wild-type C57Bl6J mice treated with DEHP (100 and 1000 mg/kg body mass per day) after weaning at 3 weeks of age were protected from diet-induced obesity via PPARα-dependent activation of hepatic fatty acid catabolism (Feige et al., 2010). By using genetically modified mice in which the normal mouse PPARα gene was replaced with the human gene, it was observed that DEHP treatment did not induce expression of genes involved in fatty acid oxidation and was not effective in preventing weight gain of the "humanized mice" when placed on a high fat diet. In fact, the humanized mice treated with DEHP gained more weight and had an increase in epididymal white adipose mass compared to the wild-type animals (Feige et al., 2010). In another study in female C3H/N mice exposed to DEHP (0.05, 5, or 500 mg/kg of body weight per day), F0 generation had a significant increase in body weight, food intake, and visceral adipose tissue compared with controls (Schmidt et al., 2012). Similar metabolic changes were also observed in F1 offspring after *in utero* and lactational exposure. At weaning, exposed F1 offspring in both sexes had significantly increased body weight in the 5-mg DEHP group, and it remained elevated even after 9 weeks with standard chow without DEHP (Schimdt et al., 2012).

6.3   ARYL HYDROCARBON RECEPTOR (AhR) AGONISTS

AhR is an orphan receptor and not a member of the nuclear hormone receptor superfamily. It is a key player in the cellular defense against xenobiotic substances. AhR regulates enzymes that are important to the metabolism of both endogenous substances (e.g., hormones) and exogenous substances involved in both the detoxification and bioactivation of xenobiotics (Werck-Reichhart and Feyereisen, 2000). AhR can bind numerous chemicals and can indirectly affect metabolism of xenobiotics as well as steroid synthesis and metabolism. Crosstalk is thought to exist between AhR and ER and AR as well as other nuclear receptors. Several studies have documented that activated AhR inhibits the expression of E2-induced genes displaying anti-estrogenic effects (Safe and Wormke, 2003; Ohtake et al., 2011). The AhR has a constricted binding pocket of a 6.8 × 13.7 A° planar rectangle, and it has been shown that molecules that are nonplanar and/or do not fit in these dimensions are generally poor inducers of CYP450 via this receptor (Osimitz and Nelson, 2012).

AhR is an important mediator of the effects of polychlorinated dibenzo-*p*-dioxins (PCDDs, dioxins) and other planar dioxin-like aryl hydrocarbons. Other xenobiotics demonstrating a high affinity for AhR with similar toxic effects include polychlorinated dibenzofurans (PCDFs) substituted in the 2,3,7,8 lateral positions, and non-ortho and mono-ortho polychlorinated biphenyls (PCBs) such as dioxin-like 3,3′,4,4′,5-pentachlorobiphenyl (PCB126). PCDDs, PCDFs, and PCBs (Fig. 6.5) are ubiquitous environmental compounds.

6.3.1   Polychlorinated-Dibenzodioxins (PCDDs) and -Dibenzofurans (PCDFs)

PCDDs and PCDFs are unintentional byproducts of industrial or combustion processes involving chlorine, such as waste incineration, chemical manufacturing, and

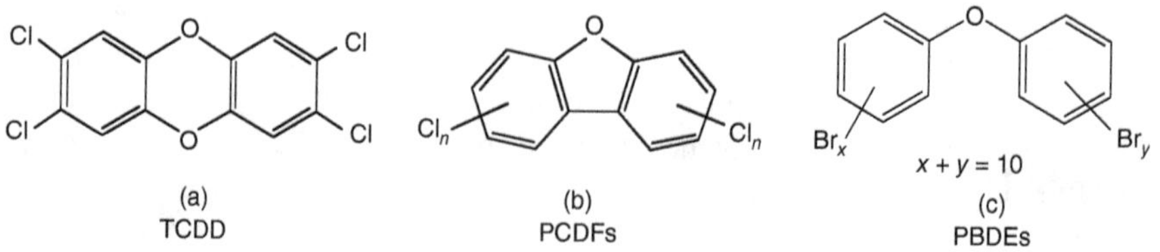

(a)	(b)	(c)
TCDD	PCDFs	PBDEs

Figure 6.5   AhR agonist polychlorinated dibenzodioxins, dibenzofurans, and biphenyls.

pulp or paper bleaching. These chemicals have been called the most toxic of all manmade chemicals, based on animal studies that show effects at extremely low doses—in the parts per trillion—and causally linked to developmental/reproductive toxicity in humans and wildlife species. The environmental contaminant TCDD has one of the lowest known LD_{50} (0.6 µg/kg of body weight) and it is also among the most potent agonists of AhR so far characterized. Exposures to these compounds have the potential to disrupt multiple endocrine pathways and induce toxic responses.

TCDD is an endocrine disrupter that acts on multiple components of the endocrine axis. TCDD exposure alters the levels of many hormones and growth factors, as well as their receptors, and has shown adverse effects in testicular function, including reduced sperm counts and motility. Agonists of the AhR form a complex with the receptor that acts as a transcription factor by binding to specific DREs (dioxin response elements) on specific genes. Most, if not all, of the toxicity of TCDD and dioxin-like compounds is thought to result from activation of the AhR. For example, three research groups independently produced AhR-null mice, deleting different exons of the AhR gene; these animals did not show TCDD-inducible toxicities (Yoshioka et al., 2011).

An explosion at a trichlorophenol manufacturing plant near Seveso, Italy, in July 1976 released up to 30 kg of TCDD. The relationship between serum TCDD concentrations and semen quality and male reproductive hormones was investigated in 135 males exposed 22 years later. The results demonstrated a reduction in E2 and a permanent effect on semen quality in human males after exposure especially in infancy/prepuberty, less in puberty, and not in adulthood, at levels seen in the general population of many industrialized countries. This has been attributed to disruptive action of low concentrations of TCDD on the endocrine system (Mocarelli et al., 2008).

In addition to reproductive, neurobehavioral, and immunological toxicities, TCDD is also thought to affect thyroid functions by AhR-mediated attenuation of sodium iodide symporter (NIS), negatively interfering with iodine uptake by the thyroid (Pocar et al., 2006). A single dose of TCDD decreased T4 and FT4 dose-dependently and increased thyroid-stimulating hormone (TSH) in adult rats (Boas et al., 2009). Given to pregnant rats, TCDD decreased T4 and increased TSH in male offspring. In Vietnam War veterans, the group with the highest exposure to TCDD had significantly higher TSH levels (Boas et al., 2009). Exposure of mouse

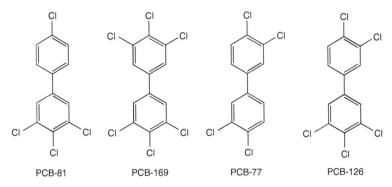

Figure 6.6 Structures of coplanar/non-ortho-substituted PCB congeners.

preimplantation embryos to TCDD was found to inhibit fetal growth in a response characterized by hypermethylation of the imprinted genes (Wu et al., 2004).

6.3.2 Coplanar Polychlorinated Biphenyls

PCBs have been frequently used in a variety of commercial applications, such as coolants and lubricants in transformers, capacitors, and other electrical equipments. Some PCBs act in a manner mechanistically similar to that of TCDD; these PCBs are usually referred to as *dioxin-like PCBs* (DL-PCBs). The four dioxin-like coplanar or non-ortho-substituted congeners of PCBs (PCB 77, -81, -126, and -169) (Fig. 6.6) and all eight mono-ortho-substituted analogs of the coplanar PCBs are structurally similar to PCDDs and PCDFs, and act in the same way as these molecules as an agonist of the AhR in organisms. TCDD and PCB 126 (3,3',4,4',5-pentachlorobiphenyl) treatment induced AhR signaling response by significant downregulation in the expression of NIS, which would restrict iodine intake by the thyroid (Pocar et al., 2006). Among the most potent PCB congeners, PCB-126 is about 100 times less potent than TCDD for inducing AhR-regulated enzyme activity in the Wistar rat (Safe, 1990).

Noncoplanar PCBs, with chlorine atoms at the ortho positions, have not been found to activate the AhR (Safe, 2001). Depending on the specific congeners, these PCBs are reported to act as estrogens or anti-androgens, or to change steroid and thyroid hormone levels through mechanisms such as displacing the natural hormones from their plasma-binding globulins or via the modulation of hormone metabolism in the liver (Kato et al., 2010).

6.3.3 Substituted Urea and Anilide Herbicides

Substituted urea herbicides diuron and linuron and the acetanilide herbicide propanil with a common chemical structure (Fig. 6.7) have been identified as potent AhR agonists in a sensitive reporter gene assay using a cell line that stably

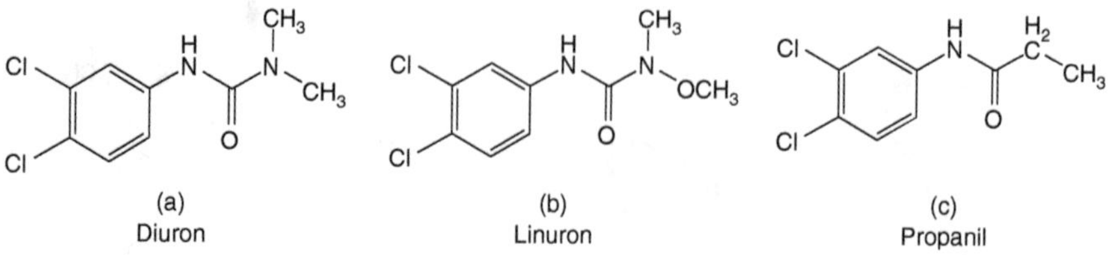

(a)   (b)   (c)
Diuron   Linuron   Propanil

Figure 6.7   AhR agonist herbicides with a common chemical structure.

expressed AhR-responsive luciferase reporter gene construct into mouse heptoma Hepa1c1c7 cells (Kojima et al., 2010). These chemicals were also found to be *in vivo* inducers of *CYP1A* genes in the mouse liver.

6.4   STEROIDOGENESIS MODULATOR (AROMATASE EXPRESSION INDUCER)

SF1 (NR5A1), a member of the orphan nuclear receptor superfamily, is an important regulator of downstream steroidogenic enzymes such as aromatase expression, and is a critical factor in vertebrate endocrine organ development, including male sexual differentiation (Hoivik et al., 2010).

6.4.1   Atrazine

Atrazine (2-chloro-4-ethylamino-6-isopropylamino-1,3,5-triazine) (Fig. 6.8) is a chlorinated-*s*-triazine group herbicide that effectively inhibits photosynthesis in broadleaf weeds and grasses. It has been extensively employed in the production of corn, sugarcane, and other crops in the United States. It is estimated that farmers apply more than 80 million pounds yearly to crops, most of it on corn in the Midwest (Chevrier et al., 2011). Atrazine is also used on golf courses, Christmas tree lots, and public lands. As a result, it is a most common pesticide contaminant of ground, surface, and drinking water (Benotti et al., 2009). A 2006 study by the US Geological Survey found atrazine in approximately 75% of stream water and about 40% of all groundwater supplies of Midwestern and southern agricultural areas of United States, where the pesticide is primarily applied. Individual drinking water samples collected under the Atrazine Monitoring Program have occasionally exceeded the

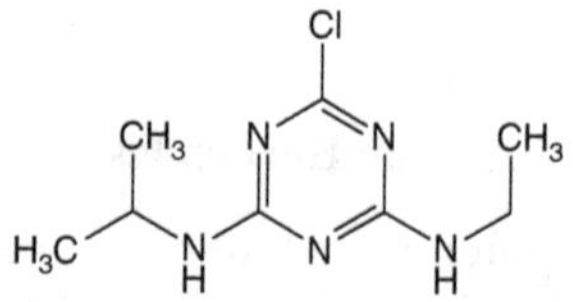

Figure 6.8   Atrazine.

maximum contaminant level (MCL) for long-term exposure of 3 ppb; in 2009 and 2010, 4% and 7% of the samples, respectively, were above the MCL (EPA, 2011).

Atrazine is found to be a potent endocrine disruptor that is active at low ecologically relevant concentrations. The EU banned it in 2001 because of health concerns and the inability to keep concentrations at safe levels in drinking water supplies. Atrazine was found to be resistant to chlorine or ozone oxidation and was detected in more than half of finished drinking waters tested in 19 US drinking water treatment plants (DWTPs) during 2006–2007 (Benotti et al., 2009). The EPA considers an atrazine concentration of ≤3 ppb in drinking water safe for consumption. The EPA is currently reevaluating the safety of atrazine because of a growing body of scientific literature linked to reproductive abnormalities in fish and amphibians that raise concerns about the chemical's safety.

Exposure to atrazine levels found in the environment affects hormone signaling and endocrine transcriptional networks in fish and in mammalian cells with reduced immune function as well as sex organ development and function. Atrazine at exposure levels of 0.1–25 µg/l (doses 30 times lower than allowed by the EPA of 3 ppb) caused tadpoles to develop both male and female sex characteristics, turning them into hermaphrodites (Hayes et al., 2002a, 2002b). It also lowered testosterone levels in adult male frogs below the level found in females. The reproductive consequences of atrazine exposure in adult male frogs often showed signs of feminization with lower testosterone levels and decreased fertility. Some were chemically castrated and grew female sex organs (Hayes et al., 2010). Hayes and colleagues further demonstrated that atrazine exposure during development induced demasculization and feminization of male gonads consistently across vertebrate classes including fish, amphibians, reptiles, and mammals (Hayes et al., 2011).

A study found that atrazine's affects are often nonmonotonic, indicating that there may be physiological effects at low doses and that these effects may be different from those observed at high doses. It showed an "inverted-U" shaped dose–response curve in the anti-androgen screen, whereby effects were observed at high and low concentrations, but not middle concentrations (Orton et al., 2009). For example, atrazine affected how fish swam, and the exposures increased hyperactivity at the lower concentrations but not at higher levels. Atrazine has been found to be both agonistic and antagonistic at different concentrations in the anti-androgen screen (androgenic: 3.9–31.3 µM, µg/l; anti-androgenic: 125–1000 µM). Atrazine had a stimulatory effect in the anti-androgen screen (i.e., yeast androgen screen, YAS) but it did not behave as AR agonists in the absence of testosterone (Orton et al., 2009).

Recent *in vitro* data suggest that one mechanism by which atrazine exerts its endocrine disrupting effects is by enhancing the activity or expression of the enzyme aromatase (Cyp19A), by binding to and inhibiting phosphodiesterase, causing reduction in androgen levels by increased conversion of testosterone to estrogen (Hayes et al., 2011; Holloway et al., 2008; Fan et al., 2007; Sanderson et al., 2001). At low doses, atrazine (0.1–3 µg/l) significantly activated the endogenous levels of gonadal aromatase in zebrafish embryos and adversely influenced normal hormone signaling, posing a potential risk to the reproductive health of young fish (Suzawa and Ingraham, 2008). Atrazine treatment increased aromatase activity in tumor cell lines, increasing local tissue estrogen levels in estrogen-sensitive target tissues (Holloway et al., 2008). It has been shown to alter the developing mammary gland, and makes it susceptible to mammary tumors in Fischer 344 rats and increased plasma levels of estradiol in female Sprague–Dawley rats (Wetzel et al., 1994).

Enhancing the activity or expression of aromatase may increase rates of estrogen synthesis, thereby mediating estrogenic effects. However, atrazine is not estrogenic and does not directly interface with classic estrogen signaling, and therefore its precise mechanism of action remains controversial. Nevertheless, atrazine activates the orphan nuclear receptor SF-1 (NR5A1) and it has been shown that the induction of aromatase by atrazine is dependent upon SF-1 related regulatory pathways (Fan et al., 2007; Suzawa and Ingraham, 2008).

In another study to explore biological pathways and mechanism of toxicity of developmental atrazine exposures, zebrafish embryos exposed to atrazine at environmental levels showed changes in their genes. These genes were associated with neuroendocrine and reproductive system development, and function in the fish and work in similar ways in humans (Weber et al., 2013).

6.5 CONCLUSIONS AND FUTURE PROSPECTS

Although EDCs can affect every possible cellular hormonal pathway, most information is available about interference of EDCs with the steroid hormone receptors as well as thyroid hormone receptors. There is emerging evidence that exposure to several environmental chemicals is associated with obesity and related diseases, even though a cause–effect relationship between the two events has still to be demonstrated. Until the 1990s, fat cells or adipocytes were considered to be just storage depots for excess metabolic fuel. However, following the discovery of an adipocyte-derived hormone leptin which communicates energy reserve information from adipocytes to other organs of the body including the central nervous system, a new appreciation has emerged that these fat storage cells actually function as an endocrine organ (Collins, 2005). Agonist ligands for nuclear receptors RXR and PPARγ play pivotal roles in lipid homeostasis and adipogenesis. Particularly, PPARγ is considered a master regulator of adipogenesis (Tontonoz and Spiegelman 2008). PPARs and RXR have been shown to be targets for EDC action. Several studies suggest a role in obesity for the organotins TBT and TPT, which are potent agonists of PPARγ and RXR, influencing lipid biosynthesis and storage.

About 35% of US adults are categorized as clinically obese, that is, at least 20% heavier than their ideal weight, and 68% are overweight, more than double the worldwide average (Flegal et al., 2012). The obesity is defined as (i) BMI $\geq 30 \, kg/m^2$ and (ii) waist circumference (WC) ≥ 102 cm in men and ≥ 88 cm in women (NCEP, 2002). A recent trend is seen in the increasing rate of obesity in very young children and even in infants, with nearly 17% of children aged 2–9 years are obese (Ogden et al., 2012). Increased obesity has been observed in animals (pets such as cats and dogs, laboratory animals such as rats, mice, and primates, and feral rats) living in proximity to humans in industrialized societies (Klimentidis et al., 2011). The onset of obesity involves extensive remodeling of adipose tissue at the cellular level and is dependent on the coordinated interplay between adipocyte hypertrophy (increase of fat cell size) and hyperplasia (increase of fat cell number). Chemical "obesogens," a term coined by Bruce Blumberg at the University of California, Irvine, may alter human metabolism and predispose some people to gain weight. Fetal and early-life exposures to certain obesogens may alter some individuals' metabolism and fat-cell makeup for life. However, the molecular mechanisms behind a possible involvement of EDCs, so called obesogens, in obesity are poorly understood.

There is emerging evidence that exposure to several environmental chemicals is associated with obesity and related diseases, even though a cause–effect relationship between the two events has still to be demonstrated. Until the 1990s, fat cells or adipocytes were considered to be just storage depots for excess metabolic fuel. However, following the discovery of an adipocyte-derived hormone leptin, which communicates energy reserve information from adipocytes to other organs of the body including the central nervous system, a new appreciation has emerged that these fat storage cells actually function as an endocrine organ (Collins, 2005). Agonist ligands for nuclear receptors retinoid X receptor (RXRα, RXRβ, and RXRγ) and PPARγ play pivotal roles in lipid homeostasis and adipogenesis. Particularly, PPARγ is considered a master regulator of adipogenesis (Tontonoz and Spiegelman, 2008).

REFERENCES

Abbott, B. D. Review of the expression of peroxisome proliferator-activated receptors alpha (PPAR alpha), beta (PPAR beta), and gamma (PPAR gamma) in rodent and human development, *Reprod. Toxicol.* **2009**, 27(3–4), 246–257.

Abbott, B. D.; Wolf, C. J.; Schmid, J. E., et al., Perfluorooctanoic acid-induced developmental toxicity in the mouse is dependent on expression of peroxisome proliferator-activated receptor-alpha, *Toxicol. Sci.* **2007**, 98(2), 571–581.

Asakawa, A.; Toyoshima, M.; Harada, K. H.; Fujimiya, M.; Inoue, K.; Koizumi, A. The ubiquitous environmental pollutant perfluorooctanoic acid inhibits feeding behavior via peroxisome proliferator-activated receptor-alpha, *Int. J. Mol. Med.* **2008**, 21, 439–445.

Benotti, M. J.; Trenholm, R. A.; Vanderford, B. J.; Holady, J. C.; Stanford, B. D.; Snyder, S. A. Pharmaceuticals and endocrine disrupting compounds in U.S. drinking water, *Environ. Sci. Technol.* **2009**, 43(3), 597–603.

Berger, J.; Moller, D. E. The mechanisms of action of PPARs, *Annu. Rev. Med.* **2002**, 53, 409–435.

Bility, M. T.; Thompson, J. T.; McKee, R. H.; David, R. M.; Butala, J. H., Heuvel, J. P. V.; Peters, J. M. Activation of mouse and human peroxisome proliferator-activated receptors (PPARs) by phthalate monoesters, *Toxicol. Sci.* **2004**, 82, 170–182.

Blumberg, B. Obesogens, stem cells and the maternal programming of obesity, *J. Develop. Orig. Health Disease* **2011**, 2(1), 3–8.

Boas, M.; Main, K. M.; Feldt-Rasmussen, U. Environmental chemicals and thyroid function: an update, *Curr. Opin. Endocrinol. Diabet. Obes.* **2009**, 16(5), 385–391.

Boberg, J.; Metzdorff, S.; Wortziger, R.; Axelstad, M.; Brokken, L.; Vinggaard, A. M.; Dalgaard, M.; Nellemann, C. Impact of diisobutyl phthalate and other PPAR agonists on steroidogenesis and plasma insulin and leptin levels in fetal rats, *Toxicology* **2008**, 250(2–3), 75–81.

Butt, C. M.; Berger, U.; Bossi, R.; Tomy, G. T. Levels and trends of poly- and perfluorinated compounds in the arctic environment, *Sci. Total Environ.* **2010**, 408, 2936–2965.

Calafat, A. M.; Wong, L. Y.; Kuklenyik, Z.; Reidy, J. A.; Needham, L. L. Polyfluoroalkyl chemicals in the U.S. population: data from the National Health and Nutrition Examination Survey (NHANES) 2003–2004 and comparisons with NHANES 1999–2000, *Environ. Health Perspect.* **2007**, 115, 1596–1602.

Chamorro-García, R.; Sahu, M.; Abbey, R. J.; Laude J.; Pham, N.; Blumberg, B. Transgenerational inheritance of increased fat depot size, stem cell reprogramming, and hepatic steatosis elicited by prenatal exposure to the obesogen tributyltin in mice, *Environ. Health Perspect.* **2013**, 121, 359–366.

Chevrier, C.; Limon, G.; Monfort, C.; Rouget, F.; Garlantézec, R., et al. 2011 urinary biomarkers of prenatal atrazine exposure and adverse birth outcomes in the PELAGIE birth cohort. *Environ. Health Perspect.* **2011**, 119(7), 1034–1041.

Collins, S. Overview of clinical perspectives and mechanisms of obesity, *Birth Defects Res. A Clin. Mol. Teratol.* **2005**, 73(7), 470–471.

D'eon, J. C.; Mabury, S. A. Is indirect exposure a significant contributor to the burden of perfluorinated acids observed in humans? *Environ. Sci. Technol.* **2011**, 45, 7974–7984.

Desvergne, B.; Wahli, W. Peroxisome proliferator-activated receptors: nuclear control of metabolism, *Endocr. Rev.* **1999**, 20(5), 649–688.

Desvergne, B.; Feige, J. N.; Casals-Casas, C. PPAR-mediated activity of phthalates: a link to the obesity epidemic? *Mol. Cell. Endocrinol.* **2009**, 304 (1–2), 43–48.

EPA, *Water Contaminant Candidate List 3–CCL*, 2009. Available at http://water.epa.gov/scitech/drinkingwater/dws/ccl/ccl3.cfm (accessed October 10, 2009).

EPA. *Atrazine post-RED results: Office of Pesticide Programs' Monitoring in Community Water Systems, 2011 atrazine monitoring program (AMP) drinking water data*, 2011. Available at http://www.epa.gov/opp00001/reregistration/atrazine/atrazine_update.htm #cws (accessed May 11, 2011).

Eveillard, A.; Mselli-Lakhal, L.; Mogha, A.; Lasserre, F.; Polizzi, A.; Pascussi, J. M.; Guillou, H.; Martin, P. G.; Pineau, T. Di-(2-ethylhexyl)-phthalate (DEHP) activates the constitutive androstane receptor (CAR): a novel signalling pathway sensitive to phthalates, *Biochem. Pharmacol.* **2009**, 77(11), 1735–1746.

Fan, W.; Yanase, T.; Morinaga, H.; Gondo, S.; Okabe, T., Nomura, M.; Komatsu, T.; Morohashi, K.; Hayes, T. B.; Takayanagi, R.; Nawata, H. Atrazine-induced aromatase expression is SF-1 dependent: implications for endocrine disruption in wildlife and reproductive cancers in humans, *Environ. Health Perspect.* **2007**, 115(5), 720–727.

Feige, J. N., Gelman, L.; Rossi, D.; Zoete, V.; Métivier, R.; Tudor, C.; Anghel, S. I.; Grosdidier, A.; Lathion, C.; Engelborghs, Y.; Michielin, O.; Wahli, W.; Desvergne, B. The endocrine disruptor mono-ethyl-hexyl-phthalate is a selective peroxisome proliferator-activated receptor gamma modulator that promotes adipogenesis, *J. Biol. Chem.* **2007**, 282(26), 19152–19166.

Feige, J. N.; Gerber, A.; Casals-Casas, C.; Yang, Q.; Winkler, C., Bedu, E.; Bueno, M.; Gelman, L.; Auwerx, J.; Gonzalez, F. J.; Desvergne, B. The pollutant diethylhexyl phthalate regulates hepatic energy metabolism via species-specific PPARα-dependent mechanisms, *Environ. Health Perspect.* **2010**, 118(2), 234–241.

Flegal, K. M., Carroll, M. D.; Kit, B. K.; Ogden, C. L. Prevalence of obesity and trends in the distribution of body mass index among US adults, 1999–2010, *JAMA* **2012**, 307(5), 491–497.

Grün, F.; Blumberg, B. Endocrine disrupters as obesogens. *Mol. Cell. Endocrinol.* **2009**, 304, 19–29.

Grün, F.; Blumberg, B. Environmental obesogens: organotins and endocrine disruption via nuclear receptor signaling, *Endocrinology* **2006**, 147, S50–S55.

Grün, F.; Watanabe, H.; Zamanian, Z.; Maeda, L.; Arima, K.; Cubacha, R.; Gardiner, D. M.; Kanno, J.; Iguchi, T.; Blumberg, B. Endocrine-disrupting organotin compounds are potent inducers of adipogenesis in vertebrates, *Mol. Endocrinol.* **2006**, 20(9), 2141–2155.

Hatch, E. E.; Nelson, J. W.; Qureshi, M. M., et al. Association of urinary phthalate metabolite concentrations with body mass index and waist circumference: a cross-sectional study of NHANES data, 1999–2002, *Environ. Health* **2008**, 7, article 27.

Hayes, T.; Haston, K.; Tsui, M.; Hoang, A.; Haeffele, C., et al. Herbicides: feminization of male frogs in the wild, *Nature* **2002a**, 419, 895–896.

Hayes, T.; Collins, A.; Lee, M.; Mendoza, M.; Noriega, N., et al. Hermaphroditic, demasculinized frogs after exposure to the herbicide atrazine at low ecologically relevant doses, *Proc. Natl. Acad. Sci. U. S. A.* **2002b**, 99, 5476–5480.

Hayes, T. B.; Khoury, V.; Narayan, A.; Nazir, M.; Park, A.; Brown, T.; Adame, L.; Chan, E.; Buchholz, D.; Stueve, T.; Gallipeau, S. Atrazine induces complete feminization and chemical castration in male African clawed frogs (Xenopus Laevis), *Proc. Natl. Acad. Sci. U. S. A.* **2010**, 107(10), 4612–4617.

Hayes, T. B.; Anderson, L. L.; Beasley, V. R.; de Solla, S. R.; Iguchi, T.; Ingraham, H.; Kestemont, P.; Kniewald, J.; Kniewald, Z.; Langlois, V. S.; Luque, E. H.; McCoy, K. A.; Muñoz-de-Toro, M.; Oka, T.; Oliveira, C. A.; Orton, F.; Ruby, S.; Suzawa, M.; Tavera-Mendoza, L. E.; Trudeau, V. L.; Victor-Costa, A. B.; Willingham, E. Demasculinization and feminization of male gonads by atrazine: consistent effects across vertebrate classes, *J. Steroid Biochem. Mol. Biol.* **2011**, 127, 64–73.

Hines, E. P.; White, S. S.; Stanko, J. P.; Gibbs-Flournoy, E. A.; Lau, C.; Fenton, S. E. Phenotypic dichotomy following developmental exposure to perfluorooctanoic acid (PFOA) in female CD-1 mice: low doses induce elevated serum leptin and insulin, and overweight in mid-life, *Mol. Cell. Endocrinol.* **2009**, 304(1–2), 97–105.

Hiromori, Y.; Nishikawa, J.; Yoshida, I.; Nagase, H.; Nakanishi, T. Structure-dependent activation of peroxisome proliferator-activated receptor (PPAR) gamma by organotin compounds, *Chem. Biol. Interact.* **2009**, 180(2), 238–244.

Hoivik, E. A.; Lewis, A. E.; Aumo, L.; Bakke, M. Molecular aspects of steroidogenic factor 1 (SF-1), *Mol. Cell. Endocrinol.* **2010**, 315, 27–39.

Holloway, A. C.; Anger, D. A.; Crankshaw, D. J.; Wu, M.; Foster, W. G. Atrazine-induced changes in aromatase activity in estrogen-sensitive target tissues, *J. Appl. Toxicol.* **2008**, 28(3), 260–270.

Hurst, C. H.; Waxman, D. J. Activation of PPARalpha and PPARgamma by environmental phthalate monoesters, *Toxicol. Sci.* **2003**, 74, 297–308.

Jacobson, A. H.; Willingham, G. L. Sea-Nine antifoulant: an environmentally acceptable alternative to organotin antifoulants, *Sci. Total Environ.* **2000**, 258(1-2), 103–110.

Janesick, A.; Blumberg, B. Minireview: PPARγ as the target of obesogens, *J. Steroid Biochem. Mol. Biol.* **2011a**, 127, 4–8.

Janesick, A.; Blumberg, B. Endocrine disrupting chemicals and the developmental programming of adipogenesis and obesity, *Birth Defects Res. C Embryo Today* **2011b**, 93(1), 34–50.

Kanayama, T.; Kobayashi, N.; Mamiya, S.; Nakanishi, T.; Nishikawa, J. Organotin compounds promote adipocyte differentiation as agonists of the peroxisome proliferator-activated receptor-γ/retinoid X receptor pathway, *Mol. Pharmacol.* **2005**, 67, 766–774.

Kato, Y.; Haraguchi, K.; Ito, Y.; Fujii, A.; Yamazaki, T.; Endo, T.; Koga, N.; Yamada, S.; Degawa, M. Polychlorinated biphenyl-mediated decrease in serum thyroxine level in rodents, *Drug Metab. Dispos.* **2010**, 38(4), 697–704.

Klimentidis, Y. C., et al. Canaries in the coal mine: a cross-species analysis of plurality of obesity epidemics, *Proc. Biol. Sci.* **2011**, 278, 1626–1632.

Kojima, H.; Takeuchi, S.; Nagai, T. Endocrine-disrupting potential of pesticides via nuclear receptors and aryl hydrocarbon receptor, *J. Health Sci.* **2010**, 56(4), 374–386.

Kwintkiewicz, J.; Nishi, Y.; Yanase, T.; Giudice, L. C. Peroxisome proliferator–activated receptor-γ mediates bisphenol A inhibition of FSH-stimulated IGF-1, aromatase, and estradiol in human granulosa cells, *Environ. Heath Perspect.* **2010**, 118(3), 400–406.

Lau, C.; Thibodeaux, J. R.; Hanson, R. G.; Rogers, J. M.; Grey, B. E.; Stanton, M. E.; Butenhoff, J. L.; Stevenson, L. A. Exposure to perfluorooctane sulfonate during pregnancy in rat and mouse. II. Postnatal evaluation, *Toxicol. Sci.* **2003**, 74, 382–392.

Lau, C.; Abbott, B. D.; Corton, J. C.; Cunningham, M. L. PPARs and xenobiotic-induced adverse effects: relevance to human health, *PPAR Res.* **2010**, 95463; doi: 10.1155/2010/954639.

Luebker, D. J.; York, R. G.; Hansen, K. J.; Moore, J. A.; Butenhoff, J. L. Neonatal mortality from in utero exposure to perfluorooctanesulfonate (PFOS) in Sprague-Dawley rats: dose-response, and biochemical and pharamacokinetic parameters. *Toxicology* **2005**, 215, 149–169.

le Maire, A.; Bourguet, W., Balaguer, P. A structural view of nuclear hormone receptor: endocrine disruptor interactions, *Cell. Mol. Life Sci.* **2010**, 67, 1219–1237.

Mocarelli, P.; Gerthoux, P. M.; Patterson, D. G. Jr.,; Milani, S.; Limonta, G.; Bertona, M.; Signorini, S.; Tramacere, P.; Colombo, L.; Crespi, C.; Brambilla, P.; Sarto, C.; Carreri, V.; Sampson, E. J.; Turner, W. E.; Needham, L. L. Dioxin exposure, from infancy through puberty, produces endocrine disruption and affects human semen quality, *Environ. Health Perspect.* **2008**, 116(1), 70–77.

NCEP, Third report of the National Cholesterol Education Program (NCEP) expert panel on detection, evaluation, and treatment of high blood cholesterol in adults (Adult Treatment Panel III) final report, *Circulation* **2002**, 106, 3143–3421.

Nishikawa, J. Imposex in marine gastropods may be caused by binding of organotins to retinoid X receptor, *Marine Biol.* **2006**, 149, 117–124.

Nishikawa, J.; Mamiya, S.; Kanayama, T.; Nishikawa, T.; Shiraishi, F.; Horiguchi, T. Involvement of the retinoid X receptor in the development of imposex caused by organotins in gastropods, *Environ. Sci. Technol.* **2004**, 38, 6271–6276.

Oberdörster, E.; McClellan-Green, P. Mechanisms of imposex induction in the mud snail, Ilyanassa obsoleta: TBT as a neurotoxin and aromatase inhibitor, *Mar. Environ. Res.* **2002**, 54, 715–718.

Oehlmann, J.; Di Benedetto, P.; Tillmann, M.; Duft, M.; Oetken, M.; Schulte-Oehlmamm, U. Endocrine disruption in prosobranch molluscs: evidence and ecological relevance, *Ecotoxicology* **2007**, 16(1), 29–43.

Ogden, C. L., Carroll, M. D.; Kit, B. K.; Flegal, K. M. Prevalence of obesity and trends in body mass index among US children and adolescents, 1999–2010, *JAMA* **2012**, 307(5), 483–490.

Ohtake, F.; Fujii-Kuriyama, Y.; Kawajiri, K.; Kato, S.; Cross-talk of dioxin and estrogen receptor signals through the ubiquitin system, *J. Steroid Biochem. Mol. Biol.* **2011**, 127, 102–107.

Olsen, G. W.; Burris, J. M.; Ehresman, D. J.; Froehlich, J. W.; Seacat, A. M.; Butenhoff, J. L.; Zobel, L. R. Half-life and serum elimination of perfluorooctanesulfonate, perfluorohexane-sulfonate, and pefluorooctanoate in retired fluorochemical production workers, *Environ. Health Perspect.* **2007**, 115, 1298–1305.

Olsen, G. W.; Chang, S. C.; Noker, P. E.; Gorman, G. S.; Ehresman, D. J.; Lieder, P. H.; Butenhoff, J. L. A comparison of the pharmacokinetics of perfluorobutanesulfonate (PFBS) in rats, monkeys, and human, *Toxicology* **2009**, 256, 65–74.

Orton, F.; Lutz, I.; Kloas, W.; Routledge, E. J. Endocrine disrupting effects of herbicides and pentachlorophenol: in vitro and in vivo evidence, *Environ. Sci. Technol.* **2009**, 43(9), 2144–2150.

Osimitz, T. G.; Nelson, J. L. Understanding mechanisms of metabolic transformations as a tool for designing safer chemicals, in *Handbook of Green Chemistry Volume 9: Designing Safer Chemicals*, Boethling, R. and Voutchkova, A., eds., Wiley-VCH Verlag GmbH, **2012**, pp. 47–75.

Pocar, P.; Klonisch, T.; Brandsch, C.; Eder, K.; Frohlich, C.; Hoang-Vu, C.; Hombach-Klonisch, S. AhR-Agonist-induced transcriptional changes of genes involved in thyroid function in primary porcine thyrocytes, *Toxicol. Sci.* **2006**, 89(2), 408–414.

Pyper, S. R.; Viswakarma, N.; Yu, S.; Reddy, J. K. PPARα: energy combustion, hypolipidemia, inflammation and cancer, *Nucl. Recept. Signal.* **2010**, 8, e002.

Safe, S. Polychlorinated biphenyls (PCBs), dibenzo-p-dioxins (PCDDs), and related compounds: Environmental and mechanistic considerations, which support the development of toxic equivalency factors (TEFs), *Crit. Rev. Toxicol.* **1990**, 21, 51–88.

Safe, S. PCBs as aryl hydrocarbon receptor agonists: implications for risk assessment, in *PCBs: Recent Advances in Environmental Toxicology and Health Effects*, Robertson, L. W. and Hansen, L. G., eds., The University Press of Kentucky, **2001**, pp. 171–175.

Safe, S.; Wormke, M. Inhibitory aryl hydrocarbon receptor-estrogen receptor α cross-talk and mechanisms of action, *Chem. Res. Toxicol.* **2003**, 16, 807–816.

Sanderson, J. T.; Letcher, R. J.; Heneweer, M., et al. Effects of chloro-S-triazine herbicides and metabolites on aromatase activity in various human cell lines and on vitellogenin production in male carp hepatocytes, *Environ. Health Perspect.* **2001**, 109, 1027–1031.

Schmidt, J. S.; Schaedlich, K.; Fiandanese, N.; Pocar, P.; Fischer, B. Effects of di(2-ethylhexyl) phthalate (DEHP) on female fertility and adipogenesis in C3H/N Mice, *Environ. Health Perspect.* **2012**, 120(8), 1123–1129.

Shearer, B. G.; Hoekstra, W. J. Recent advances in peroxisome proliferator-activated receptor science, *Curr. Med. Chem.* **2003**, 10, 267–280.

Smith, B. S. Male characteristics on female mud snails caused by antifouling bottom paints, *J. Appl. Toxicol.* **1981**, 1, 22–25.

Sousa, A.; Laranjeiro, F.; Takahashi, S.; Tanabe, S.; Barroso, C. M. Imposex and organotin prevalence in a European post-legislative scenario: temporal trends from 2003 to 2008, *Chemosphere* **2009**, 77, 566–573.

Sousa, A. C. A.; Barroso, C. M.; Tanabe, S.; Horiguchi, T. Involvement of retinoid X receptor in impox development in *Nucella lapillus* and *Nassarius reticulates*–preliminary results, in *Biological Responses to Contaminants: from Molecular to Community Level*, Hamamura, N., Suzuki, S., Mendo, S., Barrospo, C. M., Iwata, H., S. Tanabe, eds., TERRAPUB, Tokyo, Japan, **2010**, pp. 189–196.

Stahlhut, R. W.; van Wijgaarden, E.; Dye, T. D.; Cook, S.; Swan, S. H. Concentrations of urinary phthalate metabolites are associated with increased waist circumference and insulin resistance in adult U.S. males, *Environ. Health Perspect.* **2007**, 115, 876–882.

Sternberg, R. M.; Gooding, M. P.; Hotchkiss, A. K.; LeBlanc, G. A. Environmental-endocrine control of reproductive maturation in gastropods: implications for the mechanism of tributyltin-induced imposex in prosobranchs, *Ecotoxicology.* **2010**, 19(1), 4–23.

Suzawa, M.; Ingraham, H. A. The herbicide atrazine activates endocrine gene networks via non-steroidal NR5A nuclear receptors in fish and mammalian cells, *PLoS ONE* **2008**, 3(5), e2117, 11 pages.

Tontonoz, P.; Spiegelman, B. M.; Fat and beyond: the diverse biology of PPARgamma, *Annu. Rev. Biochem.* **2008**, 77, 289–312.

Weber, G. J.; Sepúlveda, M. S.; Peterson, S. M.; Lewis, S. S.; Freeman, J. L. Transcriptome alterations following developmental atrazine exposure in zebrafish are associated with disruption of neuroendocrine and reproductive system function, cell cycle, and carcinogenesis, *Toxicol. Sci.* **2013**, 132(2), 458–466.

Werck-Reichhart, D.; Feyereisen, R. Cytochromes P450: a success story, *Genome Biol.* **2000**, 1(6), Article ID REVIEWS3003, 2000.

Wetzel, L. T.; Luempert, L. G. III,; Breckenridge, C. B.; Tisdel, M. O.; Stevens, J. T.; Thakur, A. K.; Extrom, P. J.; Eldridge, J. C. Chronic effects of atrazine on estrus and mammary tumor formation in female Sprague–Dawley and Fischer 344 rats, *J. Toxicol. Environ. Health* **1994**, 43, 169–182.

White, S. S.; Fenton, S. E.; Hines, E. P. Endocrine disrupting properties of perfluorooctanoic acid, *J. Steroid Biochem. Mol. Biol.*, **2011**, 127(1–2), 16–26.

Wolf, C. J.; Takacs, M. L.; Schmid, J. E.; Lau, C.; Abbott, B. D. Activation of mouse and human peroxisome proliferator-activated receptor alpha by perfluoroalkyl acids of different functional groups and chain lengths, *Toxicol. Sci.* **2008**, 106(1), 162–171.

Wu, Q.; Ohsako, S.; Ishimura, R.; Suzuki, J. S.; Tohyama, C. Exposure of mouse preimplantation embryos to 2,3,7,8-tetrachlorodibenzop-dioxin (TCDD) alters the methylation status of imprinted genes H19 and Igf2, *Biol. Reprod.* **2004**, 70(6), 1790–1797.

Xu, H. E.; Lambert, M. H.; Montana, V. G.; Parks, D. J.; Blanchard, S. G.; Brown, P. J.; Sternbach, D. D.; Lehmann, J. M.; Wisely, G. B.; Willson, T. M.; Kliewer, S. A.; Milburn, M. V. Molecular recognition of fatty acids by peroxisome proliferator-activated receptors, *Mol. Cell* **1999**, 3, 397–403.

Yang, C.; Tan, Y. S.; Harkema, J. R.; Haslam, S. Z. Differential effects of peripubertal exposure to perfluorooctanoic acid on mammary gland development in C57Bl/6 and Balb/c mouse strains. *Reprod. Toxicol.* **2009**, 27, 299–306.

Yoshioka, W.; Peterson, R. E.; Tohyama, C. Molecular targets that link dioxin exposure to toxicity phenotypes, *J. Steroid Biochem. Mol. Biol.* **2011**, 127, 96–101.

Zhao, Y.; Tan, Y. S.; Haslam, S. Z.; Yang, C. Perfluorooctanoic acid effects on steroid hormone and growth factor levels mediate stimulation of peripubertal mammary gland development in C57Bl/6 mice, *Toxicol. Sci.* **2010**, 115(1), 214–224.

Zoete, V.; Grosdidier, A.; Michielin, O. Peroxisome proliferator-activated receptor structures: ligand specificity, molecular switch and interactions with regulators, *Biochim. Biophys. Acta* **2007**, 1771, 915–925.

Zuo, Z.; Chen, S.; Wu, T.; Zhang, J.; Su, Y.; Chen, Y.; Wang, C. Tributyltin causes obesity and hepatic steatosis in male mice, *Environ. Toxicol.* **2011**, 26(1), 79–85.

7

EFFECTS OF EDC MIXTURES

7.1 INTRODUCTION

When individuals and populations are exposed to an endocrine disruptor chemical (EDC), it is likely that other environmental pollutants are involved because contamination of environments is rarely due to a single compound (Diamanti-Kandarakis et al., 2009). As a result, the field of "mixtures toxicology" is emerging as an area of increasing scientific and regulatory focus. A view has persisted that combination effects do not occur when each chemical is present at doses equal to their no-observed-adverse-effect-levels (NOAELs), or lower (COT, 2002; VKM, 2008). NOAEL is the highest tested dose at which no statistically or biologically adverse effects can be identified and is used for establishing "acceptable" exposures for humans (Christiansen et al., 2009). Now there is good evidence to show that the combined effects of endocrine disruptors (EDs) belonging to the same category (e.g., estrogenic-, anti-androgenic-, or thyroid-disrupting agents) can be predicted by using dose addition (DA; US EPA, 2000). This is true for a variety of endpoints representing a wide range of organizational levels and biological complexity. Combinations of EDCs are able to produce a significant effect even when each chemical is present at low doses that individually do not induce observable effects.

7.2 COMBINED EFFECT OF EXPOSURE TO MULTIPLE CHEMICALS

For predicting the effects of chemical mixtures, most models used the concepts of dose and effect addition. Dose or concentration addition is the widely accepted reference model in environmental toxicology and applies to all mixtures of compounds

Endocrine Disruptors in the Environment, First Edition. Sushil K. Khetan.

that act according to a common mode of action (US EPA, 2000). Kortenkamp (2007) has proposed that EDs should be grouped according to their ability to induce similar effects (as opposed to similar mechanisms) until better mechanistic information is forthcoming. Dose (concentration) additivity means that mixture effects are to be expected even when each chemical is present below zero-effect levels, because it is assumed that all toxicants in the mixture behave as if they were a dilution of one another. DA assumes that each chemical contributes to the mixture's toxicity in direct proportion to the individual toxic unit, that is, its concentration and potency, and that the response to the mixture is the same as that expected from an equivalent dose of an index chemical. The equivalent dose is the sum of compound doses scaled by their toxic potency relative to the index chemical (US EPA, 2000). The concept of DA can be mathematically formulated as follows:

$$ECx_{mix} = \left(\sum_{i=1}^{n} \frac{p_i}{ECx_i} \right)^{-1} \tag{7.1}$$

where ECx_{mix} is the total concentration of the mixture provoking $x\%$ effect, n denotes the number of mixture components, p_i is the concentration of chemical i in the total mixture concentration (i.e., $p_i = c_i/c_{mix}$), and ECx_i is the effective concentration of the ith compound in the mixture which on its own produces the same quantitative effect x as the mixture. The individual effect concentrations are derived from the concentration–response functions for the chemicals by using their inverse functional form (Kortenkamp et al., 2010; Ermler et al., 2011).

The other type of additivity, independent action (IA) (also termed as *effect addition*), predicts the effectiveness of a mixture of chemicals that effect the same endpoint but act independently (biological activity through different target cells or tissues or through dissimilar modes of action) (US EPA, 2000). The equation for IA is based on probability theory and is expressed as follows:

$$E(c_{mix}) = 1 - \prod_{i=1}^{n}[1 - E(c_i)] \tag{7.2}$$

where $E(c_{mix})$ is the total effect of the mixture concentration based on the effects of the chemicals that they generate at concentrations at which they are present in the mixture $E(c_i)$ (Ermler et al., 2011).

Both concepts require data for the individual components and are based on the assumption that chemicals in a mixture do not influence each other's toxicity, that is, they do not interact with each other at the biological target site. This is thought to be the case where effects are generally assumed to be additive with chemicals with common modes of action, but additivity is not expected for chemicals that act through different modes of action. As IA uses individual effects of the mixture components to calculate the expected mixture effect, this concept predicts that no-effect doses of individual chemicals will also produce no effect when combined.

This central tenet of IA is commonly taken to mean that exposed subjects are protected from mixture effects as long as the doses of all agents in the combination do not exceed their NOAELs (Kortenkamp et al., 2007).

There is now good evidence demonstrating significant mixture effects from low dose multiple exposures of combinations of chemicals well below their individual NOAELs, both with mixtures composed of similarly and dissimilarly acting agents. Again, it has been seen that criteria should focus on common adverse outcomes rather than common mechanisms. The widely held view that mixtures of dissimilarly acting chemicals are "safe" at levels below NOAELs is based on the erroneous assumption that NOAELs can be equated with zero-effect levels (Kortenkamp et al., 2007). Thus, a disregard of combination effects of chemicals with similar action may lead to considerable underestimations of the risks associated with exposures to EDCs. Additionally, the quantity, chemical combinations, and metabolism/clearance are all important components, but the timing of exposure may also be relevant.

In the following paragraphs, various studies on the mixture effects of estrogenic, anti-androgenic, and thyroid-disrupting chemicals are reviewed. Mixture effects of estrogenic chemicals, estrogens and anti-estrogens, estrogens and anti-androgens, anti-androgens with common mechanism of action and with different modes of action, and a comparative profile of chronic exposure of low dose mixture of anti-androgens and acute exposure to high dose individual compounds are discussed. The effects of a combination of thyroid-disrupting chemicals and chemicals acting via the aromatic (aryl) hydrocarbon receptor (AhR) are also reviewed.

7.3   MIXTURE EFFECTS OF ESTROGENIC CHEMICALS

Estrogenic chemicals, which include both the natural and synthetic steroidal estrogens as well as a wide range of synthetic chemicals that mimic the actions of endogenous estrogen, are known to mediate their effects by binding with the estrogen receptor (ER). Thus, estrogenicity can mean affinity to the ER (ERα or β), the ability to activate expression of estrogen-dependent genes, or stimulation of cell proliferation of ER-competent cells (Kortenkamp, 2007). The potencies of these different types of estrogenic chemicals vary over several orders of magnitude. The chemicals that mimic the actions of estrogen, such as alkylphenols, exhibit much lower potencies and rarely occur at concentrations that are individually effective in the environment, thus posing negligible risk. However, this approach does not consider the potential of estrogenic chemicals to act in combination and may lead to underestimation of hazard that exists in real exposure situations. Similar estrogenic loads may be generated through exposure to mixtures of different estrogenic chemicals, and similar effects may be generated through exposure to chemicals with varied mechanisms.

The assessment of mixture effects in combinations of two, three, and four estrogenic chemicals *in vitro*, using the yeast estrogenicity screen (YES) assay, was reported by Payne et al. (2000). Individual dose–response curves for *o,p'*-DDT, genistein, 4-nonylphenol, and 4-n-octylphenol were obtained, and this informa-tion was used to successfully predict the combination effects for the mixtures by employing the concentration addition model (Payne et al., 2000). Similarly, the effects of a mixture containing E2 and 7 and 11 low potency estrogenic chemicals, respectively, at low effect concentrations were demonstrated *in vitro* using the YES and the human breast cancer cell proliferation assay (E-SCREEN) (Rajapakse et al., 2002; Silva et al., 2002). In both cases, the mixtures' responses seen using the YES agreed excellently with the effects predicted by using concentration addition.

A few studies indicated antagonisms in the joint effects of estrogenic agents (Charles et al., 2007; Rajapakse et al., 2004) but these deviations were rather small. Estrogenicity caused by the combined exposure to a six-component estrogenic chemicals mixture containing 17β-estradiol, 17α-ethinylestradiol, BPA, 4-nonyl-phenol, 4-*tert*-octylphenol, and genistein showed a minor deviation from expected concentration additivity determined by measuring cell proliferation in breast cancer cell lines treated with human adipose tissue samples (the E-SCREEN assay). All six estrogenic chemicals individually bind to and activate the ER and all induce cell proliferation in the E-SCREEN. By excluding one or more of the chemicals from the six-component mixture, it was observed that the presence of 4-nonyl-phenol and 4-*tert*-octylphenol was associated with the antagonisms observed with the six-component mixture and thus negatively affected the predictability of mixture effects (Rajapakse et al., 2004). The sensitive nature of E-SCREEN assay with regard to the growth restricting influence of these chemicals was attributed as contributing to the observed deviation from additivity.

Another study evaluated the impact of low level exposure to a mixture of six synthetic chemicals, namely methoxyclor, o,p'-DDT, octylphenol, BPA, β-hexachlorocyclohexane (β-HCH), and 2,3-bis(4-hydroxy-phenyl)-propionitrile, under conditions of co-exposure to various levels of phytoestrogens using an *in vitro* human ER transcriptional activation assay and an *in vivo* immature rat uterotrophic assay (Charles et al., 2007). Both *in vitro* and *in vivo*, while relatively high levels of a putative synthetic estrogen mixture increased the estrogenic action of common dietary phytoestrogens, low levels were without effect. *In vitro*, interactions between high doses of synthetic estrogens and phytoestrogens were greater than additive, whereas mixtures of synthetic estrogens in the absence of phytoestrogens interacted in a less than additive manner. *In vivo*, the synthetic estrogens and phytoestrogens mixture responses were consistent with additivity (Charles et al., 2007).

Combined effects of five estrogenic chemicals, namely E2, EE2, 4-nonylphenol, 4-*tert*-octylphenol, and BPA, were determined on the egg yolk protein vitellogenin (VTG) induction in the freshwater fish fathead minnows (*Pimephales promelas*) as an endpoint (Brian et al., 2005). The induction of VTG is an established *in vivo* assay for analyzing estrogenic effects in fish. This protein is normally induced in the livers of female fish in response to stimulation by endogenous estrogen. However, it can be induced in both male and female fish exposed to extremely low concentrations of estrogenic chemicals. A master stock containing each of the chemicals at their EC_{50} concentrations was prepared. This was diluted to give a range of mixture concentrations of 100%, 50%, 30%, 20%, 10%, and 5%, which corresponded with relative VTG responses between 0% and 100%, according to the concentration addition expectations. The observed effects were comparable to the predicted effects with the concentration addition of the mixture. Mixture effects at low effect concentrations, determined by exposing the fish based on one-fifth of the EC_{50} of each chemical at which individual chemicals did not induce a significant response when exposed to the same dose of all five chemicals in combination, showed that VTG was significantly induced and matched the DA expectation (Brian et al., 2005). A similar observation on vitellogenesis in the marine fish European sea bass (*Dicentrarchus* labrax) was reported on concentration addition effect of a mixture of three estrogenic chemicals E2, EE2, and BPA (Correia et al, 2007).

The potential for estrogenic mixture effects *in vivo* has been also explored using an assay based on an increase in rat uterotrophic weight (Charles et al., 2002; Tinwell and Ashby, 2004). The additive effect of a mixture of E2, EE2, and DES was observed at three dose levels using uterine proliferation in immature CD-1 mice as the endpoint (Charles et al., 2002). In another study, concentrations that individually induced low effects were determined for seven estrogenic chemicals, namely nonylphenol, BPA, methoxychlor, genistein, E2, DES, and EE2. Equipotent concentrations were tested, both individually and in combination, at different concentrations. The highest concentration of the mixture induced a significant increase in uterine weight in relation to the effects produced by the individual chemicals (although this difference was marginal). At 5- and 10-fold dilutions, a few of the individual chemicals induced a significant response, but at a 50-fold dilution no significant responses were observed. However, the same dilutions of the mixture were found to induce a significant response, demonstrating the potential for mixture effects of different ER agonists acting simultaneously to evoke an ER-regulated response even when the effects of each individual chemical could not be detected (Tinwell and Ashby, 2004).

The mixture effect of four UV filters was evaluated by measuring estrogenicity using estrogen-regulated pS2 gene transcription in the human cancer cell line MCF-7. An equipotent binary mixture of 2-hydroxy-4-methoxy benzophenone (BP-3) and its metabolite 2,4-dihydroxy benzophenone (BP-1), as well as an equipotent mixture of BP-1, BP-3, octyl methoxy cinnamate (OMC), and 3-(4-methylbenzylidene) camphor (4-MBC), was evaluated for their ability to induce pS2 gene transcription. The increased pS2 gene transcription in MCF-7 cells after exposure to mixture of UV filters was found to be dose additive (Heneweer et al., 2005).

The combined effects of a mixture of four organochlorine pesticides o,p'-DDT, p,p'-DDT, p,p'-DDE, and β-HCH were assessed in the induction of cell proliferation in MCF-7 cells (E-SCREEN) (Payne et al., 2001). All four compounds show similarities, inducing cell proliferation in estrogen-dependent breast cancer cells, as receptor agonists (o,p'-DDT and p,p'-DDT), anti-androgenic (p,p'-DDE), or some independent pathways (β-HCH). Although the concentration–response plots showed marked differences in shape and position, the combined effect could be predicted on the basis of the concentration–response relationships of the single compounds (Payne et al., 2001). The combination effects were stronger than those of the most potent compound, so the combined effects may be called *additive* or *synergistic*.

Additivity of estrogenic and anti-androgenic chemicals was explored in an *in vivo* study on the feminization of male fish downstream of some wastewater treatment plants (WWTPs). Associations between modeled concentrations and activities of estrogenic and anti-androgenic chemicals in 30 UK rivers using additive statistical modeling demonstrated that feminizing effects in wild fish could be best modeled as a function of their predicted exposure to both anti-androgens and estrogens or to anti-androgens alone (Jobling et al., 2009).

7.4 MIXTURE EFFECTS OF ESTROGENS AND ANTI-ESTROGENS

It is supposed that the estrogenic effects of estrogenic chemicals will be balanced by the presence of other EDCs with anti-estrogenic activities. This assumption was tested in a study by assessing 17β-estradiol (E2) and the anti-estrogens letrozole (an aromatase inhibitor) and tamoxifen, individually and in combination, using a 21-day reproduction *in vivo* assay with the Japanese medaka (*Oryzias latipes*) (Sun et al., 2009). Exposure to E2 (200 ng/l) alone resulted in significant biological changes in paired fish, including impaired reproductive capacity and plasma VTG induction. Upon coexposure with tamoxifen or letrozole (10, 50, and 250 μg/l), the effects of estrogen on some biomarkers (e.g., plasma VTG concentration) could be partially neutralized, but the impairments in reproductive performance were hardly ameliorated, or even became more severe. The outcome created a question mark on the basic assumption that the effects of estrogenic chemicals can be cancelled out by the presence of anti-estrogens in aquatic organisms, as reproductive performance is a more holistic parameter with population-level relevance (Sun et al., 2009).

The effects of a mixture of EE2 with the potent anti-estrogen ZM189,154 (Fig. 7.1) was investigated by exposing adult male fathead minnow (*P. promelas*) to aqueous doses of EE2, ZM, and to mixtures of EE2 and ZM. ZM189,154 functions as a "pure" anti-estrogen, meaning that it will bind to and inhibit activation of the ERs in all tissues. The study was aimed to detect whether the ZM in the mixture would block the action of EE2 on soluble ERs in the fathead minnow gonad and effectively block gene expression changes observed with EE2 alone (Garcia-Reyero et al., 2009). ZM (100 ng/l) treatment alone or in the mixture with EE2 (2, 5, and 10 ng/l) for 48 h decreased plasma T levels, but alone it did not induce plasma VTG concentrations, nor did it inhibit the increase in VTG induced by EE2 in the mixture in males. It was concluded that response to estrogens occurs via multiple mechanisms, including binding to ERs, membrane receptors enacting immediate changes in signaling via nongenomic pathways or some other potential mechanisms, escaping antagonism, and may not be blocked by even pure anti-estrogens (Garcia-Reyero et al., 2009).

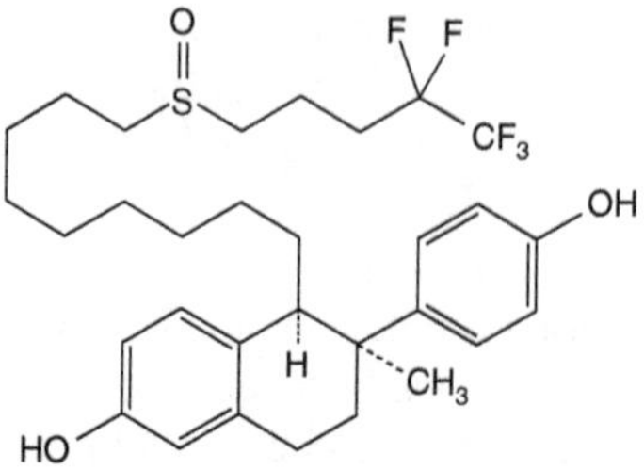

Figure 7.1 Anti-estrogen ZM 189,154; 2-(4-hydroxyphenyl)-2-methyl-1-[9-(4,4,5,5,5-penta-fluoropentane-1-sulfinyl)nonyl]-1,2,3,4-tetra-hydro-naphth-6-ol.

In another study, the sensitivity and utility of the early life stages of fathead minnow were evaluated as a model to measure the effects of estrogenic and anti-estrogenic EDCs on physiological and gene expression endpoints relative to growth and reproduction (Johns et al., 2011). Embryos (<24 h post fertilization) were exposed to EE2 (2, 10, and 50 ng/l); to a weak estrogen, mycotoxin zearalenone (ZEN) (same concentrations as above); to an antiestrogen, ZM 189,154 (40, 250, and 1000 ng/l); and to mixtures of EE2 and ZM until swim-up stage (~170 h post fertilization). There was a significant increase in the frequency of abnormalities (mostly edema) in larvae exposed to all concentrations of EE2, high ZEN, and EE2 + ZM mixture groups. Expression of growth hormone was upregulated by most of the conditions tested. Exposure to 50 ng/l ZEN caused an induction of insulin-like growth factor 1, whereas exposure to 40 ng/l ZM caused a downregulation of this gene. Expression of steroidogenic acute regulatory protein gene was significantly upregulated after exposure to all concentrations of EE2, and luteinizing hormone expression increased significantly in response to all treatments tested. As expected, EE2 induced VTG expression; however, ZEN also induced expression of this gene to similar levels as EE2. Overall, exposure to EE2 + ZM mixture resulted in a different expression pattern compared to single exposures. The results of this study suggest that an early life stage 7-day exposure is sufficient to recognize and evaluate effects of estrogenic compounds on gene expression in this fish model (Johns et al., 2011).

7.5 MIXTURE EFFECTS OF ANTI-ANDROGENS

7.5.1 Anti-Androgens with Common Mechanism of Action

Exposure to anti-androgenic chemicals during gestation can disrupt the action of androgens and induce irreversible demasculinization and malformations of sex organs among male offspring. Anti-androgenic chemicals with the same mechanism of toxicity were found to conform to a model of DA. Several case studies are presented below.

Additive effects of similar acting compounds have been observed for a binary mixture composed of the dicarboximide fungicides vinclozolin and procymidone *in vitro* in the AR reporter gene assay, finding that both AR antagonists additively inhibited testosterone binding to the AR (Nellemann et al., 2003) and consistently followed a dose additive antagonistic effect on the AR-inducing malformations in castrated, testosterone-treated male rats exposed *in utero* (Rider et al., 2009). A mixture of vinclozolin and iprodione also produced anti-androgenic dose additive effect on Sprague–Dawley rats on several endpoints, including reproductive and nonreproductive organ weights. However, iprodione antagonized the vinclozolin-induced increase in serum testosterone (Blystone et al., 2009).

A mixture of three AR antagonists, namely vinclozolin, procymidone, and flutamide, displayed dose additive effect *in vitro* in the AR reporter gene assay (Kjærstad et al., 2010) and *in vivo* for various endpoints in pregnant Wistar rats. The additive effects were observed for changes in the anogenital distance (AGD), nipple retention (NR), reproductive organ weights, and androgen-regulated gene changes in prostates in male offspring rats (Hass et al., 2007; Metzdorff et al., 2007). Severe dysgenesis of external genitals resulted in 50% of animals with the mixture at doses for which the individual compounds caused no effects (Metzdorff et al., 2007).

Similar results were reported in experiments with rats; with a mixture of two phthalates DBP and DEHP, which act through a common mode of action by suppressing testosterone synthesis, the combined effects were additive (Howdeshell et al., 2007). There was a significant decrease in fetal testicular testosterone levels observed in animals exposed to DBP or the phthalate mixture. However, no significant changes were observed in AGD and NR, which are variables that are used to indicate possible anti-androgenic effects (Martino-Andrade et al., 2009). Testosterone plays a critical role during sexual differentiation of the male fetus in all mammals including rodents and humans, and therefore fetal testicular testosterone levels seem to be the most sensitive markers of prenatal phthalate exposure as the critical endpoint. Similarly, administration of a mixture of five anti-androgenic phthalate esters, namely *n*-butyl benzylphthalate (BBP), di-*n*-butylphthalate (DBP), di(2-ethylhexyl)phthalate (DEHP), DiBP (diisobutyl phthalate), and DPP (dipentyl phthalate), to pregnant Sprague–Dawley rats, adjusted for their individual potency in a manner that each contributed equally, exerted significant reductions in fetal testosterone production in a dose additive manner (Howdeshell et al., 2008). BBP, DBP (Fig. 3.1), and DiBP were found to be of equivalent potency to DEHP ($ED_{50} = 440 \pm 16$ mg/kg/day) in reducing fetal testosterone production, whereas DPP was three times as potent ($ED_{50} = 130$ mg/kg/day) as DEHP (Howdeshell et al., 2008). Thus, the DA approach seems to be able to provide a solid basis for the prediction of joint effects of multicomponent mixtures of receptor-mediated anti-androgenic action. Owing to cumulative effect of phthalates, recently Denmark has proposed a ban on four commonly used phthalates DEHP, DBP, BBP, and DIPB, which individually and in small concentrations do not rise to the level of being considered harmful to health (Miljøministeriet, 2011).

A mixture of parabens (methyl-, ethyl-, propyl-, butyl- and isobutyl-paraben) exhibited AR antagonistic effects *in vitro*, which were markedly higher than expected. The predicted effect was based solely on the effect of one-fifth of the parabens, as isobutyl-paraben was the only AR antagonist in the assay. The effect of isobutyl-paraben was statistically significant at concentration of 25 μM and above, while the mixture of all five parabens antagonized the AR at concentrations of 2 μM and above (Kjærstad et al., 2010).

7.5.2   Anti-Androgens with Different Modes of Action

Two *in utero* studies with mixtures of pairs of chemicals with different mechanisms of action found cumulative dose additive effects of the mixtures. For example, a mixture of the phthalate BBP (fetal testosterone inhibitor) and the thiourea herbicide linuron (anti-androgen), which disrupt the androgen-signaling pathway via diverse mechanisms of toxicity, produced dose additive effects on reproductive tract development (Hotchkiss et al., 2004). In another study, pregnant rats dosed with individual compounds DBP and the AR antagonist procymidone or their binary mixture, at a dose level of one-half of the ED_{50} value for malformations, indicated that the interaction was at least dose additive (Rider et al., 2009).

Similar observations were made when rats were dosed during pregnancy with a combination of seven anti-androgenic chemicals with different mechanisms of action, that is, AR antagonist or inhibition of testosterone synthesis, including three testosterone synthesis inhibitor phthalates (DBP, BBP, and DEHP), two AR antagonist fungicides (vinclozolin and procymidone), and two mixed-mechanism chemicals that bind to the AR and decrease testosterone production (linuron and prochloraz) (Rider et al., 2008). The observed effects were cumulative and dose additive on androgen-dependent reproductive development (Rider et al., 2008). Some of the toxicants lowered testosterone levels in the tissues, whereas others prevented testosterone from activating the androgen receptor, reduced expression of androgen-dependent genes, and altered differentiation of the tissues. An inference could be drawn that chemicals that do not act via a common cellular mechanism of action may result in dose additive effects on common downstream endpoints.

In vivo study involving gestational exposure to a mixture of three anti-androgenic chemicals, namely vinclozolin, flutamide and procymidone, in rats markedly increased frequencies of hypospadias, compared to administration of the three chemicals alone (Christiansen et al., 2008). These anti-androgens function dose-additively together and bring about adverse effects at their established no-adverse-effect levels when administered together. In another study, gestational exposure to a mixture of four anti-androgenic chemicals with differing mechanisms, such as the phthalate DEHP, the fungicides vinclozolin and prochloraz, and the pharmaceutical finasteride, was investigated for effects on male sexual development in the rat. The combined effects were additive for the investigated developmental endpoints, including reduced AGD, NR, and sex organ weights in male rats (Christiansen et al., 2009). Strikingly, however, the combined effect was synergistic for malformations of external sex organs such as hypospadias, such that the observed responses were greater than would be predicted from the toxicities of the individual chemicals. Prochloraz, one of the chemicals in the mixture, induces an elevated testicular progesterone concentration, thereby increasing the risk of hypospadias, and it is presumed to have a role in the observed synergism with severe hypospadias. Although in comparison to typical environmental exposures the doses were high, the observations give rise to concerns about possible synergism with mixtures of these chemicals, which may have important implications for human risk assessment (Christiansen et al., 2009). The additive effects of the same mixture – finasteride, prochloraz, vinclozolin, and MEHP (DEHP metabolite) – were demonstrated in the AR reporter gene assay (Kjærstad et al., 2010). However, MEHP is a known inhibitor of androgen biosynthesis and had no effect on the AR (Kjærstad et al., 2010).

A large multicomponent mixture of 17 chemicals comprising varied structural features with AR antagonist activity was tested in an *in vitro* AR-dependent luciferase reporter gene assay based on human breast cancer MDA-kb2 cells. The mixture's effect could be predicted well using the concept of CA, supporting the idea that it is a good model for approximating the *in vitro* effects of multicomponent mixtures of AR antagonists with widely differing chemical properties (Ermler et al., 2011).

Mixture effects of five endocrine-disrupting fungicides, namely procymidone, mancozeb, epoxyconazole, tebuconazole, and prochloraz, were investigated on the pregnancy length and pup survival at low doses. Mancozeb (Fig. 7.2c) acts mainly via disruption of the thyroid hormones and is suspected to disrupt brain development. The triazole fungicides tebuconazole (Fig. 7.2a) and epoxyconazole (Fig. 7.2b) induce high plasma concentration of progesterone in the dams, which may cause an increase in gestation length and the virilizing effect on female pups (Taxvig et al., 2007). The mixture ratio was chosen according to the doses of each individual pesticide that produced no observable effects on pregnancy length and pup survival, and the dose levels used ranged from 25% to 100% of this mixture. All dose levels caused increased gestation length above 25% and caused impaired parturition leading to markedly decreased number of live born offspring and high pup perinatal mortality. The sexual differentiation of the pups was affected at 25% and higher; AGD was affected in both male and female offspring at birth; and the male offspring exhibited malformations of the genital tubercle, increased NR, and decreased prostate and epididymis weights at pup day 13. The results show that doses of endocrine disrupting pesticides, which appear to induce no effects on gestation length, parturition, and pup mortality when judged on their own, induced marked adverse effects on these endpoints in concert with other pesticides. In addition, the sexual differentiation of the offspring was significantly affected (Jacobsen et al., 2010).

The reproductive toxic effects of a mixture of five dissimilarly acting pesticides, namely deltamethrin (Fig. 7.3a), methiocarb (Fig. 7.3b), prochloraz, tribenuron-methyl (Fig. 7.3c), and simazine (Fig. 7.3d), after exposure during gestation were analyzed for anti-androgenic effects *in vitro* and *in vivo* (Birkhuj et al., 2004). The

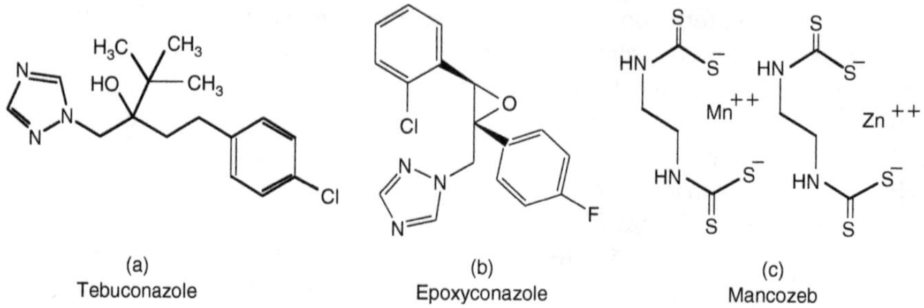

(a)	(b)	(c)
Tebuconazole	Epoxyconazole	Mancozeb

Figure 7.2   Fungicides that exhibit endocrine disrupting characteristics.

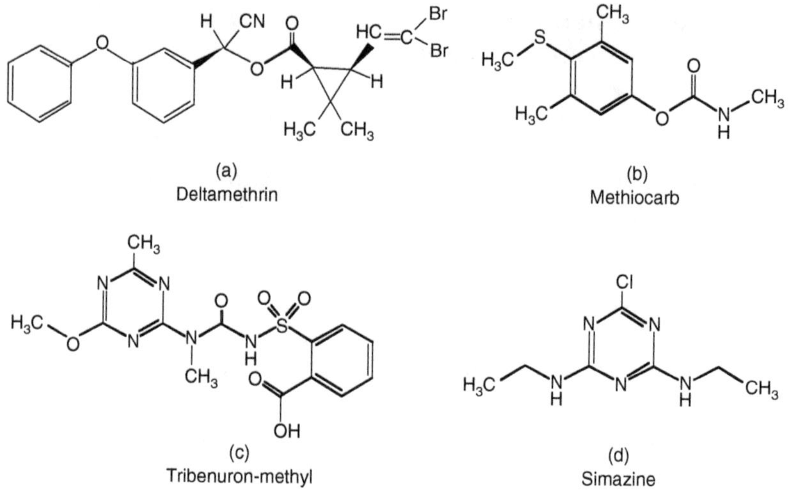

(a)	(b)
Deltamethrin	Methiocarb

(c)	(d)
Tribenuron-methyl	Simazine

Figure 7.3   Pesticidal compounds with potential ED properties.

IC_{25} values for the inhibition of the AR for deltamethrin, methiocarb, prochloraz, and their mixture were 5.8, 5.8, 3.5, and 7.5 µM, respectively, while simazine and tribenuron-methyl were found to be ineffective. An isobole coefficient of 0.94 at IC_{25} for the effect of the mixture was obtained by applying the isobole method, indicating additive effects of the pesticides *in vitro*. *In vivo*, the organ weight changes indicated that the pesticides had an accumulating effect which was not observed for the individual pesticides (Birkhuj et al., 2004). Thus, taken together, there is good evidence that similarly acting EDCs produce combination effects in a dose additive manner.

7.5.3   Chronic Exposure of Low Dose Mixture of Anti-Androgens Versus Acute Exposure to High Dose Individual Compounds

Humans and wild animals are exposed to various environmental and food EDCs simultaneously, generally at low levels, throughout their lives. The effects of a chronic exposure to low doses of EDCs on the reproductive axis, such as life-time exposures to low (environmental) doses of estrogenic "feminizing" and anti-androgenic "de-masculinizing" EDCs on male reproductive function, compared to acute exposure to non-environmental high doses of single compounds in isolation have been determined (Eustache et al., 2009). The effects of a chronic exposure of male Wistar Han rats to low combined doses of genistein and vinclozolin were close to those of high dose vinclozolin alone, evoking a synergistic androgenic effect. The male Wistar Han rat's reproductive health was affected by inducing reproductive developmental anomalies, alterations in sperm production and quality, and fertility disorders. The low genistein dose is able to potentiate the effects of vinclozolin, possibly through activation by genistein of specific receptors of protein ligands induced by low dose vinclozolin. Genistein exhibited *in vitro* anti-androgenic activity in addition to its well-established estrogenic activity (Rosenberg Zand et al., 2000).

7.6 MIXTURE EFFECTS OF THYROID DISRUPTING CHEMICALS

The variety of mechanisms by which TDCs alter thyroid homeostasis raises a question as to whether the cumulative effects in a mixture are chemical-class-specific or related to downstream consequence (e.g., circulating hormone levels, brain biochemistry, and behavior) which would be mechanism independent. A small numbers of studies that reported effects of mixtures of TDCs were conducted without concurrent experimental characterization of the effects of the individual chemicals and lacked the ability to test for additivity (Desaulniers et al. 2003; Khan et al. 2005; McLanahan et al. 2007; Wade et al. 2002).

For example, the additive effects of a mixture of coplanar PCBs, polychlorinated dibenzodioxins (PCDDs), and polychlorinated dibenzofurans (PCDFs) on circulating thyroxine (T4) concentrations in neonatal rats could be predicted by using toxic equivalents of 2,3,7,8-tetrachlorodibenzo-*p*-dioxin (TCDD) (Desaulniers et al., 2003). A binary mixture of perchlorate and sodium chlorate showed enhanced toxicity on thyroid hormone and pathology indicators caused by the individual chemicals in adult male F344 rats (Khan et al., 2005). A binary mixture containing PCB126, a congener of PCB, and perchlorate, known to cause hypothyrodism by different modes of action, administered by addition to drinking water of adult Sprague–Dawley rats produced a less than additive effect on the hypothalamic–pituitary–thyroid (HPT) axis, including a pretreatment with a high dose of PCB126 (McLanahan et al., 2007).

A mixture of 18 polyhalogenated aromatic hydrocarbons (PHAHs) (containing 2 dioxins, 4 dibenzofurans, and 12 PCBs) was tested on young female Long–Evans rats by dosing via gavage for 4 consecutive days for their effects on serum T4. Individually, these chemicals were each known to decrease circulating concentrations of T4 (Crofton et al., 2005). The mechanisms by which these chemicals alter THs involved upregulation of hepatic catabolic enzymes via at least two paths. TCDD, dibenzofurans, and dioxin-like PCBs bind to AhR, activating one set of liver enzymes. The non-dioxin-like PCBs activated a different set of liver enzymes that metabolize THs via binding to PXR and the constitutive androstane receptor (CAR). These differences in mechanisms of action (i.e., AhR agonists and CAR/PXR agonists) suggest that DA theory might not predict the effects of the mixture. The exposure at the highest mixture dose was at or below the no-observed-effect levels (NOELs) of the individual components for serum thyroxin concentration. Dilutions ranged to 100-fold lower levels. It was found that the mixture had a dose additive effect on T4 at environmentally relevant doses but a greater-than-additive effect on T4 at higher doses. Thus, the limited data from the TDC mixture studies suggest that DA is reasonably accurate in predicting the effects on serum T4 concentrations (Crofton, 2008).

Further increasing the complexity of the exposure, when female Long–Evans rats were dosed for 4 consecutive days with a mixture of all the 18 PHAHs cited above and a mixture of three pesticides (thiram, pronamide, and mancozeb) that inhibit TH synthesis, 45% decrease in serum T4 was experienced. The dose additive method could predict the effect of the combination of all 21 chemicals (Flippin et al., 2009). Thus, in the regulatory context, DA as a default option is precautionary without implying massive and costly overprotection.

7.7   MIXTURE EFFECTS OF CHEMICALS ACTING VIA AhR

The potency-adjusted dose additivity for induction of increased tumor incidence has been observed in a mixture of dioxin-like compounds with a common mechanism of action as aryl hydrocarbon receptor (AhR) agonists (Walker et al., 2005). In a 2-year chronic rodent carcinogenicity bioassay with female Harlan Sprague–Dawley rats, treated by gavage (2.5 ml/kg in corn oil), 5 days per week, with TCDD, 3,3′,4,4′,5-pentachlorobiphenyl (PCB-126), 2,3,4,7,8-pentachlorodibenzofuran (PCDBF), or a mixture of the three compounds, the combined effect could be predicted from a combination of the potency-adjusted doses of individual compounds (Walker et al., 2005).

Hamm et al. (2003) studied a mixture of nine dioxins, furans, and coplanar PCBs and looked at developmental reproductive endpoints in time-pregnant Long–Evans rats, comparing the results of the mixture to that of 2,3,7,8-TCDD alone. The results showed that the mixture causes a similar spectrum of effects seen with TCDD, and the slightly lowered degree of response based on administered dose was attributed to decreased transfer of the mixture components to the offspring.

Some of the significant results of estrogenic, anti-androgenic, thyroid disrupting chemicals, and AhR agonist mixture effects are summarized in Table 7.1.

7.8   CONCLUSIONS AND FUTURE PROSPECTS

In natural ecosystems, EDCs occur in complex mixtures and therefore we are all exposed simultaneously to low doses of a large number of chemicals, many with the capacity to alter a range of reproductive outcomes. Significant progress has been

TABLE 7.1   Significant Mixture Effects of EDCs in Dose Additive Manner

Mixture Components	Species/Endpoint	Individual Dose or Concentration.	Mixture Effect	Reference
Estrogenic mixtures				
Eight estrogenic chemicals	YES – Recombinant yeast estrogen screen	43–100% of NOEC	Significant estrogenic activity	Silva et al. (2002)
Eight estrogenic chemicals	Immature female AP rat, uterotrophic assay, uterine weight reduction	≤NOEL	Significant utertophic activity	Tinwell and Ashby (2004)
Five estrogenic chemicals	Fish, vitellogenin induction	NOEC	Significant vitellogenin induction	Brian et al. (2005)
Anti-androgenic mixtures				
Three androgen receptor antagonists	Male rats exposed *in utero*, feminization of anogenital distance	NOEL	Significant feminization	Hass et al. (2007)
	Male rats exposed *in utero*, dysgenesis of genitals	NOEL	Severe dysgenesis	Metzdorff et al. (2007)
	Male rats exposed *in utero*, incidence of hypospadias	NOEL	Significantly increased incidence	Christiansen et al. (2008)

(continued)

TABLE 7.1 (Continued)

Mixture Components	Species/Endpoint	Individual Dose or Concentration.	Mixture Effect	Reference
Five phthalates	Rats exposed in utero/suppression of fetal testosterone levels	NOEL	Significant suppression	Howdeshell et al. (2008)
Thyroid disrupting chemical mixture				
Eighteen thyroid disrupting chemicals	Female Long–Evans rat, Decrease of serum total thyroxine (T4) levels	NOEL	Significant T4 decrease	Crofton et al. (2005)
Twenty-one thyroid disrupting chemicals (18 PHAHs and 3 pesticides)	Female Long–Evans rat, 45% decrease in serum T4		Significant T4 decrease	Flippin et al. (2009)
Aryl hydrocarbon receptor agonists mixture				
Three AhR agonists	Female Harlan Sprague–Dawley rats, induction of tumor incidence	2.5 ml/kg in corn oil	Tumor incidence increased	Walker et al. (2005)
Nine AhR agonists	Long–Evans rats, developmental effects of offspring		Puberty time increased	Hamm et al. (2003)

made with mixture studies, and it has been shown that these effects are dose additive. The mixture led to toxic effects at doses of the components that individually did not induce observable effects. These observations are of great importance for the regulation of EDCs. The experimental doses that are used as a basis for deriving health-based exposure standards (e.g., acceptable daily intakes) cannot be considered safe under all circumstances if exposure is to a large number of chemicals that also produce the effect of interest. Although research on mixture exposures and potential health effects is scant, developmental effects of *in utero* exposure to phthalates (Howdeshell et al., 2008) is a notable exception.

There is strong evidence that steroid and thyroid hormone disrupting chemicals of the same class produce combination effects in a dose additive manner. Where deviations from expected additivity occurred, the differences between anticipated and observed effects were small. The scientific committee of the European Commission has commented on the scientific review on the problem of chemical cocktails (Kortenkamp et al., 2010). It has supported the DA approach for mixtures of chemicals with similar modes of action (SCHER, SCENIHR, SCCS, 2012). For mixtures of chemicals with dissimilar modes of action, it has found that current evidence does not show significant mixture toxicity at exposures at or below zero-effect levels of the individual components. The Commission, while acknowledging that this is not the same as a true "zero-effect" level, has opined that it can be considered to be the same because safety thresholds include 100-fold uncertainty factors as a buffer (SCHER, SCENIHR, SCCS, 2012). Toxicologically significant interactions of chemicals in mixtures are difficult to foresee, particularly for long-term effects. More data on risk assessments are required than are available from conventional methods; in particular, data from exposures to EDC mixtures are needed. Research is needed to define criteria that predict potentiation or synergy.

For years, toxicologists have tended to avoid studying cumulative effects because it was considered an intractable problem. This was especially so for endocrine active agents because of the vast array of ligands and multiplicity of sources, which includes not only manmade chemicals but also compounds in plants, endogenous hormones, and even nonchemical stressors. However, because of the availability of new high throughput tools, refined statistical methods, and economical experimental designs for mixture studies, questions about combined exposures to hormonally active agents can now be addressed in a scientifically rigorous and efficient manner.

REFERENCES

Birkhuj, M.; Nellemann, C.; Jarfelt, K.; Jacobsen, H.; Andersen, H. R.; Dalgaard, M.; Vinggaard, A. M. The combined antiandrogenic effects of five commonly used pesticides, *Toxicol. Appl. Pharmacol.* **2004**, 201(1), 10–20.

Blystone, C. R.; Lambright, C. S.; Cardon, M. C.; Furr, J.; Rider, C. V.; Hartig, P. C.; Wilson, V. S.; Gray, L. E., Jr., Cumulative and antagonistic effects of a mixture of the antiandrogens vinclozolin and iprodione in the pubertal male rat, *Toxicol. Sci.* **2009**, 111(1), 179–188.

Brian, J. V.; Harris, C. A.; Scholze, M.; Backhaus, T.; Booy, P.; Lamoree, M.; Pojana, G.; Jonkers, N.; Runnalls, T.; Bonfà, A.; Marcomini, A.; Sumpter, J. P. Accurate prediction of the response of freshwater fish to a mixture of estrogenic chemicals, *Environ. Health Perspect.* **2005**, 113(6), 721–728.

Charles, G. D.; Gennings, C.; Zacharewski, T. R.; Gollapudi, B. B.; Carney, E. W. An approach for assessing estrogen receptor-mediated interactions in mixtures of three chemicals: a pilot study, *Toxicol. Sci.* **2002**, 68, 349–360.

Charles, G. D.; Gennings, C.; Tornesi, B.; Kan, H. L.; Zacharewski, T. R.; Bhaskar, G. B.; Carney, E. W. Analysis of the interaction of phytoestrogens and synthetic chemicals: an in vitro/in vivo comparison, *Toxicol. Appl. Pharmacol.* **2007**, 218(3), 280–228.

Christiansen, S.; Scholze, M.; Axelstad, M.; Boberg, J.; Kortenkamp, A.; Hass, U. Combined exposure to anti-estrogens causes markedly increased frequencies of hypospadias in the rat, *Int. J. Androl.* **2008**, 31, 241–248.

Christiansen, S.; Scholze, M.; Dalgaard, M.; Vinggaard, A. M.; Axelstad, M.; Kortenkamp, A.; Hass, U. Synergistic disruption of external male sex organ development by a mixture of four antiandrogens, *Environ. Health Perspect.* **2009**, 117(12), 1839–1846.

Correia, A. D.; Freitas, S.; Scholze, M.; Gonçalves, J. F.; Booj, P.; Lamoree, M. H., et al. Mixtures of estrogenic chemicals enhance vitellogenic response in sea bass, *Environ. Health Perspect.* **2007**, 115(1), 115–121.

COT, *Risk assessment of mixtures of pesticides and similar substances*, FSA/0691/0902, UK: Committee on the Toxicity of Chemicals in Food, Consumer Products and the Environment, 2002.

Crofton, K. M. Thyroid disrupting chemicals: mechanisms and mixtures, *Int. J. Androl.* **2008**, 31(2), 209–223.

Crofton, K. M.; Craft, E. S.; Hedge, J. M.; Gennings, C.; Simmons, J. E.; Carchman, R. A.; Carter, W. H. Jr.; DeVito, M. J. Thyroid-hormone-disrupting chemicals: evidence for dose-dependent additivity or synergism, *Environ. Health Perspect.* **2005**, 113, 1549–1554.

Desaulniers, D.; Leingartner, K.; Musicki, B.; Yagminas, A.; Xiao, G. H.; Cole, J., et al. Effects of postnatal exposure to mixtures of non-ortho-PCBs, PCDDs, and PCDFs in prepubertal female rats, *Toxicol. Sci.* **2003**, 75(2), 468–480.

Diamanti-Kandarakis, E.; Bourguignon, J.P.; Giudice, L.C.; Hauser, R.; Prins, G.S.; Soto, A.M.; Zoeller, R.T.; Gore, A.C. Endocrine-disrupting chemicals: an Endocrine Society scientific statement, *Endocr. Rev.* **2009**, 30(4), 293–342.

Ermler, S.; Scholze, M.; Kortenkamp, A. The suitability of concentration addition for predicting the effects of multi-component mixtures of up to 17 anti-androgens with varied structural features in an in vitro AR antagonist assay, *Toxicol. Appl. Pharmacol.* **2011**, 257(2), 189–197.

Eustache, F.; Mondon, F.; Canivenc-Lavier, M. C.; Lesaffre, C.; Fulla, Y.; Berges, R.; Cravedi, J. P.; Vaiman, D.; Auger, J. Chronic dietary exposure to a low-dose mixture of genistein and vinclozoline modifies the reproductive axis, testis transcriptome, and fertility, *Environ. Health Perspect.* **2009**, 117(8), 1272–1279.

Flippin, J. L.; Hedge, J. M.; DeVito, M. J.; LeBlanc, G. A.; Crofton, K. M. Predictive modeling of a mixture of thyroid hormone disrupting chemicals that affect production and clearance of thyroroxine, *Int. J. Toxicol.* **2009**, 28(5), 368–381.

Garcia-Reyero, N.; Kroll, K. J.; Liu, L.; Orlando, E. F.; Watanabe, K. H.; Sepúlveda, M. S.; Villeneuve, D. L.; Perkins, E. J.; Ankley, G. T.; Denslow, N. D. Gene expression responses in male fathead minnows exposed to binary mixtures of an estrogen and antiestrogen, *BMC Genomics* **2009**, 10, 308, 17 pages.

Hamm, J. T.; Chen, C. Y.; Birnbaum, L. S. A mixture of dioxins, furans, and non-ortho PCBs based upon consensus toxic equivalency factors produces dioxin-like reproductive effects, *Toxicol. Sci.* **2003**, 74, 182–191.

Hass, U.; Scholze, M.; Christiansen, S.; Dalgaard, M.; Vinggaard, A. M.; Axelstad, M., et al. Combined exposure to anti-androgens exacerbates disruption of sexual differentiation in the rat, *Environ. Health Perspect.* **2007**, 15, 122–128.

Heneweer, M.; Muusse, M.; van den Berg, M.; Sanderson, J. T. Additive estrogenic effects of mixtures of frequently used UV filters on pS2-gene transcription in MCF-7 cells, *Toxicol. Appl. Pharmacol.* **2005**, 208(2), 170–177.

Hotchkiss, A. K.; Parks-Saldutti, L. G.; Ostby, J. S.; Lambright, C.; Furr, J.; Vandenbergh, J. G.; Gray, L. E. Jr., A mixture of the "antiandrogens" linuron and butyl benzyl phthalate alters sexual differentiation of the male rat in a cumulative fashion, *Biol. Reprod.* **2004**,71(6), 1852–1861.

Howdeshell, K. L.; Furr, J.; Lambright, C. R.; Rider, C. V.; Wilson, V. S.; Gray, L. E., Jr., Cumulative effects of dibutyl phthalate and diethylhexyl phthalate on male rat reproductive tract development: altered fetal steroid hormones and genes, *Toxicol. Sci.* **2007**, 99, 190–202.

Howdeshell, K. L.; Wilson, V. S.; Furr, J.; Lambright, C. R.; Rider, C. V.; Blystone, C. R., et al. A mixture of five phthalate esters inhibits fetal testicular testosterone production in the Sprague-Dawley rat in a cumulative, dose-additive manner, *Toxicol. Sci.* **2008**, 105, 153–165.

Jacobsen, P. R.; Christiansen, S.; Boberg, J.; Nellemann, C.; Hass, U. Combined exposure to endocrine disrupting pesticides impairs parturition, causes pup mortality and affects sexual differentiation in rats, *Inter. J. Androl.* **2010**, 33(2), 434–442.

Jobling, S.; Burn, R. W.; Thorpe, K.; Williams, R.; Tyler, C. Statistical modeling suggest that antiandrogens in effluents from wastewater treatment works contribute to widespread sexual disruption in fish living in English rivers, *Environ. Health Perspect.* **2009**, 117(5), 797–802.

Johns, S. M.; Denslow, N. D.; Kane, M. D.; Watanabe, K. H.; Orlando, E. F.; Sepúlveda, M. S. Effects of estrogens and antiestrogens on gene expression of fathead minnow (Pimephales promelas) early life stages, *Environ. Toxicol.* **2011**, 26(2), 195–206.

Khan, M. A.; Fenton, S. E.; Swank, A. E.; Hester, S. D.; Williams, A.; Wolf, D. C. A mixture of ammonium perchlorate and sodium chlorate enhances alterations of the pituitary-thyroid axis caused by the individual chemicals in adult male F344 rats, *Toxicol. Pathol.* **2005**, 33, 776–783.

Kjærstad, M. B.; Taxvig, C.; Andersen, H. R.; Nellemann, C. Mixture effects of endocrine disrupting compounds in vitro, *Int. J. Androl.* **2010**, 33(2), 425–433.

Kortenkamp, A. Ten years of mixing cocktails: a review of combination effects of endocrine-disrupting chemicals, *Environ. Health Perspect.* **2007**, 115(S-1), 98–105.

Kortenkamp, A.; Faust, M.; Scholze, M.; Backhaus, T. Low-level exposure to multiple chemicals: reason for human health concern? *Environ. Health Perspect.* **2007**, 115(S-1), 106–114.

Kortenkamp, A.; Backhaus, T.; Faust, M. *State of the art report on mixture toxicity – final report*, European Commission – Environment, **2010**. Available at: http://ec.europa.eu/environment/chemicals/pdf/report_Mixture%20toxicity.pdf (accessed 15 Jul 2012).

Martino-Andrade, A. J.; Morais, R. N.; Botelho, G. G. K.; Muller, G.; Grande, S. W.; Carpentieri, G. B.; Leão, G. M. C.; Dalsenter, P. R. Coadministration of active phthalates results in disruption of foetal testicular function in rats, *Inter. J. Androl.* **2009**, 32(6), 704–712.

McLanahan, E. D.; Campbell, J. L. Jr.; Ferguson, D. C.; Harmon, B.; Hedge, J. M.; Crofton, K. M., et al. Low-dose effects of ammonium perchlorate on the hypothalamic-pituitary-thyroid axis of adult male rats pretreated with PCB126, *Toxicol. Sci.* **2007**, 97, 308–317.

Metzdorff, S. B., Dalgaard, M., Christiansen, S., Axelstad, M., Hass, U., Kiersgaard, M. K.; Scholze, M.; Kortenkamp, A.; Vinggaard, A. M. Dysgenesis and histological changes of genitals and perturbations of gene expression in male rats after in utero exposure to antiandrogen mixtures, *Toxicol. Sci.* **2007**, 98(1), 87–98.

Miljøministeriet – *Miljøminister vil forbyde fire farlige ftalater*, 2011. Available at: http://www.mim.dk/Nyheder/Pressemeddelelser/20113004_ forbud _mod_ftalater.htm (accessed 12 Aug 2012).

Nellemann, C.; Dalgaard, M.; Lam, H. R.; Vinggaard, A. M. The combined effects of vinclozolin and procymidone do not deviate from expected additivity in vitro and in vivo, *Toxicol. Sci.* **2003**, 71(2), 251–262.

Payne, J.; Rajapakse, N.; Wilkins, M.; Kortenkamp, A. Prediction and assessment of the effects of mixtures of four xenoestrogens, *Environ. Health Perspect.* **2000**, 108(10), 983–987.

Payne, J.; Scholze, M.; Kortenkamp, A. Mixtures of four organochlorines enhance human breast cancer cell proliferation, *Environ. Health Perspect.* **2001**, 109, 391–197.

Rajapakse, N.; Silva, E.; Kortenkamp, A. Combining xenoestrogens at levels below individual no-observed effect- concentrations dramatically enhances steroid hormone action, *Environ. Health Perspect.* **2002**, 110, 917–921.

Rajapakse, N.; Silva, E.; Scholze, M.; Kortenkamp, A. Deviation from additivity with estrogenic mixtures containing 4-nonylphenol and 4-tert-octylphenol detected in the E-SCREEN assay, *Environ. Sci. Technol.* **2004**, 38(23), 6343–6352.

Rider, C. V.; Furr, J.; Wilson, V. S.; Gray, L. E., Jr., A mixture of seven antiandrogens induces reproductive malformations in rats, *Inter. J. Androl.* **2008**, 31(2), 249–262.

Rider, C. V.; Wilson, V. S.; Howdeshell, K. L.; Hotchkiss, A. K.; Furr, J. R.; Lambright, C. R.; Gray, L. E., Jr, Cumulative effects of *In utero* administration of mixtures of "antiandrogens" on male rat reproductive development, *Toxicol. Pathol.* **2009**, 37(1), 100–113.

Rosenberg Zand, R. S.; Jenkins, D. J. A.; Diamandis, E. P. Genistein: a potent natural antiandrogen, *Clin. Chem.* **2000**, 46, 887–888.

SCHER, SCENIHR, SCCS *Opinion concerning toxicity and assessment of chemical mixtures*, European Commission, Brussels, 2012. http://ec.europa.eu/health/scientific_committees/environmental_risks/docs/scher_o_155.pdf (accessed on 28 Oct 2013).

Silva, E.; Rajapakse, N.; Kortenkamp, A. Something from 'nothing' – eight weak estrogenic chemicals combined at concentrations below NOECs produce significant mixture effects, *Environ. Sci. Technol.* **2002**, 36(8), 1751–1756.

Sun, L.; Zha, J.; Wang, Z. Effects of binary mixtures of estrogen and antiestrogens on Japanese medaka (Oryzias latipes), *Aquat. Toxicol.* **2009**, 93(1), 83–89.

Taxvig, C.; Hass, U.; Axelstad, M.; Dalgaard, M.; Boberg, J.; Andersen, H. R.; Vinggaard, A. M. Endocrine disrupting activities *in vivo* of the fungicides tebuconazole and epoxiconazole, *Toxicol. Sci.* **2007**, 100(2), 464–473.

Tinwell, H., Ashby, J. Sensitivity of the rat uterotrophic assay to mixtures of estrogens, *Environ. Health Perspect.* **2004**, 112, 575–582.

US EPA. *Supplementary Guidance for Conducting Health Risk Assessment of Chemical Mixtures, 630/R-00/002*, Washington, DC: US EPA, **2000**.

VKM, *Combined Toxic Effects of Multiple Chemical Exposures. 1*, Norwegian Scientific Committee for Food Safety, Oslo, Norway, **2008**.

Wade, M. G.; Parent, S.; Finnson, K. W.; Foster, W.; Younglai, E.; McMohan, A.; Cyr, D. G.; Hughes, C. Thyroid toxicity due to subchronic exposure to a complex mixture of 16 organochlorines, lead and cadmium, *Toxicol. Sci.* **2002**, 67, 207–218.

Walker, N. J.; Crockett, P. W.; Nyska, A.; Brix, A. E.; Jokinen, M. P.; Sells, D. M.; Hailey, J. R.; Easterling, M.; Haseman, J. K.; Yin, M.; Wyde, M. E.; Bucher, J. R.; Portier, C. J. Dose-additive carcinogenicity of a defined mixture of "dioxin-like compounds," *Environ. Health Perspect.* **2005**, 113, 43–48.

8

ENVIRONMENTALLY INDUCED EPIGENETIC MODIFICATIONS AND TRANSGENERATIONAL EFFECTS

8.1 INTRODUCTION

Mammalian development begins with a single cell, the zygote. Zygote is a totipotent cell that has the ability to develop into a complete organism. This cell divides and differentiates into many different cell types, ultimately giving rise to an organism. In multicellular organisms, all the cells that make up an individual originate from the same fertilized egg that creates a single totipotent cell and share the same genome; however, cells might perform vastly different functions. Cell differentiation occurs without change in the DNA sequence. Different cell types are the result of the type and number of active genes. Cellular development requires the silencing and activation of specific gene sequences in a well-orchestrated manner on their way to specialization. There are over 200 different types of cells in the human body, and the human genome consists of approximately 21,000 genes (Bernstein et al., 2012) but only a fraction of them are used in each cell. Each cell type maintains a unique cellular identity represented by the specific sets of genes they transcribe. For example, skin cells and brain cells have different forms and functions, despite having exactly the same DNA. Thus, there are mechanisms, other than DNA, that make sure that skin cells stay skin cells when they divide. It is the epigenome that tells our cells what sort of cells they should be. Cells in the skin, liver, and heart, all have same genome, and their epigenomes silence the unneeded genes or express the needed ones to make cells different from one another.

Genetic information in DNA is stored as a code made up of the sequence of four chemical bases, adenine (A), guanine (G), cytosine (C), and thymine (T), which determines an organism's genotype, or genetic makeup, and does not

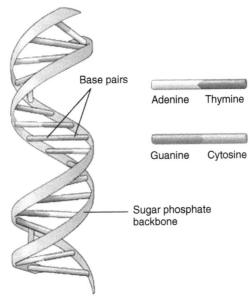

Base pairs

Adenine   Thymine

Guanine   Cytosine

Sugar phosphate
backbone

Figure 8.1   Structure of DNA. Source: U.S. National Library of Medicine.

change (Fig. 8.1). Genetic control has been shown to be essential but insufficient to accommodate the requirements for sustained differential gene expression. Additional regulatory mechanisms exist to meet the need for differential patterns of gene expression to specify diverse types of tissues from a single genome in multicellular organisms' cells. These ensure that, for example, cellular identity is faithfully maintained through cell divisions for a lifetime, despite differentiation occurring earlier during embryonic development. The plasticity of cellular differentiation and the stability of cellular memory represent epigenetic phenomena wherein inherited changes in phenotype occur independently of changes in the underlying DNA sequence (Gardner et al., 2011).

Whereas the genome remains constant in all cell types, the epigenome is distinct in different cell types of the body. As cellular differentiation is based on differential gene expression, and epigenetic mechanisms program different patterns of gene expression characteristic of each different cell type, it is the epigenome of a cell that determines its identity (McCarrey, 2012).

During development, cells acquire epigenetic changes – principally through different types of modifications to DNA and nucleosomal histone proteins, which can affect the accessibility of gene regulatory regions to the gene expression machinery. This affects which genes will be active in which cells at a given time and which will be silent. At the molecular level, one mechanism by which long-term repression of gene expression and gene silencing is achieved chemically is by the methylation of the nucleotide cytosine (C) at the 5-position of the base (Münzel et al., 2011).

The methylation pattern is a crucial part of the epigenetic information and a critical marker that distinguishes cells. Chromatin structure and packaging is largely determined by DNA methylation or various covalent modifications to histone proteins, and these are the major epigenetic mechanisms that control gene expression. Epigenetic markers transmitted through cell division control differentiation in multicellular organisms. Cell differentiation is based on the establishment of differential expression of genes and provides specific identity to each cell type. The process that allows cell-type-specific gene expression is called *epigenetic gene regulation* (Reik, 2007).

Because of the stable nature of genome, and mechanisms in place to ensure fidelity, most environmental chemical exposures do not have the ability to alter DNA sequence or promote genetic mutations (Skinner and Guerrero-Bosagna, 2009). However, some environmental chemicals can alter the epigenome rather than mutate the genome, and thus alter cellular phenotype without altering the genotype. This can result in a better match between adult phenotype and selective environment, and thus represents a potential solution to problems posed by environmental fluctuation. The phenomenon is called *adaptive developmental plasticity* (Beldade et al., 2011).

8.2 REGULATORY EPIGENETIC MODIFICATIONS

Epigenetic mechanisms for regulation of the gene expression are based on a set of molecular processes that can activate, reduce, or completely disable the activity of particular genes. Epigenetic mechanisms have many layers of complexity in structural regulation of the chromatin, such as methylation of cytosine residues in the sequences of DNA and modifications on the histones surrounding DNA, in particular acetylation or methylation of histone proteins, and post-transcriptional gene regulation, such as mediated repression of gene expression (Fig. 8.2). The different classes of processes are not independent from each other but often regulate gene activity in a complex and interactive manner (Berger, 2007). Interactions between these epigenetic mechanisms generate diversity of cell types during development and then maintain the expression profiles of the different cell types throughout life.

8.2.1 Methylation of Cytosine Residues in the DNA and Impact on Gene Expression (Transcriptional Silencing)

The addition of a small methyl molecule to cytosine, one of the four bases of DNA, is a repressive, epigenetically propagated DNA modification. It is a potent way of transcriptionally silencing genes and one of the best characterized epigenetic modifications (LeBaron et al., 2010). A methyl group gets added to the 5'-ring carbon position of the cytosine pyrimidine ring in individual bases in cytosine–guanine (CpG) dinucleotides, and forms one of the multiple layers of epigenetic mechanisms controlling and modulating gene expression through the chromatin structure

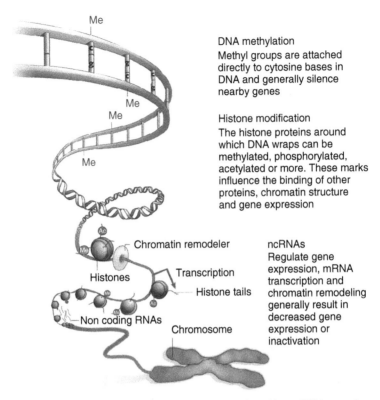

DNA methylation
Methyl groups are attached
directly to cytosine bases in
DNA and generally silence
nearby genes

Histone modification
The histone proteins around
which DNA wraps can be
methylated, phosphorylated,
acetylated or more. These marks
influence the binding of other
proteins, chromatin structure
and gene expression

ncRNAs
Regulate gene
expression, mRNA
transcription and
chromatin remodeling
generally result in
decreased gene
expression or
inactivation

Chromatin remodeler

Transcription

Histones

Histone tails

Non coding RNAs

Chromosome

Figure 8.2 Epigenetic mechanisms include, among other things, DNA cytosine methylation, histone modification, positioning of histone variants, nucleosome remodeling, and noncoding RNAs susceptible to transcription. Source: Adapted from Jones et al. (2008). Reprinted with permission from Macmillan Publishers Ltd © 2008.

(Amato, 2009). Along the linear DNA chain, there are sites of DNA where a cytosine is followed by and linked via a phosphate to guanine, another nucleotide. These sites are called *CpG sites*, and regulatory regions of DNA that have a high density of CpG sites are called *CpG islands* (CGI). CpG dinucleotides are underrepresented (1–2%) in the mammalian genome overall, and those that do not exist as CpG clusters are usually methylated. The exceptions are short stretches of CGI, predominantly located in the promoter regions of genes, which are hypomethylated (Illingworth and Bird, 2009). In other words, isolated CpG sites are methylated but CpG clusters (CGI) are not methylated. DNA methylation occurs predominately on the CGI, the rest being typically located in functional promoter regions, such as the housekeeping genes and other essential and cell/tissue-specific genes, which are nearly always active.

Unoccupied regions along DNA not bound to proteins are accessible to methyltransferases and therefore become methylated at particular residues (cytosines).

In contrast, regions of DNA bound to proteins are inaccessible to methyltransferases. DNA methylation involves multiple DNA methyltransferase (DNMT) proteins – DNMT1, which is primarily responsible for maintaining previously extant DNA methylation, and the DNMT3a/DNMT3b complex which establishes *de novo* DNA methylation (Rottach et al., 2009).

Given its location in the promoters, cytosine methylation in CGI serves a regulatory function in gene expression. The methyls serve as a kind of switch that renders genes active or inactive by affecting interactions between DNA and the cell's protein-making machinery. The number and pattern of methylated cytosines affect the expression of specific genes. By turning genes on and off, the methyls have been found to have a profound impact on the form and function of cells and organisms, without changing the underlying DNA sequence. In most studies, increased DNA methylation is implicated for chromatin compaction and gene silencing, and decreased methylation is associated with chromatin relaxation and gene activation (Fig. 8.3) (Crews and McLachlan, 2006). DNA methylation, which reduces gene expression – so the proteins whose synthesis they encode are not produced – is linked to key developmental events, as well as many types of cancer-causing aberrant repression of tumor suppressor genes.

The epigenome is likely to be most vulnerable to environmental factors during embryogenesis because the DNA synthetic rate is high and the elaborate DNA methylation patterning for normal tissue development is established during this period. Embryonic stem (ES) cells can develop into any type of cell in the body. After fertilization, and at a certain point of the embryonic development, a large number of the methylation marks are erased, which allows ES cells to differentiate into any possible specialized cell. The amount of methylation of genes occurring early in life may have profound effects years later, causing lasting functional changes in specific organs and tissues and increased susceptibility to disease that may even be transgenerationally inherited (Dolinoy et al., 2006).

8.2.2 Remodeling of Chromatin Structure through Post-Translational Modifications of Histone Tails (Determinants of Accessibility)

Epigenetic regulation is possible because DNA in every cell is packaged within a specialized dynamic structure called *chromatin*, which consists of DNA wrapped around histone proteins (see Fig. 8.3b). Epigenetic modifications of DNA and histones, the core components of chromatin, constitute an additional layer of information that influences the expression of the underlying genes. The packaging of the DNA is just as important in determining the expression of that DNA into proteins that make an organism's observable traits or phenotype. The environment is a critical factor in the control of these packaging processes. When the chromatin structure around a genomic region is tightly packed, regardless of DNA sequence, gene expression is repressed. In contrast, a more open chromatin configuration, in which DNA and histones loosely interact, allows access of transcription factors and general transcriptional machinery to the gene regulatory region, leading to the initiation of gene expression (Fig. 8.4) (Li et al., 2007).

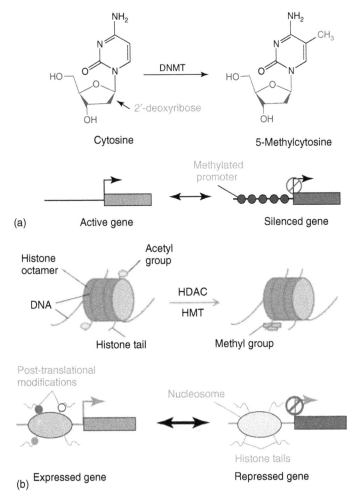

Figure 8.3 Epigenome modification includes enzymatically modified cytosine ring in DNA to 5-methylcytosine. Histone deacetylation and histone methylation represent histone tail modifications for transcriptional regulation. DNMT, DNA methyl transferase; HDAC, histone deacetylase; HMT, histone methyl transferase. (a) DNA methylation. (b) Histone modifications. Source: (a) Adapted from Vandegehuchte and Janssen (2011); figure 1A,B. Reprinted with permission from Springer Science+Business Media; (b) Adapted from Zaidi (2011). Reprinted with permission from The American Society for Biochemistry and Molecular Biology.

Histones are globular proteins with a flexible N-terminus (the so-called tail), which, together with the DNA, make up the nucleosome – the fundamental repeating unit of chromatin that consists of DNA wrapped around an octamer of histones (Fig. 8.4). In multicellular eukaryotes, DNA must be highly compacted to fit within the confines of the nuclear space; however, chromatin is much more than a passive

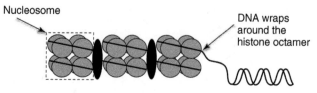

Figure 8.4   DNA in chromatin is wrapped around histone proteins, in units referred to as *nucleosomes*. Source: Adapted from Choudhuri et al. (2010). Reproduced with permission from Academic Press.

way to package the genome. It is a critical player in controlling the accessibility of DNA for transcription.

Histones significantly influence the levels of chromatin compaction by creating a generally condensed "heterochromatin" or more open "euchromatin" region, providing a means by which rapid and localized access to DNA can be accomplished. Most of the chemical modifications of the histones are made to the flexible amino-terminal tails protruding out of the nucleosomal core histones. These tails are subject to post-translational modifications, including phosphorylation and ubiquitination (the addition of a small protein called *ubiquitin*), as well as the more common acetylation and methylation of lysine residues (Fig. 8.3), which are associated with specific transcriptional states of the associated DNA (Jenuwein and Allis, 2001).

The modifications change the charge of the histone tails. For example, of the many possible modifications, lysine residues in histones can be acetylated by histone acetyltransferases (HATs), adding a negatively charged acetyl group to a positively charged lysine, thereby neutralizing the basic charge of the residue on which it occurs. This change has an effect of disrupting histone contacts with other histones and/or DNA and, in turn, chromatin compaction, which in some cases can free up DNA from histones, making activator binding sites accessible. This can lead to changes in chromatin conformation, precipitating an epigenetic effect on transcription (Choudhuri et al., 2010). Altered chromatin conformation, in turn, can limit or enhance the accessibility and binding of the transcription machinery, thereby allowing the underlying gene to be activated or repressed. In general, acetylation of lysine residues is associated with the relaxation of chromatin (euchromatin), facilitating increased gene expression. Thus, histone acetylation is considered the best hallmark by which to predict chromatin activity. Histone acetylation can be reversed by deacetylation by histone deacetylases (HDACs), which remove the acetyl groups from the lysine residues leading to the formation of a condensed (heterochromatin) and transcriptionally silenced chromatin (Fig. 8.5).

Methylation of histones is associated with either repression or activation of transcription, depending on the site of lysine methylation (Yan and Boyd, 2006). Since there are different states of methylation (mono-, di-, or trimethylation) possible for one lysine residue, the biological consequences of methylation may differ. Improper modifications of histones cause genes to not be expressed when they normally would be, or vice versa.

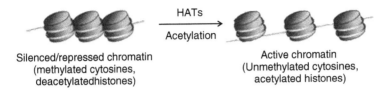

Silenced/repressed chromatin
(methylated cytosines,
deacetylatedhistones)

Active chromatin
(Unmethylated cytosines,
acetylated histones)

Figure 8.5 Activation and repression of transcription involve chromatin remodeling and post-translational modification of the histone tails (chromatin modification). Acetylation of lysine residues in histones is associated with chromatin transcriptional activation.

An "epigenetic code" is defined by combinations of histone modifications that are predictive of, and necessary for, expression patterns of differentiation and developmental-specific genes (Gardner et al., 2011). It is known that there is interaction between histone modifications and DNA methylation, although the precise mechanism is not known. Generally speaking, DNA methylation must work in concert with histone deacetylation and histone methylation to create a repressed chromatin state for gene silencing (Zhang and Ho, 2011). A recent finding indicates that HDACs are also recruited by methyl-CpG-binding domain proteins (MBPs) to methylated CGI, resulting in the deacetylation of neighboring promoters. This association creates a combinatorial effect of transcriptional repression of certain genes in mammals.

8.2.3   Regulation of Gene Expression by Noncoding RNAs

Genes are made of DNA, and produce an intermediate molecule called messenger RNA (mRNA) that is then translated into a protein. Gene expression can be changed as a response to exogenous stressors such as environmental chemicals. Such changes may be regulated by specific endogenous, small (20–25 nucleotides long), noncoding RNAs (ncRNAs) that are also encoded by DNA. ncRNAs act as a cellular rheostat for fine-tuning gene expression by playing a role in the epigenetic regulation during development and differentiation. The term *noncoding* is employed for RNA that does not encode a protein. They interact with the mRNAs of protein coding genes with which they share partial sequence complementarity, leading to post-transcriptional gene silencing through a variety of mechanisms, including translational repression of mRNA, mRNA degradation, DNA methylation, and chromatin modification.

Understanding of small ncRNA-mediated epigenetic regulation has expanded with the discovery of microRNAs (miRNAs) as regulators of developmental genes and small interfering RNAs (siRNAs) as defenders of genome integrity in response to foreign or invasive nucleic acids such as viruses. Both are broadly distributed, characterized by the double-stranded nature of their precursors, double-stranded RNA (dsRNA) or hairpin RNA, cleaved by a biological scissor, the ribonuclease (RNase) III enzyme (Dicer). Argonaute effector proteins can bind single-stranded forms of both miRNAs and siRNAs and are found to be associated with effector

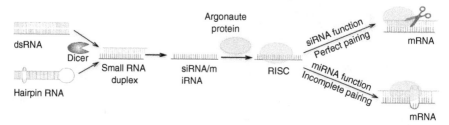

Figure 8.6 Noncoding RNA-mediated pathways. ncRNA molecules such as microRNA (miRNA) and small interfering RNA (siRNA) are snipped from longer double-stranded RNA (dsRNA) or hairpin RNA chains by an enzyme called *Dicer*. A strand of the siRNA is used by an RNA-induced silencing complex (RISC) to target messenger RNAs (mRNAs), which results in post-translational repression leading to gene silencing. Source: Adapted from Vandegehuchte and Janssen (2011); figure 1C. Reprinted with permission from Springer Science+Business Media.

assemblies known as *RNA-induced silencing complexes* (RISCs). It is thought that Dicer processing is coupled with unwinding of the duplex, as only one strand is incorporated into the RISC. RISC is targeted to mRNA through sequence complementarity (Watson/Crick base pairing), which results in cleavage and degradation of mRNA or translational repression of the target mRNA and subsequently in decreased gene expression (Carthew and Sontheimer, 2009). When an miRNA has complete sequence complementarity with a target mRNA, it instead directs cleavage of the transcript; without its mRNA, a gene is essentially inactive (Fig. 8.6). miRNAs have newly emerged as a gene expression regulatory factor that may link environmental chemicals and their related diseases.

Through DNA methylation, histone tail modifications, and small regulatory RNAs, the epigenome systematically controls gene expression during development both *in utero* and throughout life. Its labile nature allows it to respond and adapt to environmental perturbations to ensure survival during fetal growth.

8.2.4 DNA Demethylation

As DNA methylation is directly involved in the modulation of gene expression and cellular identity, DNA demethylation is important for cleaning the genomic slate during embryogenesis or achieving rapid reactivation of previously silenced genes. Thus, one very important aspect of epigenetic methylation is its reversibility, which is creating a promising field of epigenetic therapy. However, the enzymes responsible for demethylation have been elusive for a long time. A recent study indicated that in mouse ES cell genomic DNA, the TET (ten-eleven translocation) family of dioxygenases could catalyze the oxidative conversion of 5-methylcytosine (5mC) of DNA to 5-hydroxymethylcytosine (5hmC) and also to 5-formylcytosine (5fC) (Pfaffeneder et al., 2011) and 5-carboxylcytosine (5caC), the molecular entities thought to play a role in DNA demethylation (Ito et al., 2010, 2011). Although this

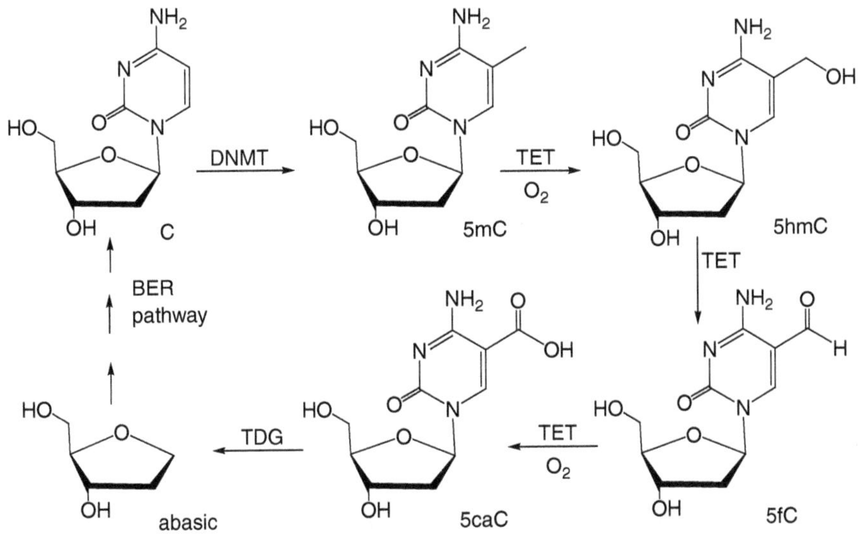

Figure 8.7 DNA demethylation. Cytosine (C), which is modified to 5-methylcytosine (5mC) by DNA methyltransferases (DNMTs), is oxidized by TET family of oxygenases to 5-hydroxymethyl C (5hmC), and subsequently to the higher oxidation substituents 5-formyl C (5fC) and 5-carboxyl C (5caC), thought to be the putative demethylation intermediates (Ito et al., 2011). Removal of the entire caC nucleobase by thymine-DNA glycosylase (TDG), and subsequent repair of the resulting abasic site restores unmodified C (He et al., 2011).

hypothetic pathway for DNA demethylation is appealing, the enzyme that is capable of decarboxylating 5caC-containing DNA has not been found (Ito et al., 2011). 5caC is also stated to be chemically stable and does not spontaneously decarboxylate to cytosine under physiological conditions (He et al., 2011). Recently, direct removal of the entire caC nucleobase by the DNA-repair enzyme thymine DNA glycosylase (TDG) has been suggested, by excising the mismatched thymine formed from the resulting G:T base pairs. The resulting abasic site can then be repaired by the base excision repair (BER) pathway to incorporate cytosine bases, resulting in replacement of 5-mc with unmodified cytosine (He et al., 2011) (Fig. 8.7).

8.2.5 Assays for Epigenetic Modification

There are many assays used to assess the effects of epigenetic modifications. Bisulfite modification tracks changes in DNA methylation by employing the relative resistance of the conversion of methylcytosine to uracil compared with cytosine (Fig. 8.8) (Herman et al., 1996). Chromatin immunoprecipitation (ChIP) is another commonly used technique that serves to monitor changes in chromatin structure (DeAngelis et al., 2008). A conventional ChIP uses formaldehyde to cross-link chromatin-associated proteins to DNA, followed by immunoprecipitation of DNA–protein complexes with specific antibodies. Once the crosslinks

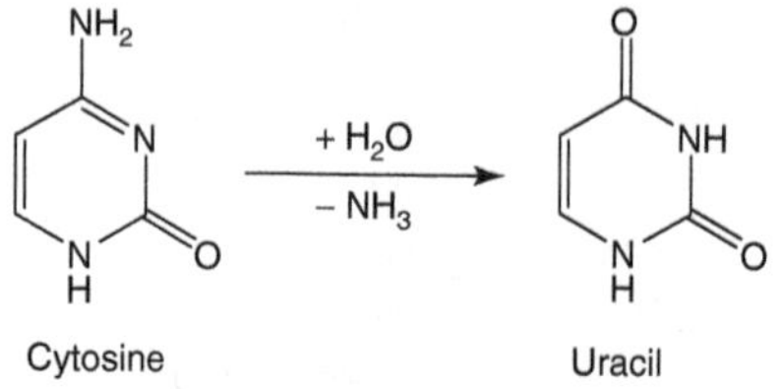

Figure 8.8   Treatment of DNA with bisulfite at pH 5 followed by alkaline desulfonation leads to conversion of cytosines to uracil, but 5-methylcytosines are protected.

with formaldehyde are reversed, the recovered DNA can then be analyzed using polymerase chain reaction (PCR) to determine whether specific DNA sequences are associated with the protein of interest.

8.3   EPIGENETIC DYSREGULATION EFFECTS OF ENDOCRINE DISRUPTION

Most man-made synthetic compounds have not been present in our biosphere until very recently in human and vertebrate evolutionary history. Therefore, biological evolution has not had enough time to evolve mechanisms against the adverse effects of the disruption caused by these chemicals. Hormones are chemical messengers that travel through the blood to target cells where they interact with receptors, which, in turn, directly influence gene activity, including likely via epigenetic mechanisms. Any endocrine disruption may therefore have epigenetic consequences at the molecular level such as DNA methylation and histone modification (Foley et al., 2009).

Epigenetic events play a critical role in normal physiological responses to environmental stimuli by changing gene expression patterns without altering the genetic code and modify adult disease susceptibility in various ways. Environmental contaminants can cause some genes to be methylated at times during development when methylation would not normally occur. Low levels of methylation correspond to genes that could potentially be expressed; high methylation areas correspond to low gene activity. Environmental modifications of gene expression can affect embryonic imprinting, cellular differentiation, and phenotypic expression (Weinhold, 2006). These epigenetic modifications can also be detrimental, both in later life and to future generations. Effects of environmental influences on the epigenome not only depend on the dose but also on the critical developmental timing such as *in utero*, during puberty, and during pregnancy, which are times of great tissue differentiation.

Recent studies have demonstrated the ability of EDCs to have epigenetic effects (Newbold et al., 2006; Anway et al., 2005). The first to report the epigenetic effect of an EDC most likely was Barrett et al. (1982), who proposed that diethylstilbestrol (DES) could transform cells by a mechanism other than point mutations, frame-shift mutations, or small deletions. With the current knowledge of epige-netic mechanisms, it is likely that such transformations reported by them were the products of epigenetic processes (Guerrero-Bosagna and Valladares, 2007).

The epigenome is susceptible to dysregulation throughout life; however, it is thought to be most vulnerable to environmental factors during embryonic devel-opment, which is a period of rapid cell division and epigenetic remodeling. This change is mediated by inappropriate activation or deactivation of receptors that act as transcription factors. The classical model of receptor activation is that, in the absence of a ligand, co-repressors are bound, chromatin is condensed, and transcription is minimal at target genes. Ligand binding triggers a conformational change in the receptor, which favors binding of co-activators and release of co-repressors, chromatin decondensation, and transcriptional activation (Janesick and Blumberg, 2011).

Most diseases have no known genetic basis but are thought to have an environ-mental basis. Most environmental agents are, nonetheless, not mutagenic. Research into a number of chemicals including vinclozolin, methoxychlor, and BPA is show-ing the potential to cause epigenetic effects related to various diseases including cancer, diabetes and obesity, infertility, respiratory diseases, allergies, and neurode-generative disorders such as Parkinson's and Alzheimer's diseases (Edwards and Myers, 2007). These effects stack up over a lifetime. Studies involving monozy-gotic twins have shown that they accrue differences in methylation patterns as they age, with the greatest differences found between older twins living farther apart (Fraga et al., 2005). Given that twins who begin life are genetically and epigeneti-cally identical, something is modifying the supra-genetic mechanisms that control when their genes are turned on and off, which may result in one twin developing a disease such as cancer while the other twin does not.

Several reviews have dealt with the subject, including all-inclusive reviews on endocrine disruption and epigenetics, implications for ecotoxicology, molecular targets of epigenetic mechanisms, transgenerational inheritance, and adverse envi-ronmental impacts in mammals (Choudhuri et al., 2010; Jablonka and Raz, 2009; Bollati and Baccarelli, 2010; LeBaron et al., 2010; Vandegehuchte and Janssen, 2011; Zhang and Ho, 2011; Greally, 2011).

8.3.1 Bisphenol A (BPA): A Case Study

A number of compounds can be used to demonstrate epigenetic mechanisms via environmental EDCs, such as BPA, which provides a highly illustrative example of long-lasting effects. BPA is an industrial chemical used in polycarbonate plastic production and in epoxy resin linings in metal-based food and beverage cans. An NIH (National Institutes of Health) sponsored expert panel determined that BPA alters epigenetic programming of genes in experimental animals and wildlife and that this results in persistent effects that are expressed later in life (vom Saal et al., 2007). Specifically, *in utero* or neonatal exposures to low doses of BPA are associ-ated with increased breast and prostate cancer, altered reproductive function and behavior of laboratory animals, and obesity. Agouti viable yellow (A^{vy}) mouse is a sensitive reporter of epigenetic changes for environmental effects on fetus (Waterland, 2006). *Agouti* gene is normally expressed in skin and gives the normal coat color of agouti mice, ranging from pure yellow (hypomethylation) to pseudo-agouti brown (hyper-methylation) (Kundakovic and Champagne, 2011). Evidence that epigenetic patterning during early stem-cell development is sensitive to BPA exposure was provided by maternal exposure of A^{vy} mouse with BPA (10 mg/kg body weight/day), which led to significant shift in the offspring's coat color toward yellow. This was an indication of epigenetic dysregulation due to hypomethylation of the gene. In contrast, dietary exposure to phytoestrogen genistein in A^{vy} mice induced gene hypermethylation, shifting offspring coat color toward pseudo-agouti brown (Dolinoy et al., 2006). The maternal nutritional supplementation rich with methyl donors such as folic acid or genistein also counteracted the DNA hypomethylating effect of BPA, resulting in a controlled coat color distribution in the BPA-induced offspring (Dolinoy et al., 2007; Bernal and Jirtle, 2010). These alterations in the coat color are also associated with the overall health of the animals, with pseudo-agouti being healthy and yellow being obese, diabetic, and susceptible to tumor development (Fig. 8.9). This also demonstrated how diet could protect against deleterious effects of chemical compounds, at least in this specific case.

BPA exposure of fetal mice during pregnancy led to epigenetic changes that caused permanent reproduction problems for both male and female offspring. The altered methylation has been identified as a novel mechanism of BPA-induced altered developmental programming. The study showed that BPA exposure

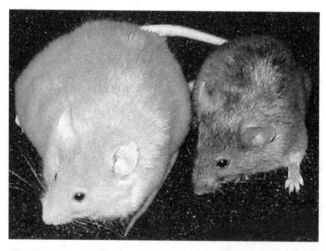

Figure 8.9 The two Agouti mice are genetically identical and are of the same age. The different appearances of these offspring result from alterations in the epigenome. The mother of the mouse at left (yellow coat) was fed a normal diet, while the mother of the mouse at right (brown coat) was fed a diet supplemented with methyl donors (i.e. choline, folic acid, betaine and vitamin B12), which turned the gene off. Source: Reprinted with permission from Dr. Randy Jirtle.

permanently affected the uterus by decreasing regulation of gene expression. These epigenetic changes caused the mice to overrespond to estrogen throughout adulthood, long after the BPA exposure (Bromer et al., 2010). It has been suggested that exposure to BPA during the critical development window genetically "programmed" the uterus to be hyper-responsive to estrogen. Extreme estrogen sensitivity can lead to fertility problems, advanced puberty, and altered mammary development and reproductive function, as well as higher incidence of hormone-related breast and prostate cancers. Although the estrogenic function has been described in adults, adult exposure did not lead to epigenetic alterations in DNA methylation. Permanent epigenetic alteration of estrogen response element (ERE) sensitivity to estrogen may be a general mechanism through which endocrine disruptors exert their action (Bromer et al., 2010).

The effect of xenoestrogens on DNA methylation and embryonic development may be independent of their function. For example, *in utero*, BPA exposure to pregnant mice led to decreased methylation and consequently increases in adult *Hoxa10* gene expression. *Hoxa10* is an estrogen-regulated gene that is necessary for uterine development and pregnancy. A similar *in utero* DES exposure was seen to lead to increased methylation. This difference in epigenetic alterations may also explain the distinct set of developmental consequences seen after exposure to these two estrogenic compounds (Bromer et al., 2010). A more direct evidence linking epigenetic reprogramming via DNA methylation and aberrant gene expression in adult tissues and altered disease susceptibility was provided by a study showing increased prostate cancer risk in rats exposed neonatally to bisphenol A or estradiol (Ho et al., 2006).

8.3.2 DEHP

The anti-androgenic di-2-(ethylhexyl) phthalate (DEHP) administered to gravid (Kunming) female mice (an outbred colony in China) resulted in testicular function abnormalities in offspring. A global increase in DNA methylation in testes was observed in the exposed fetal and newborn mice, with increases in DNMT gene expression and protein levels, suggesting an epigenetic contribution to the male reproductive tract (Wu et al., 2010).

8.4 ENVIRONMENTAL EPIGENETIC EFFECTS OF HEAVY METALS EXPOSURE

Heavy metals are widespread environmental contaminants. Arguably, heavy metals are also endocrine disruptors, but since their mechanisms of action are frequently different from those organic EDCs, they are often considered to be a separate category. Several studies have established an association between DNA methylation and heavy metals, including nickel, cadmium, lead, and, particularly, arsenic. Metal-induced oxidative stress is proposed to represent a unifying process to account for these findings across different metals. Metals are known to catalyze and increase the production of reactive oxygen species (ROS), which may induce oxidative DNA damage. This can interfere with the ability of methyltransferases to interact with DNA, thus resulting in a generalized altered methylation of cytosine residues at CpG sites (Baccarelli and Bollati, 2009).

8.4.1 Cadmium

Cadmium (Cd) exposure for 1 week caused hypomethylation in a rat liver cell line, while a 10-week exposure period induced DNA hypermethylation (Takiguchi et al., 2003). It was shown that Cd inhibited DNMT activity, possibly as a result of binding with the DNA binding domain of the enzyme, which can explain the initial hypomethylation. However, prolonged exposure was shown to lead to DNA hypermethylation in the same experiment, likely a compensatory effect due to the initial inhibition of the enzyme DNMT genes being overexpressed. This is consistent with other studies, in which short-term (24–48 h) and long-term (2 months) Cd exposure induced hypomethylation and hypermethylation, respectively, in human cells (Huang et al., 2008; Jiang et al., 2008).

8.4.2 Arsenic

Arsenic (As) is another metal associated with epigenetic effects. Exposure to As alters DNA methylation patterns, possibly as a result of competition for methyl donors since As is methylated during metabolic process of detoxification. Association of long-term exposure to low levels of arsenic-containing compounds has been shown with global DNA hypomethylation (Zhao et al., 1997; Reichard et al., 2007) and hypermethylation of tumor suppressor genes in subjects exposed to higher levels of arsenic (Chanda et al., 2006). In a study with rat liver cell lines chronically exposed to As, global hypomethylation was observed and shown to be dose and time dependent (Zhao et al., 1997). On the other hand, a study from India on human subjects exposed to toxic level of arsenic showed significant hypermethylation of blood DNA compared to controls. In this study, a dose–response relationship was observed with arsenic measured in drinking water (Chanda et al., 2006). Arsenic exposure has also been shown to increase histone acetylation by inhibiting the activity of HDACs (Ramirez et al., 2008).

8.4.3 Nickel

Nickel ion exposure has been shown to increase DNA methylation and long-term gene silencing and also to interfere with the removal of histone methylation *in vivo*. Broday et al. (2000) studied nickel effects, at nontoxic levels, on yeast and mammalian cells and found a decrease in histone H4 acetylation (Broday et al., 2000). Similarly, a recent study has shown that nickel ions can inhibit the activity of the histone demethylase enzyme JMJD1A by replacing iron ions within the enzyme's catalytic domain (Chen et al., 2010). Human lung cells exposure to soluble nickel compound caused histone modifications, including loss of acetylation, increased demethylation, and increased ubiquitinylation (Ke et al., 2006).

8.4.4 Lead

Lead is among the most prevalent toxic environmental metals, and has substantial oxidative properties. Exposure to lead during the first 400 days of the lives of 23-year-old monkeys led to decreased DNMT activity in their brain cells (Wu et al., 2008). Similar inhibitory effect of Pb was demonstrated in a study on a group of Mexican population, showing an inverse relationship between Pb concentrations in maternal bone tissue, a good bioindicator of Pb exposure, and global DNA methylation in umbilical cord blood samples (Pilsner et al., 2009).

8.5 TRANSGENERATIONAL INHERITANCE OF ENVIRONMENTALLY INDUCED EPIGENETIC ALTERATIONS

Epidemiological studies have indicated the associations of environmental factors in childhood, such as stress or poor nutrition, which could induce epigenetic changes that last into adulthood or into the next generation (Neel, 1962). A body of research suggests that the health consequences of fetal exposure to environmental chemicals might also be passed to future generations. The transmission of epigenetic information between generations in the absence of any direct environmental exposures is termed as *transgenerational epigenetic inheritance*. Many of the EDCs exert significant epigenetic action, causing adverse effects that may persist and even be transgenerational (Zhang and Ho, 2011). DNA in primordial germ cells is demethylated and then remethylated in a sex-specific manner during gonadal sex determination. The mechanism involved in the transgenerational phenotypes is the reprogramming of the germ line (sperm) during male sex determination. This altered sperm epigenome appears to be permanently reprogrammed and escapes the DNA methylation programming at fertilization to allow transgenerational transmission of the altered sperm epigenome, which then promotes all tissues developed from that sperm to have altered cell and tissue transcriptomes that can promote transgenerational disease.

It has been believed that epigenetic reprogramming events occur in primordial germ cells and early embryo that undergo genome-wide demethylation. The new organism would have the epigenetic marks acquired by the previous generation erased and would develop solely based on the inherited genetic makeup. However, there is now evidence that DNA methylation at certain loci can escape reprogramming during development, providing the basis for the hypothesis that transgenerational inheritance may occur through epigenetic mechanisms both in rodents and humans (Lange and Schneider, 2010; Reik, 2007). Although most genes get reset in early embryonic development, a subset of genes called *imprinted genes* maintain their DNA methylation pattern, which appears to be permanently programmed. The pregnant mother exposed at the time of sex determination appears to have altered remethylation of the germ line, a permanently reprogrammed imprinted pattern of DNA methylation (Anway et al., 2005). This provides a unique epigenetic mechanism to propagate environmentally induced transgenerational phenotype.

The potential of EDCs to modify the epigenome could have long-lasting effects when these epigenetic changes occur during certain stages of development; they are permanent and are heritable extending to several generations (Anway et al., 2005). The lingering effect on subsequent generations of an initial environmental disturbance in parent animals can be profound, with genes continuing to be variously silenced or expressed without an associated change in gene sequence for many generations. Epigenetic alteration of DNA methylation of imprinted genes has been shown to promote disease states such as cancer and tumor development (Skinner et al., 2010). This implicates the profound importance of epigenetic mechanisms affecting development, and suggests that contaminants altering the epigenetic control of gene expression are key to understanding fetal origins of adult disease hypothesis. The results to date suggest that a wide range of environmental conditions during embryonic development and early life determine susceptibility to disease during adult life.

8.5.1 DES

Both human and animal (Newbold et al., 2006) studies demonstrate that an embryonic exposure (F0 generation mother) can produce an impact on F2 generation phenotype (Fig. 8.10). One of the best examples of this phenomenon emerged from studies of DES. In humans, prenatal DES treatment is now known to be associated with an increased risk of reproductive anomalies and reproductive tract tumors, not only in individuals exposed to DES *in utero* but also in the subsequent generation of offspring (see Chapter 3). In mice, perinatal exposure to DES resulted in genital tract abnormalities and cancers in the first (F1) and second (F2) generation offspring. It has been suggested that these abnormalities may be associated with aberrant DNA methylation in uterine-development- and uterine-cancer-related genes, implying that epigenetic alterations might underlie transgenerational adverse effects of DES (Newbold et al., 2006).

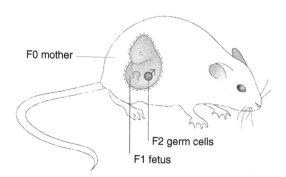

F0 mother

F2 germ cells

F1 fetus

Figure 8.10 In a gestating mother, there is a multiple-generation exposure of the F0 female, the F1 fetus, and the F2 generation germ cells to environmental factors. Source: Adapted from Jirtle and Skinner (2007). Reprinted with permission from Macmillan Publishers Ltd.

However, it is known that when mothers are exposed to a toxicant during pregnancy, the mother (F0 generation), the developing fetus (F1 generation), and the germ cells developing within those fetus, which mature into the sperm and eggs that give rise to F2 generation, experience direct exposure to the compound (Fig. 8.10) (Jirtle and Skinner, 2007). Therefore, disease phenotypes in the F1 and F2 generations might still be due to the toxicology of direct exposure to the environmental factor. Therefore, only a study with the F3 generation, the great-grandchildren of the original animal, which is the first generation not directly exposed to the environmental factor, can provide the first unequivocal signs of transgenerational inheritance. Effects that extend to the F2 generation are known as *multigenerational*, whereas those that extend to the F3 generation are known as *transgenerational* (Skinner, 2008).

Several studies have shown marked effects of environmental toxicants on the F3 generation through germline (sperm, ova) alterations in the epigenome, including the fungicide vinclozolin, methoxychlor, BPA, and dioxin. A critical factor in epigenetic transgenerational inheritance is that the phenotype be transmitted through the germ line (sperm) in the absence of direct exposure (Skinner et al., 2011). A study on rats has shown the transgenerational action of endocrine disruptors on spermatogenic capacity together with an associated change in sperm DNA methylation. The ability of an endocrine disruptor to reprogram the germ line and to promote a transgenerational disease state has been considered to have significant implications for evolutionary biology and disease etiology (Anway et al., 2005; Crews and Gore, 2012).

8.5.2   Vinclozolin

Environmental insult such as transient embryonic exposure to the estrogenic insecticide methoxychlor or the anti-androgenic fungicide vinclozolin during a critical period for testis sex differentiation in Sprague–Dawley rat (embryonic d 8–15) produced male offspring that had reduced fertility and reduced sperm development in the adult testis (Anway et al. 2005, 2006; Crews et al., 2007a, 2007b; Skinner et al., 2011). Crucially, vinclozolin led to the effect only when administered between 8 and 15 days post coitum, during the period of gonadal sex determination, and had no effect when administered later, between 15 and 20 days. This sensitive development period coincides with the epigenetic remethylation phase in the male, thus suggesting that the hormonal effect of androgens is developmentally specific (limited to this period of epigenetic programming). Remarkably, these effects could still be detected to at least the F4 generations of male progeny without diminution, with no additional exposure (Anway et al., 2005). Interestingly, the phenotype was observed in nearly all males from EDC-treated generations and was found to be associated with modulation of genome-wide DNA methylation patterns in the male germ line (sperm), triggering an epigenetic change to a genetic trait (Fig. 8.11) (Skinner et al., 2013; Anway et al., 2008; Skinner, 2007; Edwards and Myers, 2007). In the study, exposure levels in the rat were higher than a typical

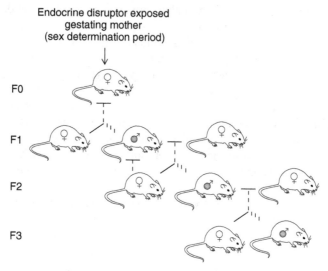

Figure 8.11 Epigenetic transgenerational actions of endocrine disruptors through the male germ line. Source: Adapted from Jirtle and Skinner (2007). Reprinted with permission from Macmillan Publishers Ltd.

environmental exposure, but the epigenetic effects on male fertility caused by these EDCs point to an important new mechanism for EDC disruption of gene expression.

Altered DNA methylation of two genes was suggested as a potential mediator of this effect. Several DNA, RNA, and histone methyltransferases were shown to be altered significantly in the testes of offspring prenatally exposed to vinclozolin, compared to controls. A subset of these genes remained altered in subsequent generations, despite the fact that vinclozolin exposure only occurred in F0 (Anway et al., 2008). Later in life, the animals developed adult onset disease states such as mammary tumors, prostate disease, kidney disease, testis abnormalities, and immune abnormalities at high (20–50%) frequencies (Anway et al., 2006).

When a female rat was caged with two different males—the F3 male offspring of vinclozolin-treated pregnant rats and a control animal—the female shunned the male descended from a treated rat. While this behavioral change because of sperm abnormalities did not affect reproductive success, it is suggested that such multigenerational effects could bias reproduction, and play a role in evolution (Crews et al., 2007a, 2007b).

Recently, two research groups (Schneider et al., 2008; Inawaka et al., 2009) failed to reproduce the reported adverse transgenerational effects, one of these employing vinclozolin administration by intraperitoneal injection using the same dosing level and regimen (100 mg/kg/day) as reported by Anway et al. (2005) (Inawaka et al., 2009; also Furr and Gray, 2009), and the other by the oral route (Schneider et al., 2008). The differences in finding are ascribed to the inbred versus outbred nature of the rat strain used in these studies (Skinner et al., 2010; Kaiser,

2014). Nevertheless, another recent study with mice administering 50 mg/kg/day vinclozolin *in utero* exposure during pregnancy confirmed the induction of transgenerational effects on DNA methylation of some imprinted genes, exhibiting decreased sperm motility in two generations of male mice but motility recovering to the level of controls by the F3 generation (F1 = 56%, F2 = 90%, F3 = 100%) (Stouder and Paoloni-Giacobino, 2010).

8.5.3 Methoxychlor

Methoxychlor exposure to fetal and neonatal rats caused adult ovarian dysfunction. This was correlated to down expression of key ovarian genes including ERβ, without affecting ERα (Zama and Uzumcu, 2009). Significant hypermethylation in the ERβ regions was observed as the case of downregulation. Administration of methoxychlor to pregnant female mice resulted in transgenerational effect, promoting a spermatogenic defect characterized by increased apoptosis and decreased cell number and motility in adult F1, which was carried over four generations. The defect was linked to altered DNA methylation of the male germ line and the induction of new imprinted-like DNA methylation sites (Stouder and Paoloni-Giacobino, 2011).

8.5.4 BPA

Recently, low levels of BPA exposure at environmentally relevant levels (1.2 and 2.4 µg/kg/day) were shown to induce transgenerational effects in rats affecting the male germ line (Salian et al., 2009a). Male offspring perinatally exposed to BPA from gestational day 12 through postnatal day 21 had impaired fertility with reduced sperm counts and sperm motility, and these phenotypes persisted through the F3 generation. The immunohistochemistry of the F1–F3 rats revealed that AR, ERβ, steroid receptor co-regulator 1, and nuclear co-repressor protein expression were decreased in their testes (Salian et al., 2009a). Steroid receptor co-regulators are known to be HATs and HDACs, implying that the early life BPA exposure may result in long-term alterations to histone modifications and chromatin remodeling in a transgenerational manner.

Exposure of female mice to low doses of BPA, in a range similar to those measured in humans, only during gestation was also found to have immediate and long-lasting, transgenerational effects on the brain and social behaviors, and related hormones, such as vasopressin, in their F4 offspring (Wolstenholme et al., 2012 et al., 2012).

8.5.5 2,3,7,8-Tetrachlorodibenzo-*p*-dioxin (TCDD)

Dioxins, which are industrial byproducts created by waste incinerators and other processes, have been linked to cancer, reproductive disorders, and other health problems. A study of TCDD exposure *in utero* in F1 C57BL/6 mice has demonstrated an increased incidence of premature birth. Also, after the gestating F0 generation was exposed to TCDD, decreased fertility was seen in F3 and F4 generation female mice (Bruner-Tran and Osteen, 2011). In another study, F0 generation pregnant rats were exposed to TCDD when their fetuses were 8 and 14 days old, and adult onset disease was evaluated in F1 and F3 generation (not directly exposed) rats (Manikkam et al., 2012a). The generation F1 offspring had prostate and ovarian diseases compared to control groups. The F3 females had increased ovarian disease and early onset of puberty, and in F3 males, kidney disease was significantly higher than in the control rats. Also, F3 generation sperm epigenome identified 50 differentially DNA methylated regions in gene promoters, providing potential epigenetic biomarkers for transgenerational disease and ancestral environmental exposures (Manikkam et al., 2012a).

8.6 TRANSGENERATIONAL ACTIONS OF EDCs MIXTURE ON REPRODUCTIVE DISEASE

Exposure of a gestating female to a mixture consisting of BPA, DEHP and DBP during the critical development period of fetal gonadal sex determination was investigated in F1 and F3 generation rats for the potential transgenerational inheritance of testis and ovary diseases, pubertal abnormalities, and obesity (Manikkam et al., 2012b, 2013). Gestating F0 generation female Sprague–Dawley rats were given <1% fraction of the oral LD_{50} dose intraperitoneally (i.p.) daily during embryonic days 8–14 of fetal development correlating with the gonadal sex determination. Significant increases in the incidence of total disease/abnormalities were observed in F3 generation animals (Manikkam et al., 2013). The onset of puberty was investigated in the F1–F3 generation rats, for females at postnatal day 30 and males at postnatal day 35 until puberty (Manikkam et al., 2012b). The F1 generation had delayed female pubertal onset, while the F2 generation had early onset of puberty for both females and males. The transgenerational F3 generation had early onset of puberty in females, with no effect on males. Therefore, this exposure promoted early onset of puberty only in females transgenerationally (Manikkam et al., 2012b).

Fertility is influenced by testis and ovary functions, which are hormone-regulated, and both produce endocrine steroids. Gonadal function for both testis and ovary were investigated in the F3 generation at postnatal 120 days of age. A transgenerational effect on the F3 generation ovary was a significant reduction in primordial follicle pool. The F3 generation males had a reduction in testosterone levels. Therefore, the endocrine system was altered transgenerationally in the males.

The F3 generation rat sperm from the control and exposure group were analyzed for genome-wide promoter DNA methylation, and 197 differentially methylated regions (DMRs) were identified as compared with control. These DMR clusters may represent "epigenetic control regions" where different exposure DMRs may commonly regulate genome activity. The identification of epigenetic alterations in specific regions of the F3 generation sperm may support a role for epigenetic transgenerational inheritance of the disease phenotypes observed (Manikkam et al., 2012b).

8.7 CONCLUSIONS AND FUTURE PROSPECTS

Epigenetics is a burgeoning field of science that studies how gene expression and function can be altered by means other than a change in the sequence of DNA, that is, a mutation. Epigenetic programming of our genes is critical for normal human development and function. For example, epigenetics is the reason why the single fertilized egg we all began as differentiates into the more than 200 different types of cells that make up our adult bodies.

Advances in our understanding of molecular epigenetics have added considerable insight into the effects of environmental stimuli during development and the significance of the timing of exposures to these stimuli on later human health. The evidence thus far is highly suggestive of a role for epigenomic dysregulation mediating the effects of exposures to environmental endocrine disruptors, having profound effects on development and fertility. Mechanistically, it is plausible that the epigenome is responsible for some or most of the phenotypic consequences of these exposures. There is evidence from rat studies that perturbations of components of the reproductive system induced in one generation by EDC exposure can be expressed at least up to the F4 generation, even in the absence of any further exposure. Currently, a handful of papers have implicated EDCs in epigenetic programming and DNA methylation and a few studies have examined the long-term consequences of embryonic exposure to EDCs in terms of reproductive fitness across generations. That epigenetic mechanisms may play a role in endocrine disruption helps explain the transgenerational effects of some hormonally active chemicals. Such transgenerational epigenetic effects of EDC exposure, yet to be demonstrated more widely, are likely to depend on the chemical, animal species, and physiological system involved.

The brisk pace of research into the intricacies of gene regulation, which includes the study of epigenetic mechanisms, is rapidly expanding our understanding of the ways in which environmental influences can affect these processes. And we are beginning to understand how acute exposure to EDCs may result in long-term epigenetic effects on the developing individual, and on subsequent generations. By identifying the molecular epigenetic mechanisms of transmission, it may be possible to reverse adverse changes in DNA methylation and histone modifications through interventions targeted to these biological pathways. Thus far, endocrine disrupting studies have mainly focused on epigenetic changes in reproductive tract tissues. However, similar effects can conceivably occur in other differentiating endocrine responsive tissues (Newbold, 2010).

Human exposures are comparable to those in wildlife, because people are exposed throughout their lives, and the cause and effect relationship between xenobiotic exposures, epigenetic changes, and physiological/pathological consequences, as well as the underlying mechanisms, can be difficult to ascertain. It is also important to note that species variation does occur, and direct linkages between wildlife and human abnormalities may or may not occur (Walker and Gore, 2011). Nevertheless, the weight of evidence to date supports a need to be concerned about EDC exposures, and to invoke the *Precautionary Principle* when new chemicals are introduced into household and food products.

Recently, Daxinger and Whitelaw (2012) considered DNA methylation being the molecular basis of transgenerational epigenetic inheritance via the gametes as counterintuitive. In their view, an inherited epigenetic mark not cleared would affect the genes' activity in all cell types of developing embryo, affecting the organism's ability to develop all the correct cell types. Citing recent evidence, they favored the role of RNA in this process (Daxinger and Whitelaw, 2012). Perhaps future studies would focus more at looking for processes (or factors) that disrupt or enhance the reestablishment of silent heterochromatin between generations rather than looking for an epigenetic mark that is retained across generations.

REFERENCES

Amato, I. Gene takes a back seat, *C&E News* **2009**, 87(14), 28–32.

Anway, M. D.; Cupp, A. S.; Uzumcu M.; Skinner, M. K. Epigenetic transgenerational actions of endocrine disruptors and male fertility, *Science* **2005**, 308, 1466–1469.

Anway, M. D.; Leathers, C.; Skinner, M. K. Endocrine disruptor vinclozolin induced epigenetic transgenerational adult-onset disease, *Endocrinology* **2006**, 147, 5515–5523.

Anway, M. D.; Rekow, S. S.; Skinner, M. K. Transgenerational epigenetic programming of the embryonic testis transcriptome, *Genomics* **2008**, 91(1), 30–40.

Baccarelli, A.; Bollati, V. Epigenetics and environmental chemicals, *Curr. Opin. Pediatr.* **2009**, 21(2), 243–251.

Barrett, J. C.; Wong, A.; McLachlan, J. A. Diethylstilbestrol induces neoplastic transformation without measurable gene mutation at two loci, *Science* **1982**, 212(4501), 1402–1404.

Beldade, P.; Mateus, A. R.; Keller, R. A. Evolution and molecular mechanisms of adaptive developmental plasticity, *Mol. Ecol.* **2011**, 20(7), 1345–1363.

Berger, S. L. The complex language of chromatin regulation during transcription, *Nature* **2007**, 447, 407–412.

Bernal, A. J.; Jirtle, R. L. Epigenomic disruption: The effects of early developmental exposures, *Birth Defects Res. A: Clin. Mol. Teratol.* **2010**, 88(10), 938–944.

Bernstein, B. E.; Birney, E.; Dunham, I.; Green, E. D.; Gunter, C.; Snyder, M. An integrated encyclopedia of DNA elements in the human genome: ENCODE Project Consortium, *Nature* **2012**, 489(7414), 57–74.

Bollati, V.; Baccarelli, A. Environmental epigenetics, *Heredity (Edinb.)* **2010**, 105(1), 105–112.

Broday, L.; Peng, W.; Kuo, M. H.; Salnikow, K.; Zoroddu, M.; Costa, M. Nickel compounds are novel inhibitors of histone H4 acetylation, *Cancer Res.* **2000**, 60, 238–241.

Bromer, J. G.; Zhou, Y.; Taylor, M. B.; Doherty, L.; Taylor, H. S. Bisphenol-A exposure in utero leads to epigenetic alterations in the developmental programming of uterine estrogen response, *FASEB J.* **2010**, 24, 2273–2280.

Bruner-Tran, K. L.; Osteen, K. G.; Developmental exposure to TCDD reduces fertility and negatively affects pregnancy outcomes across multiple generations, *Reprod. Toxicol.* **2011**, 31(3), 344–350.

Carthew, R. W.; Sontheimer, E. J. Origins and mechanisms of miRNAs and siRNAs, *Cell* **2009**, 136(4), 642–655.

Chanda, S.; Dasgupta, U. B.; Guhamazumder, D.; Gupta, M.; Chaudhuri, U.; Lahiri, S.; Das, S.; Ghosh, N.; Chatterjee, D. DNA hypermethylation of promoter of gene p53 and p16 in arsenic-exposed people with and without malignancy, *Toxicol. Sci.* **2006**, 89, 431–437.

Chen, H.; Giri, N. C.; Zhang, R.; Yamane, K.; Zhang, Y.; Maroney, M.; Costa, M. Nickel ions inhibit histone demethylase JMJD1A and DNA repair enzyme ABH2 by replacing the ferrous iron in the catalytic centers. *J. Biol. Chem.* **2010**, 285, 7374–7383.

Choudhuri, S.; Cui, Y.; Klaassen, C. D. Molecular targets of epigenetic regulation and effectors of environmental influences, *Toxicol. Appl. Pharmacol.* **2010**, 245, 378–393.

Crews, D.; Gore, A. C. Epigenetic synthesis: a need for a new paradigm for evolution in a contaminated world, *F1000 Biol. Reports* **2012**, 4, 18 (doi: 10.3410/B4-18)

Crews, D.; McLachlan, J. A. Epigenetics, evolution, endocrine disruption, health, and disease, *Endocrinology* **2006**, 147(6) (Supplement), S4–S10.

Crews, D.; Gore, A. C.; Hsu, T. S.; Dangleben, N. L.; Spinetta, M.; Schallert, T.; Anway, M. D.; Skinner, M. K. Transgenerational epigenetic imprints on mate preference, *Proc. Natl. Acad. Sci. USA* **2007a**, 104, 5942–5946.

Crews, D.; Gore, A. C.; Hsu, T. S.; Dangleben, N. L.; Spinetta, M.; Schallert, T.; Anway M. D.; Skinner, M. K. Transgenerational epigenetic imprints on mate preference, *Proc. Natl. Acad. Sci. U. S. A.* **2007b**, 104(14), 5942–5946.

Daxinger, L.; Whitelaw, E. Understanding transgenerational epigenetic inheritance via the gametes in mammals, *Nature Rev. Genetics* **2012**, 13; doi:10.1038/nrg3188

DeAngelis, J. T.; Farrington, W. J.; Tollefsbol, T. O. An overview of epigenetic assays, *Mol. Biotechnol.* **2008**, 38(2), 179–183.

Dolinoy D. C.; Weidman J. R.; Waterland R. A.; Jirtle R. L. Maternal genistein alters coat color and protects Avy mouse offspring from obesity by modifying the fetal epigenome, *Environ. Health Perspect.* **2006**, 114(4), 567–572.

Dolinoy, D. C.; Huang, D.; Jirtle, R. L. Maternal nutrient supplementation counteracts bisphenol A-induced DNA hypomethylation in early development, *Proc. Natl. Acad. Sci. U. S. A.*, **2007**, 104, 13056–13061.

Edwards, T. M.; Myers, J. P. Environmental exposures and gene regulation in disease etiology, *Environ. Health Perspect.* **2007**, 115(9), 1264–1270.

Foley, D. L.; Craig, J. M.; Morley, R.; Olsson, C. J.; Dwyer, T.; Smith, K.; Saffery, R. Prospects for epigenetic epidemiology, *Amer. J. Epidemiol.* **2009**, 169, 389–400.

Fraga, M. F.; Ballestar, E.; Paz, M. F.; Ropero, S.; Setien, F.; Ballestar, M. L.; Heine-Suñer, D.; Cigudosa, J. C.; Urioste, M.; Benitez, J.; Boix-Chornet, M.; Sanchez-Aguilera, A.; Ling, C.; Carlsson, E.; Poulsen, P.; Vaag, A.; Stephan, Z.; Spector, T. D.; Wu, Y.-Z.; Plass, C.; Esteller, M. Epigenetic differences arise during the lifetime of monozygotic twins, *Proc. Nat. Acad. Sci. U S A*, **2005**, 102(30), 10604–10609.

Furr, J.; Gray Jr., L. E. Vinclozolin treatment induces reproductive malformations and infertility in male rats when administered during sexual but not gonadal differentiation; however, the effects are not transmitted to the subsequent generations, Abstract # 1441, in *The Toxicologist*, Society of Toxicology Annual Meeting: Baltimore, MD, March 15–19, **2009**.

Gardner, K. E.; Allis, C. D.; Strahl, B. D. Operating on chromatin, a colorful language where context matters, *J. Mol. Biol.* **2011**, 409, 36–46.

Greally, J. M. Endocrine disruptors and the epigenome, *OECD Review*, July 2011. Available at: www.oecd.org/dataoecd/42/53/48435503.pdf (accessed 10 Oct 2011).

Guerrero-Bosagna, C.; Valladares, L. Endocrine disruptors, epigenetically induced changes, and transgenerational transmission of characters and epigenetic states, in *Endocrine-Disrupting Chemicals: From Basic Research to Clinical Practice*, Gore, A. C., ed., Humana: Totowa, NJ, **2007**, pp. 175–189.

He, Y. F.; Li, B. Z.; Li, Z.; Liu, P.; Wang, Y.; Tang, Q.; Ding, J.; Jia, Y.; Chen, Z.; Li, L.; Sun, Y.; Li, X.; Dai, Q.; Song, C. X.; Zhang, K.; He, C.; Xu, G. L. Tet-mediated formation of 5-carboxylcytosine and its excision by TDG in mammalian DNA, *Science* **2011**, 333(6047), 1303–1307.

Herman, J. G.; Graff, J. R.; Myohanen, S.; Nelkin, B. D.; Baylin, S. B. Methylation-specific PCR: a novel PCR assay for methylation status of CpG islands, *Proc. Natl. Acad. Sci. U S A.* **1996**, 93, 9821–9826.

Ho, S. M.; Tang, W. Y.; Belmonte D. F.; Prins, G. S.; Developmental exposure to estradiol and bisphenol A increases susceptibility to prostate carcinogenesis and epigenetically regulates phosphodiesterase type 4 variant 4, *Cancer Res.* **2006**, 66, 5624–5632.

Huang, D.; Zhang, Y.; Qi, Y.; Chen, C.; Ji, W. Global DNA hypomethylation, rather than reactive oxygen species (ROS), a potential facilitator of Cadmium-stimulated K-562 cell proliferation, *Toxicol. Lett.* **2008**, 179(1), 43–47.

Illingworth R. S.; Bird A. P. CpG islands – "a rough guide" *FEBS Lett.* **2009**, 583, 1713–1720.

Inawaka, K.; Kawabe, M.; Takahashi, S.; Doi, Y.; Tomigahara, Y.; Tarui, H.; Abe, J.; Kawamura, S.; Shirai, T. Maternal exposure to anti-androgenic compounds, vinclozolin, flutamide, and procymidone, has no effects on spermatogenesis and DNA methylation in male rats of subsequent generations, *Toxicol. Appl. Pharmacol.* **2009**, 237, 178–187.

Ito, S.; D'Alessio, A. C.; Taranova, O. V.; Hong, K.; Sowers, L. C.; Zhang, Y. Role of Tet proteins in 5mC to 5hmC conversion, ES-cell self-renewal and inner cell mass specification, *Nature* **2010**, 466(7310), 1129–1133.

Ito, S.; Shen, L.; Dai, Q.; Wu, S. C.; Collins, L. B.; Swenberg, J. A.; He, C.; Zhang, Y. Tet proteins can convert 5-methylcytosine to 5-formylcytosine and 5-carboxylcytosine, *Science* **2011**, 333(6047), 1300–1303.

Jablonka, E.; Raz, G. Transgenerational epigenetic inheritance: prevalence, mechanisms, and implications for the study of heredity and evolution, *Quart. Rev. Biol.* **2009**, 84(2), 131–176.

Janesick, A.; Blumberg, B. Minireview: PPARγ as the target of obesogenes, *J. Steroid Biochem. Mol. Biol.* **2011**, 127, 4–8.

Jenuwein, T.; Allis, C. D. Translating the histone code, *Science* **2001**, 293, 1074–1080.

Jiang, G. F.; Xu, L.; Song, S. Z.; Zhu, C. C.; Wu, Q.; Zhang, L. Effects of long-term low-dose cadmium exposure on genomic DNA methylation in human embryo lung fibroblast cells, *Toxicology* **2008**, 244, 49–55.

Jirtle, R. L.; Skinner, M. K. Environmental epigenomics and disease susceptibility, *Nat. Rev. Genet.* **2007**, 8, 253–262.

Jones, P. A., et al., Moving AHEAD with an international human epigenome project, *Nature* **2008**, 454, 711-715.

Kaiser, J. The epigenetic heretic, *Science* **2014**, 343(6169), 361–363.

Ke, Q.; Davidson, T.; Chen, H.; Kluz, T.; Costa, M.; Alterations of histone modifications and transgene silencing by nickel chloride. *Carcinogenesis*, **2006**, 27, 1481–1488.

Kundakovic, M.; Champagne, F. A. Epigenetic perspective on the developmental effects of bisphenol A, *Brain, Behav. Immun.* **2011**, 25(6), 1084–1093.

Lange, U. C., Schneider, R. What an epigenome remembers, *Bioessays* **2010**, 32, 659–668.

LeBaron, M. J.; Rasoulpour, R. J.; Klapacz, J.; Ellis-Hutchings, R. G.; Hollnagel, H. M.; Gollapudi, B. B. Epigenetics and chemical safety assessment, *Mutation Res.* **2010**, 705, 83–95.

Li, B.; Carey, M.; Workman, J. L. The role of chromatin during transcription, *Cell* **2007**, 128, 707–719.

Manikkam, M.; Tracey, R.; Guerrero-Bosagna, C.; Skinner, M. K. Dioxin (TCDD) induces epigenetic transgenerational inheritance of adult onset disease and sperm epimutations, *PLoS ONE* **2012a**, 7(9), e46249. doi:10.1371/journal.pone.0046249

Manikkam, M.; Guerrero-Bosagna, C.; Tracey, R.; Haque, Md. M.; Skinner, M. K. Transgenerational actions of environmental compounds on reproductive disease and identification of epigenetic biomarkers of ancestral exposures, *PLoS ONE* **2012b**, 7(2), e31901. doi:10.1371/journal.pone.0031901

Manikkam, M.; Tracey, R.; Guerrero-Bosagna, C.; Skinner, M. K. Plastics derived endocrine disruptors (BPA, DEHP and DBP) induce epigenetic transgenerational inheritance of obesity, reproductive disease and sperm epimutations, *PLoS ONE* **2013**, 8(1): e55387. doi:10.1371/journal.pone.0055387

McCarrey, J. R. The epigenome as a target for heritable environmental disruptions of cellular function, *Mol. Cell. Endocrinol.* **2012**, 354, 9–15.

Münzel, M.; Globisch, D.; Carell, T. 5-Hydroxymethylcytosine, the sixth base of the genome, *Angew. Chem. Intern. Ed.* **2011**, 50(29), 6460–6468.

Neel, J. V. Diabetes mellitus: a "thrifty" genotype rendered detrimental by 'progress'? *Am. J. Human Genet.* **1962**, 14, 353-362.

Newbold, R. R. Impact of environmental endocrine disrupting chemicals on the development of obesity, *Hormones* **2010**, 9(3), 206–217.

Newbold, R. R.; Padilla-Banks, E.; Jefferson, W. N. Adverse effects of the model environmental estrogen diethylstilbestrol are transmitted to subsequent generations, *Endocrinology*, **2006**, 147, S11–S17.

Pfaffeneder, T.; Hackner, B.; Truß, M.; Münzel, M.; Müller, M.; Deiml, C. A.; Hagemeier, C.; Carell, T. The discovery of 5-formylcytosine in embryonic stem cell DNA, *Angew. Chem. Intern. Ed.* **2011**, 50(31), 7008–7012.

Pilsner, J. R.; Hu, H.; Ettinger, A.; Sanchez, B. N.; Wright, R. O.; Cantonwine, D.; Lazarus, A.; Lamadrid-Figueroa, H.; Mercado-Gracia, A.; Tellez-Rojo, M. M., Hernandez,-Avila, M. Influence of prenatal lead exposure on genomic methylation of cord blood DNA, *Environ. Health Perspect.* **2009**, 117(9), 1466–1471.

Ramirez, T.; Brocher, J.; Stopper, H.; Hock, R. Sodium arsenite modulates histone acetylation, histone deacetylase activity and HMGN protein dynamics in human cells, *Chromosoma* **2008**, 117, 147–157.

Reichard, J. F.; Schnekenburger, M.; Puga, A. Long term low-dose arsenic exposure induces loss of DNA methylation, *Biochem. Biophys. Res. Commun.* **2007**, 352, 188–192.

Reik, W. Stability and flexibility of epigenetic gene regulation in mammalian development, *Nature* **2007**, 447, 425–432.

Rottach, A.; Leonhardt, H.; Spada, F. DNA methylation mediated epigenetic control, *J. Cell. Biochem.* **2009**, 108, 43–51.

vom Saal, F. S.; Akingbemi, B. T.; Belcher, S. M.; Birnbaum, L. S.; Crain, D. A.; Eriksen, M., et al. Chapel Hill bisphenol A expert panel consensus statement: Integration of mechanisms, effects in animals and potential to impact human health at current levels of exposure, *Reprod. Toxicol.* **2007**, 24(2), 131–138.

Salian, S.; Doshi, T.; Vanage, G. Perinatal exposure of rats to bisphenol A affects the fertility of male offspring, *Life Sci.* **2009a**, 85, 742–752.

Salian, S.; Doshi, T.; Vanage, G. Impairment in protein expression profile of testicular steroid receptor coregulators in male rat offspring perinatally exposed to bisphenol A, *Life Sci.* **2009b**, 85, 11–18.

Schneider, S.; Kaufmann, W.; Buesen, R.; van Ravenzwaay, B. Vinclozolin–the lack of a transgenerational effect after oral maternal exposure during organogenesis, *Reprod. Toxicol.* **2008**, 25(3), 352–360.

Skinner, M. K. Epigenetic transgenerational toxicology and germ cell disease, *Int. J. Androl.* **2007**, 30(4), 393–397.

Skinner, M. K. What is an epigenetic transgenerational phenotype? F3 or F2, *Reprod. Toxicol.* **2008**, 25(1), 2–6.

Skinner, M. K.; Guerrero-Bosagna, C. Environmental signals and transgenerational epigenetics, *Epigenomics* **2009**, 1(1), 111–117.

Skinner, M. K.; Manikkam, M.; Guerrero-Bosagna, C. Epigenetic transgenerational actions of environmental factors in disease etiology, *Trends Endocrinol. Metab.* **2010**, 21(4), 214–222.

Skinner, M. K.; Manikkam, M.; Guerrero-Bosagna, C. Epigenetic transgenerational actions of endocrine disruptors, *Reprod. Toxicol.* **2011**, 31, 337–343.

Skinner, M. K.; Haque, C. G-B. M.; Nilsson, E.; Bhandari, R.; McCarrey J. R. Environmentally induced transgenerational epigenetic reprogramming of primordial cells and the subsequent germ line. *Plos One* **2013**, 8(7), e66318.

Stouder, C.; Paoloni-Giacobino, A. Transgenerational effects of endocrine disruptor vinclozolon on the methylation pattern of imprinted genes in the mouse sperm. *Reproduction* **2010**, 139(2), 373–379.

Stouder, C.; Paoloni-Giacobino, A. Specific transgenerational imprinting effects of the endocrine disruptor methoxychlor on male gametes, *Reproduction* **2011**, 141, 207–216.

Takiguchi, M.; Achanzar, W. E.; Qu, W.; Li, G.; Waalkes, M. P. Effects of cadmium on DNA-(Cytosine-5) methyltransferase activity and DNA methylation status during cadmium-induced cellular transformation, *Exp. Cell Res.* **2003**, 286(2), 355–365.

Vandegehuchte, M. B.; Janssen, C. R. Epigenetics and its implications for ecotoxicology, *Ecotoxicology* **2011**, 20, 607–624.

Walker, D. M.; Gore, A. C. Transgenerational neuroendocrine disruption of reproduction, *Nature Rev. Endocrinol.* **2011**, 7, 197–207.

Waterland, R. A. Assessing the effects of high methionine intake on DNA methylation. *J. Nutr.* **2006**, 136, 1706S–1710S.

Waterland, R. A.; Jirtle, R. L. Transposable elements: Targets for early nutritional effects on epigenetic gene regulation. *Mol. Cell Biol.* **2003**, 23(15), 5293–5300.

Weinhold, B. Epigenetics: the science of change, *Environ. Health Perspect.* **2006**, 114, A160–A167.

Wolstenholme, J. T.; Edwards, M.; Shetty, S. R.; Gatewood, J. D.; Taylor, J. A.; Rissman, E. F.; Connelly, J. J. Gestational exposure to bisphenol a produces transgenerational changes in behaviors and gene expression, *Endocrinology* **2012**, 153(8), 3828-3838.

Wu, J.; Basha, M. R.; Brock, B.; Cox, D. P.; Cardozo-Pelaez, F.; McPherson, C. A.; Harry, J.; Rice, D. C.; Maloney, B.; Chen, D.; Lahiri, D. K.; Zawia, N. H. Alzheimer's disease (AD) like pathology in aged monkeys following infantile exposure to environmental metal lead (Pb): evidence for a developmental origin and environmental link for AD, *J. Neurosci.* **2008**, 28(1), 3–9.

Wu, S., Zhu, J., Li, Y., Lin, T., Gan, L., Yuan, X., Xiong, J., Liu, X., Xu, M., Zhao, D.; Ma, C.; Li, X.; Wei, G. Dynamic epigenetic changes involved in testicular toxicity induced by di-2-(ethylhexyl) phthalate in mice, *Basic Clin. Pharmacol. Toxicol.* **2010**, 106, 118–123.

Yan, C.; Boyd, D. D. Histone H3 acetylation and H3 K4 methylation define distinct chromatin regions permissive for transgene expression, *Mol. Cell Biol.* **2006**, 26(17), 6357–6371.

Zaidi, S. K.; Young, D. W.; Montecino, M.; van Wijnen, A. J.; Stein, J. L.; Lian, J. B.; Stein, G. S. Bookmarking the genome: maintenance of epigenetic information, *J. Biol. Chem.* **2011**, 286(21), 18355–18361.

Zama, A. M.; Uzumcu, M. Fetal and neonatal exposure to the endocrine disruptor methoxychlor causes epigenetic alterations in adult ovarian genes, *Endocrinology* **2009**, 150(10), 4681–4691.

Zhang, X.; Ho, S. M. Epigenetics meets endocrinology, *J. Mol. Endocrinol.* **2011**, 46, R11–R32.

Zhao, C. Q.; Young, M. R.; Diwan, B. A.; Coogan, T. P.; Waalkes, M. P.; Association of arsenic-induced malignant transformation with DNA hypomethylation and aberrant gene expression, *Proc. Natl. Acad. Sci. U. S. A.* **1997**, 94(20), 10907–10912.

PART II

REMOVAL MECHANISMS OF EDCs THROUGH BIOTIC AND ABIOTIC PROCESSES

The various biotic/abiotic processes usually result in new chemical entities (also called *transformation products*) with new properties. Degradation of endocrine disrupting chemicals (EDCs) involves both biotic transformation processes – mediated by microorganisms – and abiotic processes such as chemical and photochemical reactions. As long-term treatment options for removing EDCs in environmental waters, strategies focusing on microbial or abiotic degradation *in situ*, or natural attenuation, are considered. Recent findings on the potential for EDC biodegradation illustrate the potential importance of this environmental attenuation mechanism. Persistence can be viewed as the resistance of the contaminant molecule to biological or chemical transformations. Pseudo-persistence may also result in settings where the contaminant molecule is continually replenished (e.g., wastewater-impacted systems).

The following two chapters focus on metabolites of various EDCs formed biotically (microbial degradation and those excreted by humans and animals) and on the transformation products formed during abiotic processes (such as oxidation, hydrolysis, or photolysis) often employed in disinfection or advanced oxidation processes (AOPs) in water treatment. In surface waters, for example, exposure to sunlight can cause direct photodegradation or indirect oxidation via formation of reactive oxygen species.

From the evolutionary perspective, it is evident that organisms can adapt to contamination. Microbial mechanisms for degradation of historical environmental contaminants and, by extension EDCs, are fundamentally redox processes. Consequently, *in situ* redox conditions are expected to control the efficiency of EDC biodegradation. Although some local remediation of contamination has occurred, at a global level this is simply not possible. However, it is possible, and desirable, to slow the rate and nature of contamination by regulating better known EDCs.

9

BIODEGRADATIONS AND BIOTRANSFORMATIONS OF SELECTED EXAMPLES OF EDCs

9.1 INTRODUCTION

Biological processes play a major role in the removal of environmental contaminants by taking advantage of the astonishing catabolic versatility of microorganisms to degrade/convert such compounds. Organisms require energy, carbon, and other fundamental inputs from the environment for their growth and maintenance. Microorganisms (bacteria and fungi) use the chemical substrate as an energy source. In life, they manufacture enzymes, which may transform or biodegrade contaminants that have been introduced into the environment. Enzymes that are mostly specific for the reaction type and starting compound catalyze these multistep transformations. Most natural and anthropogenic chemicals are transformed to CO_2 and water in the presence of oxygen or other electron acceptors and specialized microbes. Aromatic compounds are among the most recalcitrant of these pollutants. Thus, degradation by microorganisms offers one of the most important removal processes of endocrine disruptor chemicals (EDCs) from the environment.

Biodegradation processes can undergo two pathways, either xenobiotic utilization for growth or co-metabolism, in which a compound is modified but not used for growth. Biological processes rely on nonpathogenic bacteria to degrade organic chemicals, which in turn require the presence of other compounds (primary substrates) that can support their growth. Because trace organics usually are insufficient in concentration to serve as the primary energy source for the growth of microorganisms, trace organics are co-metabolized with dissolved organic carbon (DOC) in water. Usually, the primary substrate induces production of (an) enzyme(s) that

Endocrine Disruptors in the Environment, First Edition. Sushil K. Khetan.
© 2014 John Wiley & Sons, Inc. Published 2014 by John Wiley & Sons, Inc.

fortuitously alter(s) the molecular structure of another compound. Monooxygenase enzymes are known to co-metabolize many organic compounds.

Metabolism involves a coordinated process of biotransformation and transport aimed at detoxifying and eliminating potentially harmful compounds, as well as activation and toxification of the EDCs. Exposure to EDCs not only implies exposure to its environmental degradates but also to its metabolism products. Many xenobiotics that enter the body have no nutritional or physiological value, and the study of the disposition – or fate – of xenobiotics in living systems includes the chemical and biochemical transformations they may undergo, and how and by which route(s) they are finally excreted and returned to the environment. As for "metabolism," this word has acquired two meanings, being synonymous with disposition and with biotransformation (Testa and Soine, 2003). In studies where pure bacterial cultures or enzyme extracts have been used, the transformation products could be characterized without interference from natural organic matter, proteins, and other complex macromolecules.

Metabolic studies have shown that, particularly, the hydroxy or ketone groups and aromatic moieties play an important role in the mechanism of action of EDCs. This is not unexpected because, in the steroid biosynthesis pathway, these same functional groups are involved in the conversion of cholesterol to progestins, androgens, and estrogens. On the basis of the similarity of their molecular structure to the parent compound, a significant number of biotransformation products are expected to possess comparable biological activity as their chemical precursors (Van Zelm et al., 2010). Many synthetic compounds are readily metabolized to more polar forms, often containing one or more hydroxyl groups, which increases the potential for the formation of more EDCs. The formation of several transformation products increases the complexity of the problem, notably because some of them can be more persistent, retain bioactive moieties, and/or exhibit greater toxicity than their parent compounds.

Several enzyme-catalyzed reactions are quite commonly involved in the biotransformations, such as mono- and dihydroxylation, alcohol and aldehyde oxidation, ester and amide hydrolysis, N-dealkylation, N-deacetylation, and decarboxylation. For identification of biotransformation products where only on the mass spectra (MS) have been obtained but no authentic standard is available, it might be better to view the suggested structures as "tentative identifications" unless further plausibility criteria are fulfilled confirming the proposed chemical structures (Richardson and Ternes, 2011).

The adverse health effects of EDCs in humans are increasingly getting known and have raised concerns about human exposure to these compounds. In this context, information regarding the metabolic fate of various EDCs is critical for the identification of adequate biomarkers of exposure to these chemicals that could be used for exposure and risk assessment. It is also important to understand the biotransformation mechanisms in order to be able to optimize the design and the conditions that favor effective removal of EDCs.

Biotransformations may provide a basis for the cost-effective removal of EDCs from water. We aim here not to make an exhaustive review but include only metabolites from biotic (microbial) degradation and those excreted by humans or animals of some known EDCs. Our focus is on the reaction pathways of biotransformations, and not on identification of adverse outcome pathways, and therefore we have abstained from detailed consideration of the rate of reaction (kinetics) or efficiency of transformation (total degradation or mineralization).

9.2 NATURAL AND SYNTHETIC STEROIDAL ESTROGENS

9.2.1 17β-Estradiol and Estrone

Steroid hormones participate in organ development, reproduction, body homeostasis, and stress responses. Biotransformation of the steroidal compounds is an area where the consensus is still developing and the metabolic pathway(s) of E1 and E2 are far from settled, while broad contours might be visible. For example, the degradation pathway of the natural estrogen 17β-estradiol (E2) was investigated in the supernatant of activated sludge growing on a mineral salt and high E2 concentrations. In aerobic conditions, E2 is generally oxidized on C-17 at ring D, producing E1, which is usually further degraded (Lee and Liu, 2002). Another labile metabolite with a lactone structure at the D ring of E1 was also detected at the beginning of E2 degradation (Fig. 9.1) (Lee and Liu, 2002). From this intermediate, a pathway with the initial cleavage of ring D was proposed (Lee and Liu, 2002). The degradation of E1 (produced from E2 or not) was investigated by using an activated sludge as inoculum. It was shown that E1 was quickly degraded under aerobic conditions, and no other intermediate metabolites were detected (Ternes et al., 1999).

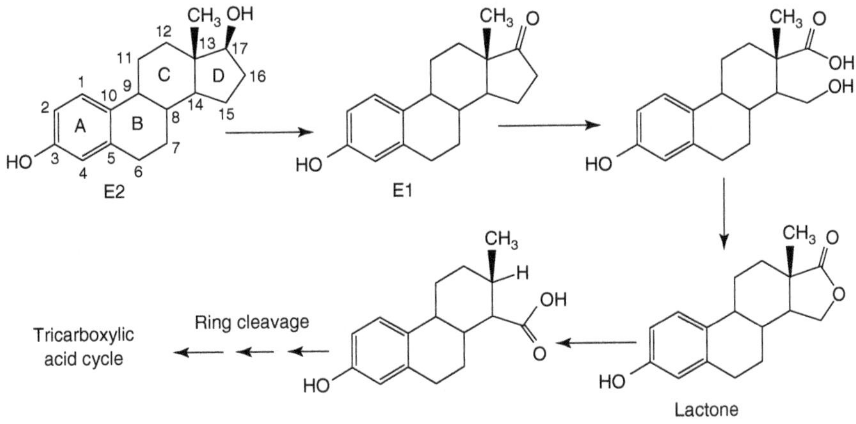

Figure 9.1   Proposed degradation pathway for 17β-estradiol by sewage bacteria under aerobic conditions (Lee and Liu, 2002).

The degradation of E2 was also studied utilizing *Sphingomonas* sp. as a model organism by incubating whole cells with E2 and 3-chlorocatechol (a meta-cleavage inhibitor) (Kurisu et al., 2010). It produced six metabolites; only two of these were positively identified, as 4-hydroxyesterone (4-OH-E1) and 4-hydroxyestradiol (4-OH-E2). None of the metabolites was detected without 3-chlorocatechol treatment, thus indicating a meta-cleavage pathway. The degradation pathway of E2 is proposed by first oxidation to E1, followed by hydroxylation of E1 at the C-4 position to form 4-OH-E1, and the ring cleavage of 4-OH-E1 between C-4 and C-5. The pathway is analogous to the reported degradation of E1 by *Nocardia* sp. E110 in a mineral salt medium, involving the cleavage of the A ring catalyzed by a dioxygenase followed by cleavage of the B ring (Fig. 9.2) (Coombe et al., 1966).

Oxidation of E2 catalyzed by the ligninolytic enzyme laccase was reported to form dimer and oligomer products by radical–radical coupling reactions with resultant elimination of estrogenic activities (Tanaka et al., 2009; Nicotra et al., 2004). A study on the removal of estrogenic compounds in a continuous enzymatic membrane reactor characterized the products of E2 laccase-catalyzed transformation as C–C and C–O dimer products and trimer products along with formation of E1 as an oxidation product of E2 (Lloret et al., 2013) (Fig. 9.3). These results are in agreement with enzyme-mediated transformation of E2 using lignin peroxidase with the formation of dimers and trimmers, as well as E1 (Mao et al., 2010).

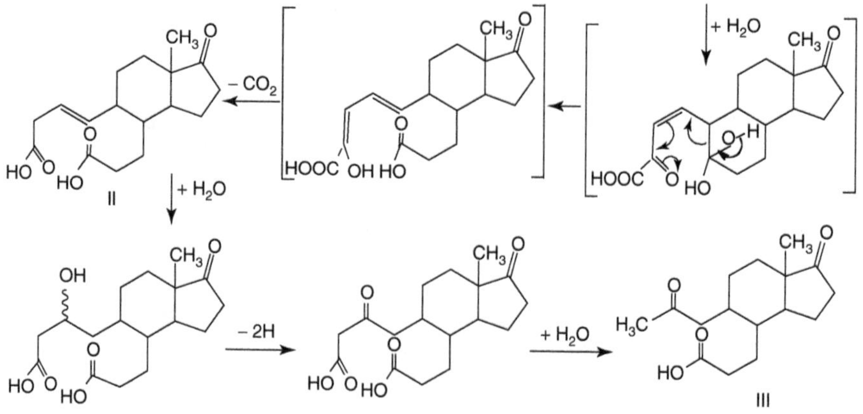

Figure 9.2   Proposed degradation pathway of estrone (E1) by *Nocardia* sp. E110 (Coombe et al., 1966).

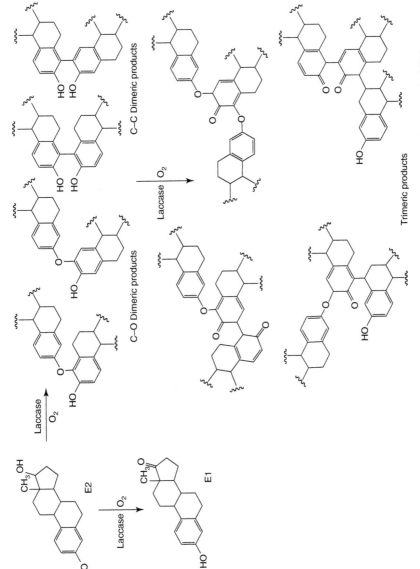

Figure 9.3 Laccase-catalyzed oxidation products of E2 (Lloret et al., 2013; Nicotra et al., 2004).

However, for peroxidase enzymes, which have demonstrated relatively high redox potentials and can achieve appreciable conversion of their target substrates, their catalytic activity requires the use of hydrogen peroxide as an oxidant. In contrast, laccase enzymes have a lower redox potential, but have the advantage of using readily available molecular oxygen as an oxidant.

9.2.2   17α-Ethynylestradiol

The synthetic hormone EE2, the active compound of the contraceptive pill, is much more resistant to biodegradation than natural ones. EE2 contains an ethinyl group at the same C atom that possesses a hydroxyl group that is normally vulnerable to microbial attack. Bacterial strains of *Rhodococcus* using enriched culture of activated sludge from wastewater treatment plant (WWTP) were reported to completely degrade estrogens. Strains *Rhodococcus zopfii* and *Rhodococcus equi* degraded E2, E1, E3, and EE2 to 1/100th of estrogenic activity level within 24 h (Yoshimoto et al., 2004).

EE2 was able to metabolize up to 87% of 30 mg/l EE2 within 10 days using a bacterial strain *Sphingobacterium* sp. JCR5 (Haiyan et al., 2007). This strain grew on EE2 as sole source of carbon and energy and was isolated from a WWTP of an oral contraceptives factory. EE2, like E2, was directly oxidized into E1 with a subsequent cleavage of the B ring by hydroxylation on C-9, and the ring A was hydroxylated to form 3,4-dihydroxy-9,10-secoandrosta-1,3,5(10)-triene-9,17-dione, leading to unsaturated acids, which were further mineralized to CO_2 and water (Fig. 9.4) (Haiyan et al., 2007). Two intermediate compounds identified were 2-hydroxy-2,4-dienevaleric acid and 2-hydroxy-2,4-diene-1,6-dioic acid (Haiyan et al., 2007).

The metabolic pathway reports have led to some apparently conflicting ideas about EE2 ring cleavage, which is a key metabolic event because it produces metabolites that are easier to biodegrade. The metabolites in EE2 degradation using enriched cultures of the ammonia oxidizing bacteria *Nitrosomonas europaea* were identified (Yi and Harper, 2007). It was suggested that the molecule is probably attacked at the aromatic ring A where the electron density is highest, producing a ring A cleavage product ETDC (3-ethynyl-3a,6,7-trimethyl-decahydro-1*H*-cyclopenta[a]naphthalene-3-ol) (Yi and Harper, 2007). In contrast to the ring A cleavage of E1 (Coombe et al., 1966), ring A of EE2 was assumed to be cleaved between C-1 and C-2 as well as between C-3 and C-4 to form ETDC. A product formed by hydroxylation adjacent to the existing hydroxyl group on ring A formed a catechol, either 2- or 4-OH-EE2 (*m/z* 311), and formation of a sulfate conjugate 3-SO$_4$-EE2 (*m/z* 375) was also identified (Fig. 9.5) (Yi and Harper, 2007; Khunjar et al., 2011). A transformation product (*m/z* 385) elucidated by LC/ion trap-MS and ^{1}H NMR was proposed to form after hydrolysis and oxidation of the ethinyl group (Skotnicka-Pitak et al., 2009).

Frontier electron density (FED) analysis supported the cleavage of ring A, which has a significantly higher electron density than in other rings, making it vulnerable to electrophilic substitutions, which may serve as initiating reactions

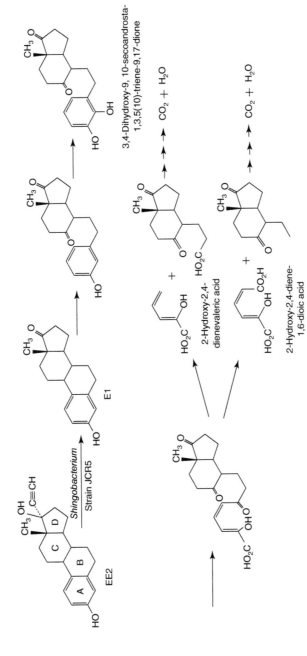

Figure 9.4 Metabolic pathway of 17α-ethinylestradiol by *Sphingobacterium* sp. JCR5. Source: Redrawn from Haiyan et al. (2007).

EE2

CH₃ OH
C≡CH

A B C D

HO

Shingobacterium
Strain JCR5

E1

CH₃ O

HO

CH₃ O

O

HO

CH₃ O

O

HO OH

3,4-Dihydroxy-9, 10-secoandrosta-
1,3,5(10)-triene-9,17-dione

CH₃ O

O

HO₂C OH

+

HO₂C OH

2-Hydroxy-2,4-
dienevaleric acid

→ → CO₂ + H₂O

CH₃ O

O

HO₂C CO₂H

+

HO₂C OH

2-Hydroxy-2,4-diene-
1,6-dioic acid

→ → CO₂ + H₂O

CH₃ O

O

HO₂C OH

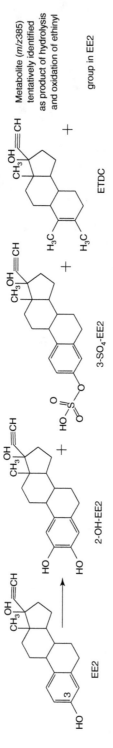

Figure 9.5 EE2 biotransformation products formed on treatment with the ammonia-oxidizing bacteria *Nitrosomonas europaea* (Yi and Harper, 2007; Skotnicka-Pitak et al., 2009; Khunjar et al., 2011).

(Yi and Harper, 2007; Barr, 2011). Thus, on the basis of the identity of metabolites produced by *Sphingobacterium* sp. JCR5 (Haiyan et al., 2007), the metabolic pathway of EE2 proposed by cleavage of ring B first appears to be an exception rather than the rule.

Algal cultures have shown their ability to transform EE2 into EE2 conjugates or more hydrophilic compounds (Fig. 9.5). Hence, *Selenastrum capricornutum* transformed EE2 into three products, namely EE2-glucoside, 3-β-D-glucopyranosyl-2-hydroxy-EE2, and 3-β-D-gluco-pyranosyl-6β-hydroxy-EE2. *Scenedesmus quadricauda* transformed EE2 into 17α-ethinyl-1,4-estradiene-10,17β-diol-3one, and *Ankistrodesmus braunii* transformed EE2 into 6-α-hydroxy-EE2 (Fig. 9.6) (Della Greca et al., 2008)

9.3 ALKYLPHENOLS

The aromatic structure of most estrogenic compounds, including alkylphenols, indicates that they have the potential to be substrates of oxidative enzymes, such as oxidases and peroxidases. The oxidation potential of bisphenol A (BPA) and *p*-nonylphenol is over 600 mV (Kuramitz et al., 2002).

9.3.1 4-*n*-Nonylphenol (4-NP$_1$)

The biotransformation of 4-NP$_1$ has been investigated in rat liver microsome and human liver microsome, which were catalyzed by CPY450 as evidenced by suppression of the formation of the oxidative metabolites on addition of CYP450 inhibitor (Tezuka et al., 2007). The metabolism of 4-NP$_1$ led to the formation of both ring-hydroxylated and side-chain-hydroxylated metabolites in Wistar rats (Zalco et al., 2003) and in rainbow trout (Thibaut et al., 2000). About 10 different metabolites were characterized. Most of them were formed by the ω- or β-oxidation of the 9-carbon side chain of 4-NP$_1$. The mechanism includes hydroxylation of the alkyl chain at the terminal carbon position as the first step, oxidation of the resulting alcohol to the corresponding carboxylic acid, and further degradation through β-oxidation losing two carbons following each loop of the β-oxidation cycle. This gives rise to products bearing a side chain with an odd number of carbon atoms, ultimately giving rise to a one-carbon side chain metabolite, 4-hydroxybenzoic acid (Fig. 9.7). All these metabolites were characterized as the corresponding sulfates and glucuronides. The second major metabolic pathway of 4-NP$_1$ was found to be the hydroxylation of the alkyl side chain, followed by the glucuronidation of the phenol moiety (Zalco et al., 2003).

Three metabolites of 4-NP$_1$ identified in a rat liver microsome reaction mixture included 4-nonyl-4-hydroxy-cyclohexa-2,5-dienone, 4'-hydroxynonano-phenone (CO-NP) as benzyl-oxidized nonylphenol, and hydroquinone. On the other hand, production of 1-(4'-hydroxyphenyl)nonan-1-ol (OH-NP), namely benzyl-hydroxylated nonylphenol, was detected in a human liver microsome reaction mixture through an ipso-substitution mechanism by which cytochrome P450 model systems, liver microsomes, and microorganisms detach various substituents

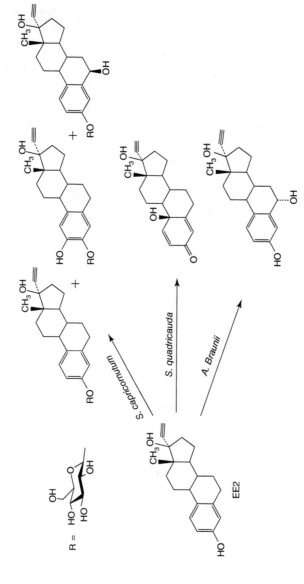

Figure 9.6 Transformation products of EE2 by microalgae cultures (Della Greca et al., 2008).

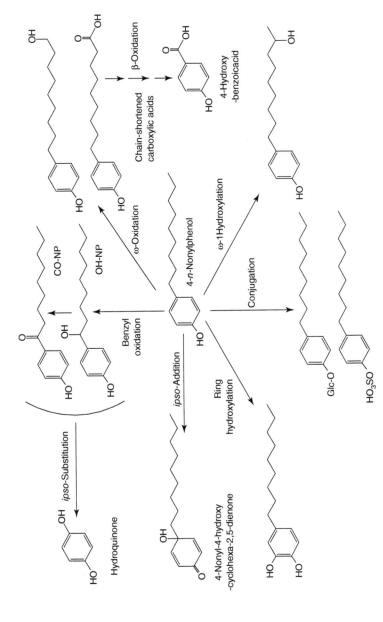

Figure 9.7 Metabolic pathways of 4-*n*-nonylphenol catalyzed by CYP450 in rat and human liver microsomes (Tezuka et al., 2007; Zalko et al., 2003).

207

in substituted phenols (Fig. 9.7). The requirement of a free hydroxy group at the para position is characteristic for the ipso-substitution reaction (Tezuka et al., 2007).

Bacterial genera of sphingomonads are known for their ability to degrade recalcitrant natural and anthropogenic compounds. The metabolic versatility of these organisms is due to the existence of multiple hydroxylating oxygenases and the conservation of specific gene clusters that adapt to quicker and/or more efficient degradation mechanisms than members of other bacterial genera (Stolz, 2009). The *Sphingobium xenophagum* Bayram, a strain isolated from activated sewage sludge, led the degradation pathway differentiated with different α-substitutions in NP isomers, indicating that NP isomers with hydrogen atoms at the benzylic position are metabolized in a way different from that of the more highly branched isomers (Kohler et al., 2008). *S. xenophagum* Bayram transformed NP isomers with hydrogen atoms at the benzylic position with an initial ipso-hydroxylation, producing 4-*n*-nonyl-4-hydroxy-cyclohexadienone intermediate (Fig. 9.8).

Horseradish peroxidase (HRP) led to free-radical oxidation of alkyl phenols, such as 4-nonylphenol and 4-octylphenol, forming almost all insoluble oligomers (Sakuyama et al., 2003). Results of the yeast estrogen screen (YES) assay demonstrated that the reaction products of HRP-catalyzed 4-nonylphenol conversion lacked estrogenic activity (Wagner and Nicell, 2005).

Biodegradation of 4-n-NP_1 by the yeast *Candida aquaetextoris* resulted in two main metabolites, namely trans-4-hydroxy-cinnamic acid and 4-hydroxy-acetophenone. The finding implied that *C. aquaetextoris* might metabolise 4-n-NP_1 via terminal oxidation of the linear alkyl chain to carboxylic acids (Vallini et al., 2001). Incubation with non-ligninolytic filamentous fungi *Gliocephalotrichum simplex* and *Aspergillus versicolor* IM 2161 effectively degraded 4-n-NP_1, whereas *A. versicolor* was seen to have about 4–5 times higher degradation efficiency (Rozalska et al., 2010; Krupinski et al., 2013). The two common end metabolites identified were 3-(4-hydroxyphenyl)propanoic acid and 4-hydroxybenzoic acid. These metabolites were also found during the metabolism of 4-n-NP_1 in Wistar rats (Zalko et al., 2003).

Even though much attention has been paid to the study of the degradation pathway of the isomer 4-NP_1 with a linear nonyl chain, the commercial nonylphenol mixtures consist of more than 85% of the isomers that possess a quaternary α-carbon on the branched alkyl chain. The linear nonyl chain NP (4-NP_1) is not reported to be present in it (Corvini et al., 2006a).

9.3.2   4-*tert*-nonylphenol isomer 4-(1-ethyl-1,4-eimethylpentyl) phenol (NP_{112})

The main metabolite of a branched chain 4-*tert*-nonylphenol isomer, namely 4-(1-ethyl-1,4-dimethylpentyl) phenol (NP_{112}), which is one of the main isomers of technical nonylphenol mixtures, was identified using rat and human liver microsomes as the ring hydroxylated product 4-(1-ethyl,1,4-dimethylpentyl) catechol. Other metabolites tentatively identified included a hydroxylated product with the alcohol functional group on the branched alkyl chain and its oxidative metabolite,

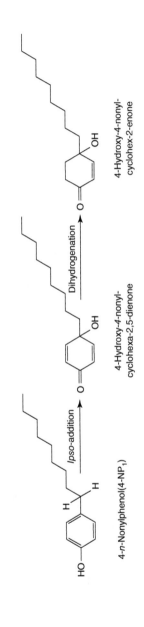

Figure 9.8 Metabolic pathway of 4-*n*-nonylphenol in *S. xenophagum* Bayram involves an initial ipso-hydroxylation to 4-hydroxy-4-nonyl-2,5-cyclohexadienone intermediate (Kohler et al., 2008).

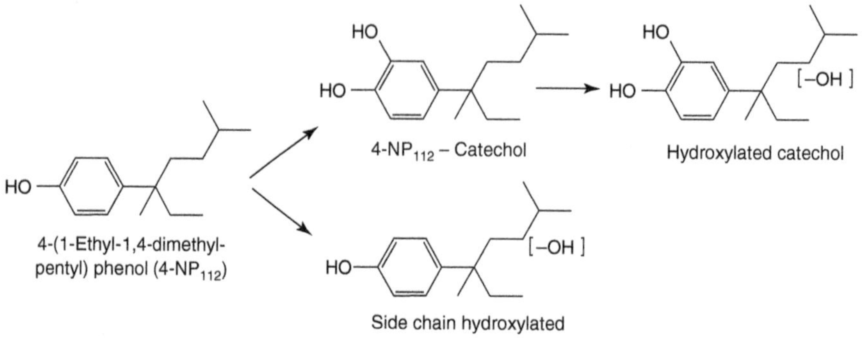

Figure 9.9   *In vitro* metabolic pathway of 4-*tert*-nonylphenol NP$_{112}$ with human and rat liver microsomes (Ye et al., 2007).

a catechol with a hydroxylated alkyl side chain (Fig. 9.9) (Ye et al., 2007). The branched-side-chain 4-NP isomers were not expected to undergo a complete breakdown of the alkyl side chain because β-oxidation could only proceed on the linear terminal part of this side chain.

Ipso-substitution is an important mechanism by which cytochrome P450 model systems, liver microsomes, and microorganisms detach various substituents in ortho- and para-substituted phenols and anilines. *S. xenophagum* Bayram transformed NP isomers with α-quaternary alkyl moieties at the benzylic position with an initial reaction of these substrates by an ipso-hydroxylation, yielding dearomatized intermediates. 4-Alkyl-4-hydroxy-cyclohexa-2,5-dien-1-ones spontaneously broke down to hydroquinone, and the α-quaternary alkyl moieties were detached as transient alkyl carbocations stabilized by α-alkyl branching as corresponding nonanol on reaction with water. On the other hand, the NP isomers with side chains containing α-hydrogens, which do not form stabilized carbocations, were not released. In the latter case, the ipso-hydroxylated intermediate proceeded to a dienone-phenol rearrangement (1,2-C,C) shift (NIH shift), leading to para-hydroxylation with retained alkyl moieties to 2-nonylhydroquinones (Fig. 9.10) (Gabriel et al., 2008; Kohler et al., 2008).

Formation of the 2-nonylhydroquinones formed during ipso-degradation of technical nonylphenol, which readily oxidized to the corresponding *p*-benzoquinone derivatives in the presence of air, has been suggested as one of the factors contributing to the incomplete degradation of technical nonylphenol observed during incubations with growing cells of strains Bayram (Gabriel et al., 2012).

9.3.3   4-*tert*-nonylphenol isomer 4-[1-ethyl-1,3-dimethylpentyl] phenol (4-NP$_{111}$)

4-[1-Ethyl-1,3-dimethylpentyl] phenol (4-NP$_{111}$) possessing a quaternary α-carbon on the branched alkyl chain is a major constituent of commercial tNP mixtures (Russ et al., 2005). A similar type II ipso-substitution mechanism is operative in the

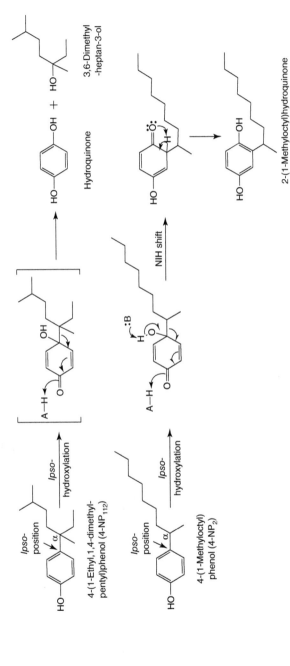

Figure 9.10 Differential degradation pathways of α-quaternary and α-tertiary NP isomers by *Sphingobium xenophagum* Bayram (Gabriel et al., 2008).

degradation pathway of NP isomers with branched side chains by *Sphingomonas* sp. TTNP3, another nonylphenol degrading bacterium, via oxidation at the quaternary α-carbon to form hydroquinone as the central metabolite and the side-chain alcohol products (Corvini et al., 2006a; 2006b). In NP metabolism, oxygen is added to the same carbon atom that harbors the alkyl substituent on the para-substituted phenol and typically results in replacement of the alkyl substituent by the oxygen atom to produce hydroquinone and an alkyl ion. Identifications were made of 3,5-dimethyl-3-heptanol as the hydroxylated alkyl chain of this NP isomer at the α-C position and, to a much smaller extent, hydroxylation of atom C-4 of the aromatic ring is followed by the migration of the alkyl chain to an adjacent C atom of the ring (NIH-shift) forming 2-[1-ethyl-1,3-dimethylpentyl]-hydroquinone. Hydroquinone is further degraded into organic acids, such as succinate and 3,4-dihydroxy butanedioic acid, while hydroquinone derivative remains a dead-end product (Fig. 9.11) (Corvini et al., 2006a).

The biotransformation of commercial nonylphenol mixtures with freshwater mitosporic fungi found in river water and sediments co-metabolically converted nonyl chain-branched isomers. The major products resulted were side-chain hydroxylated and side-chain-shortened compounds (Junghanns et al., 2005). Fungal intracellular nonylphenol biotransformation starting at branched alkyl chains is in contrast to nonylphenol utilization by bacteria where intracellular oxidative attack starts at the aromatic ring. An inference could be drawn that fungi and bacteria may cooperate in nonylphenol degradation in natural aquatic environments (Corvini et al., 2006b). Nonylphenol biotransformation in aquatic fungi also involved nonylphenol oxidation by extracellular laccases yielding polymerization (dimers to pentamers) products (Junghanns et al., 2005). In the presence of natural organic matter found in aquatic environments, such oxidative coupling reactions could lead to the removal of nonylphenol by the formation of bound residues, concomitantly eliminating its endocrine activity.

9.3.4   4-*n*- and 4-*tert*-octylphenols

Octylphenols, which are widely used in variety of detergents and plastics, are known to exhibit estrogenicity *in vivo*. Their metabolism has been elucidated in a perfused liver. Almost all 4-*n*-octylphenol was metabolized directly to glucuronide. The metabolism of the *tert*-octylphenol, which consists of only one isomer, has also been investigated. A portion of 4-*tert*-octylphenol was hydroxylated to 4-*tert*-octylcatechol and hydroxyl-*tert*-octylphenol (Fig. 9.12) and then glucuronidated by the liver microsomal fractions (Nomura et al., 2008). The differences in metabolic transformations of the two octylphenols are due to the shape of their alkyl chains. The estrogenic activity of 4-*n*-octylphenol using the YES test was found to be higher than that of 4-*tert*-octylphenol (Isidori et al., 2006).

Oxidation of 4-*tert*-octylphenol in the *Sphingomonas* sp. strain PWE1 occurs at the α-quaternary carbon, similar to branched-chain nonylphenol, resulting in a type II ipso-hydroxylation intermediate, forming hydroquinone and 2,4,4-trimethyl-1-pentene and some amount of 2,4,4-trimethyl-2-pentanol (Fig. 9.13) (Porter and Hay, 2007; Kagle et al., 2009; Tanghe et al., 2000).

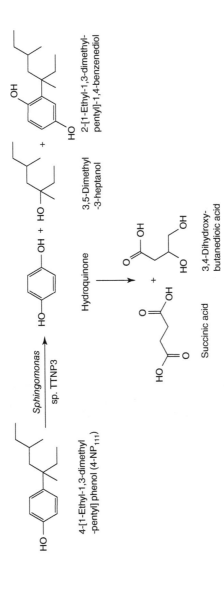

Figure 9.11 Degradation pathway of the NP isomer 4-[1-ethyl-1,3-dimethylpentyl] phenol by *Sphingomonas* sp. TTNP3 (Corvini et al., 2006a).

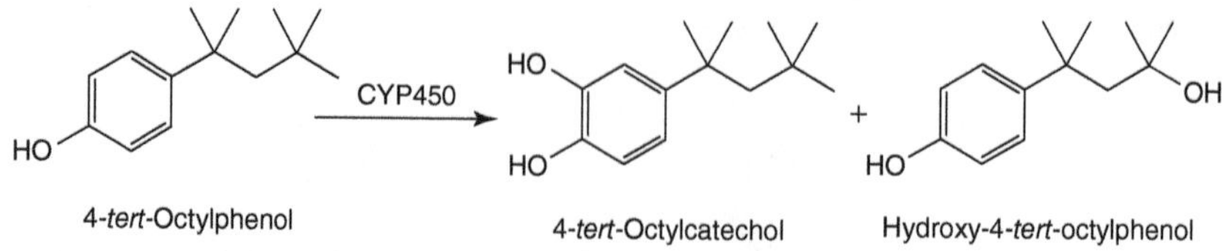

Figure 9.12 Biotransformation of 4-*tert*-octylphenol in the perfused rat liver (Nomura et al., 2008).

9.3.5 Bisphenol A

A microsomal cytochrome P450-catalyzed reaction was observed on incubation of BPA with rat or human liver microsomes. An ipso-substitution reaction generated hydroquinone and the metabolites isopropenylphenol and 4-(hydroxyisopropyl)phenol (Fig. 9.14). CYP3A4 and CYP3A5 showed higher activity for ipso-substitution. The metabolic pathway contributed to the activation of the estrogenic activity of BPA, as the ER-binding activities of 4-(hydroxyisopropyl)phenol was found to be about a hundred times greater than that of BPA and that of isopropenylphenol similar to BPA (Nakamura et al., 2011).

Incubation of BPA with rat liver S9 fraction as well as human, monkey, and mouse liver S9 fractions led to metabolic activation. The active metabolite of BPA was identified as an isopropenylphenol dimer structure, 4-methyl-2,4-bis(*p*-hydroxyphenyl)pent-1-ene (MBP) (Fig 9.15). It was suggested that the MBP formation might be the result of recombination of a radical fragment, a one-electron oxidation product of carbon–phenyl bond cleavage. MBP was found to have much more potent estrogenic activity than the parent BPA with 100–1000-fold stronger bond to the estrogen receptor than BPA (Yoshihara et al., 2004). In a study, 3D models of MBP and BPA in the human estrogen receptors were matched against estradiol in these receptors. It was observed that MBP's longer structure allowed both ends of the chemical to interact with the estrogen receptor in a way similar to estradiol. The shorter BPA molecule contacts the receptor at just one end, resulting in a weaker connection, thereby providing an explanation for BPA's lower affinity for the estrogen receptor (Baker and Chandsawangbhuwana, 2012).

BPA can be biodegraded by microorganisms distributed in the environment. BPA degradation employing soil bacteria *Sphingomonas* sp. strain AO1 has been shown to involve the cytochrome P450 monooxygenase system (Sasaki, et al., 2005). The major pathway of degradation produced two primary metabolites, namely 4-hydroxyacetophenone and 4-hydroxybenzoic acid, and the minor pathway also produced two primary metabolites, namely 2,2-bis(4-hydroxyphenyl)-1-propanol and 2,3-bis(4-hydroxyphenyl)-1,2-propanediol: the 4-hydroxybenzoic acid was formed from 4-hydroxyacetophenone by oxidative rearrangement. The addition of metyrapone, a specific inhibitor of CYP450, was found to inhibit BPA degradation (Sasaki et al., 2005). A metabolic pathway for BPA by the bacterium is shown in Figure 9.16 (Suzuki et al., 2004).

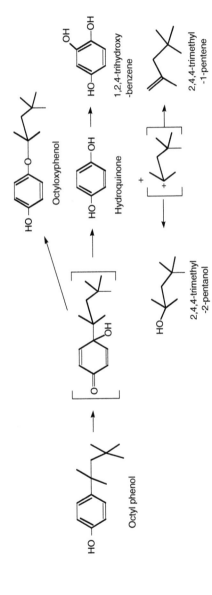

Figure 9.13 4-*tert*-Octylphenol monooxygenation in *Sphingomonas* sp. PWE1 via ipso-substitution (Porter and Hay, 2007).

Octyl phenol

Octyloxyphenol

Hydroquinone

1,2,4-trihydroxy
-benzene

2,4,4-trimethyl
-2-pentanol

2,4,4-trimethyl
-1-pentene

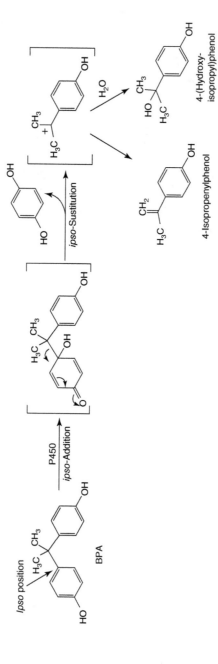

Figure 9.14 Microsomal incubation of BPA in rat and human liver microsomes leading to CPY450-catalyzed metabolic activation of BPA (Nakamura et al., 2011).

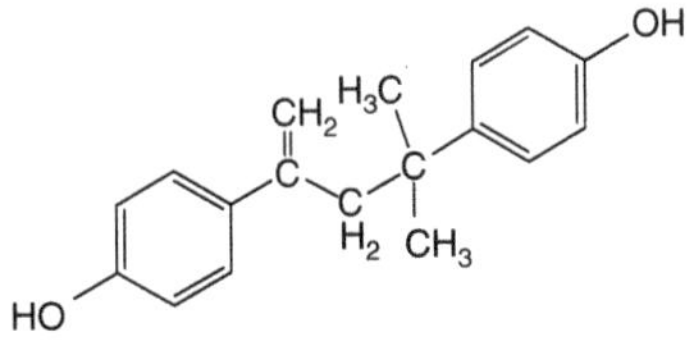

Figure 9.15 Structure of BPA's active metabolite 4-methyl-2,4-bis(4-hydroxy-phenyl)pent-1-ene (MBP).

In several other studies, a similar degradation pathway for BPA was found by different bacteria distributed in environmental waters (Suzuki et al., 2004, Masuda et al., 2007; Sakai et al., 2007, Zhang et al., 2007). Bacterial biodegradation eliminates the toxic or estrogenic effects of BPA, as among the four metabolites only 4-hydroxy-acetophenone displayed slight estrogenic activity on the yeast two-hybrid assay (Ike et al., 2002).

The degradation pathway of BPA employing *Sphingobium xenophagium* Bayram and *Sphingomonas* sp. TTNP3 proceeded via ipso-substitution involving ring hydroxylation at position C-4 followed by C–C bond breakage between the phenyl moiety and the isopropyl group. The main metabolites formed were hydroquinone (**1**) and 4-(2-hydroxypropane-2-yl) phenol (Kolvenbach et al., 2007) (Fig. 9.17). Other products identified include 4-isopropenylphenol, 4-isopropylphenol, 4-hydroxy-4-isopropenylcyclohexa-2,5-dien-1-one, and 4-hydroxy-4-isopropylcyclohexa-2,5-dien-1-one (Kolvenbach et al., 2007; Gabriel et al., 2007). Since all reported ipso-substitution-catalyzing reactions are with P450s enzymes, assays conducted in the presence of some typical cytochrome P450 inhibitors (octylamine and proadifene) inhibited the degradation of BPA by greater than 99%, in comparison to control experiments carried out without inhibitors under the same conditions (defined as 100% activity). However, in contrast to NP degradation through CYP450, neither alkylbenzenediol nor alkoxyphenol derivatives were detected in case of BPA (Kolvenbach et al., 2007).

HRP oxidation of BPA in presence of H_2O_2 at pH 8.0 resulted in the formation of mostly insoluble polymers and a minor product 4-isopropenylphenol, also produced by the reaction with laccase (Sakuyama et al., 2003) (Fig. 9.18). BPA transformation and removal from aqueous phase via oxidative coupling in HRP-mediated reaction at pH 7 in phosphate buffer involves 4-isopropenylphenol as a major intermediate (Huang and Weber, 2005; Cabana et al., 2007). The enzymatic oxidation of BPA using HRP was able to eliminate its estrogen-like activity (Sakuyama et al., 2003).

A similar reaction pathway for the degradation of BPA, removing its estrogenic activity, is caused by lignin-degrading enzymes, such as manganese peroxidase (MnP) and laccase, which are produced by white rot basidiomycetes

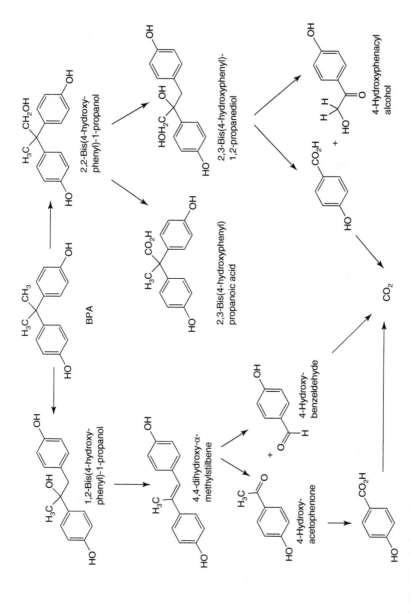

Figure 9.16 Metabolic pathways for BPA by *Sphingomonas* sp. strain AO1 distributed in environmental water (Suzuki et al., 2004; Ike et al., 2002; Spivack et al., 1994).

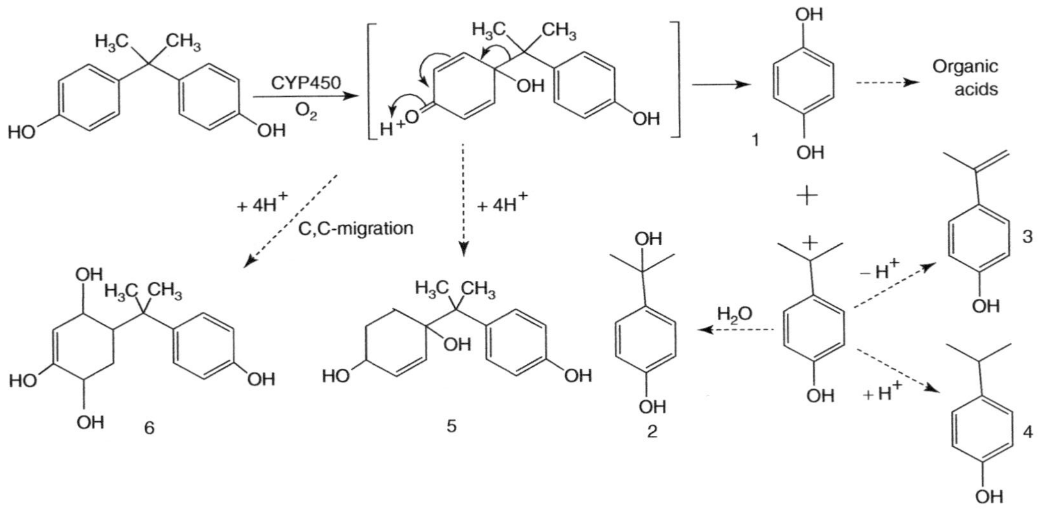

Figure 9.17 Degradation of bisphenol A in *Sphingomonas* sp. TTNP3 via an ipso-substitution (Kolvenbach et al., 2007; Gabriel et al., 2007).

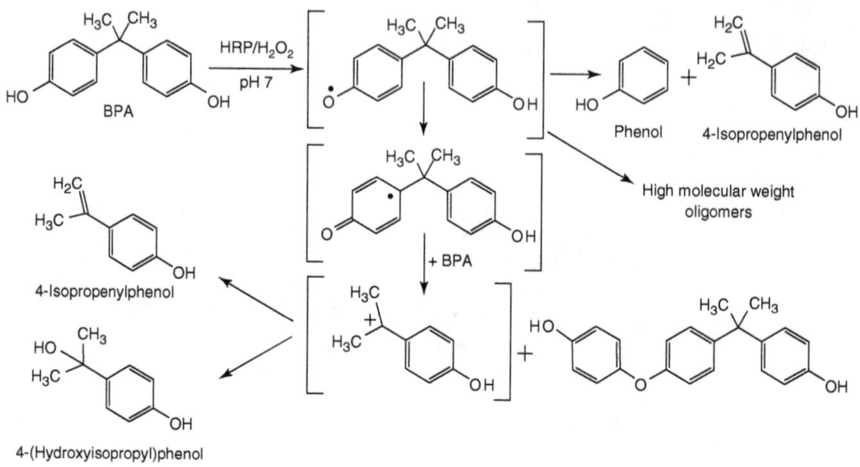

Figure 9.18   Oxidation of BPA by HRP/H$_2$O$_2$ (Huang and Weber, 2005).

fungi (Hirano et al., 2000). MnP degradation leads to the formation of phenol, 4-isopropenylphenol, 4-isopropylphenol, and hexestrol. Laccase leads to the polymerization of BPA to form a dimer and oligomers, followed by either the addition of phenol moieties or the degradation of the oligomers to release 4-isopropenylphenol (Uchida et al., 2001).

9.4   PHTHALATES

Numerous studies have demonstrated that microorganisms play major roles in phthalate degradation in the environment under various conditions. The biodegradation of phthalate diesters primarily involves the sequential hydrolysis of ester linkage, which results in monoesters. Following absorption, the monoesters are further metabolized by oxidation, mainly from ω-oxidation at the terminal or penultimate carbon, and hydroxylation reactions. Phthalic acid (PA) is a central intermediate in the biodegradation of phthalates. Under aerobic conditions, two dioxygenase-catalyzed pathways degrade PA, forming the common intermediate protocatechuate (3, 4-dihydroxy benzoate) (Eaton and Ribbons, 1982). Phthalates, known for endocrine disruption effects, with shorter ester chains, such as dibutyl phthalate (DBP) and butyl benzyl phthalate, can be readily biodegraded and mineralized, while those with longer ester chains, such as dioctyl phthalate and di-2-ethylhexyl phthalate (DEHP), are less susceptible for biodegradation. Also, the branched ester chain of phthalates is not found to be a significant factor limiting the degradation (Liang et al., 2008). Two reviews on biodegradation of phthalates have appeared covering the literature until 1997 (Staples et al., 1997) and the subsequent decade (Liang et al., 2008).

9.4.1 Di-*n*-butyl phthalate (DBP)

DBP is widely used in consumer products, such as cosmetics, toys, flooring, wallpaper, and furniture. It is also used as a plasticizer and as a solvent in polysulfide dental impression materials and as textile lubricating agent. It inhibits binding to the estrogen receptor and is an anti-androgenic (Jobling et al., 1995; Harris et al., 1997; Gray et al., 1999; Moore et al., 2001).

In humans and in rats, the primary metabolite of DBP is its hydrolytic monoester, monobutyl phthalate (MBP) (about 90%), which is further oxidized to mono 3-hydroxy-*n*-butyl phthalate (3-OH-MBP), mono 3-oxo-*n*-butyl phthalate (3-oxo-MBP), and mono 3-carboxypropyl phthalate (3-CX-MPP) (Fig. 9.19) (Silva et al., 2007).

The metabolism of phthalate esters by bacteria is considered a major fate of these widespread pollutants in environment. *Rhodococcus jostii* RHA1 is able to use monoalkyl esters including methyl, butyl, hexyl, and 2-ethylhexyl phthalates as its sole carbon and energy source. Suspensions of cells grown on phthalate could degrade dimethyl, diethyl, dipropyl, dibutyl, dihexyl, and di-(2-ethylhexyl) phthalates (Hara et al., 2010). The proposed degradation pathway of DBP by *R. jostii* RHA1 is the stepwise hydrolysis of the ester bonds, while the demethylation of the side chain to ethyl butylphthalate (EBP) and monoethyl phthalate (MEP) is a concurrent minor process (Fig. 9.20) (Hara et al., 2010). The degradation process of DBP provides an example for most reported biotransformations of phthalate esters in the natural environment.

Pseudomonas cepacia, Mycobacterium vanbaalenii PYR-1, and *Arthrobacter keyseri* 12B, all convert phthalate to a *cis*-dihydrodiol. *P. cepacia* produces the 4,5-dihydrodiol (Ballou and Batie, 1988), and *M. vanbaalenii* PYR-1 (Kim et al., 2007) and *A. keyseri* 12B (Eaton, 2001) produce the 2,3-dihydrodiol. These are transformed into the respective dihydroxy compounds, both of which can be decarboxylated to 3,4-dihydroxybenzoate (protocatechuate).

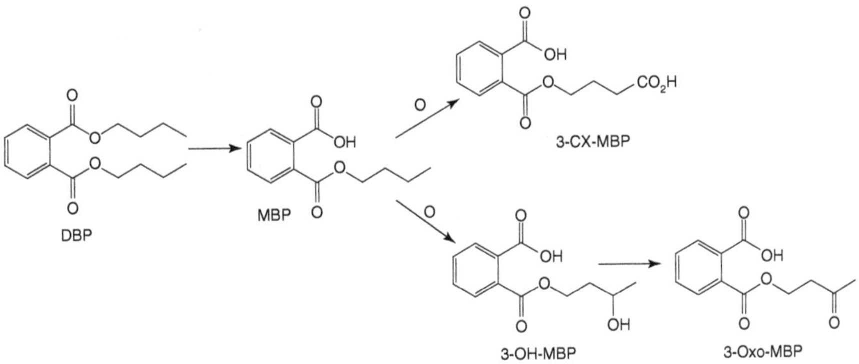

Figure 9.19 Mammalian metabolic products of di-*n*-butyl phthalate. Source: Redrawn from Silva et al. (2007).

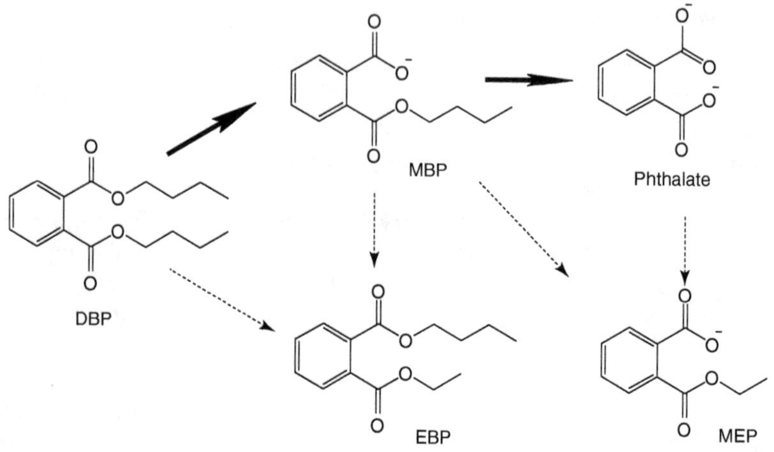

Figure 9.20 Proposed pathway for dibutyl phthalate degradation by *Rhodococcus jostii* RHA1 (Hara et al., 2010).

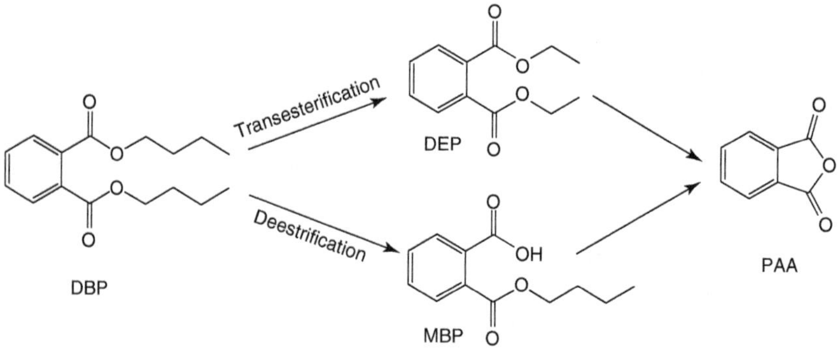

Figure 9.21 Degradation of DBP by fungus *Polyporus brumalis* (Lee et al., 2007).

The ligninolytic enzyme system from the white rot fungus *Polyporus brumalis* led the degradation of DBP, producing intermediate degradation products such as diethyl phthalate (DEP) and monobutyl phthalate (MBP) and the primary final degradation product phthalic acid anhydride (PAA), following trans-esterification and de-esterification pathways (Fig. 9.21). Trace amounts of α-hydroxyphenyl-acetic acid, benzyl alcohol, and *o*-hydroxyphenylacetic acid were also identified in the reaction mixture (Lee et al., 2007).

9.4.2   *n*-Butyl benzyl phthalate (BBP)

BBP is a plasticizer used in poly(vinyl chloride) (PVC) in food conveyor belts, carpet tiles, artificial leather, tarps, automotive trim, weather stripping, traffic cones, vinyl gloves, and cellulosic resins. BBP readily leaches from these products and is one of the important environmental contaminants. It inhibits binding to the estrogen receptor (Jobling et al., 1995).

When orally administered to female Wistar rats, six metabolites were identified. Mono-*n*-butyl phthalate (MBuP) and mono-*n*-benzyl phthalate (MBzP) represented, respectively, 29–34% and 7–12% of the total recovered metabolites. Hippuric acid, the main metabolite of benzoic acid, represented the second major metabolite (51–56%). Other metabolites identified include PA, benzoic acid, and an ω-oxidized metabolite of MBuP in small quantities (Nativelle et al., 1999).

A degradation pathway of BBP by *Pseudomonas* fluorescence B-1 is reported to cleave the ester bonds of the diester to yield phthalate monoesters, which degraded to yield PA. After decarboxylation, benzoic acid was produced, which was further metabolized to produce carbon dioxide and water (Xu et al., 2006). Recently, total degradation of BBP was achieved by employing a consortium of two bacteria, *Arthrobacter* sp. Strain WY and *Acinetobacter* sp. Strain FW, delineating the metabolic pathways of individual strains (Fig. 9.22) (Chatterjee and Dutta, 2008; Chatterjee and Karlovsky, 2010).

The *Arthrobacter* sp. strain WY utilized BBP as well as MBuP, MBzP, PA, or proto-catechuic acid as the sole source of carbon energy but not benzyl alcohol and 1-butanol. On the other hand, the *Acinetobacter* sp. strain FW utilized both benzyl alcohol and 1-butanol for growth but not BBP, MBuP, MBzP, PA, or protocatechuic acid. Besides benzyl alcohol, the strain FW also utilized benzaldehyde, benzoic acid, catechol, butyraldehyde, or butyric acid as the sole carbon source (Chatterjee and Dutta, 2008). A degradation pathway was established in which the strain WY first hydrolyzed BBP to its monoesters and then further to PA, which was metabolized to protocatechuic acid, β-carboxy-*cis*,*cis*-muconate, and ultimately leading to the tricarboxylic acid (TCA) cycle (Chatterjee and Dutta, 2008).

In addition to bacteria, fungi species such as *Fusarium oxysporum* (Kim et al., 2002) and *P. brumalis* (Lee et al., 2007) can also degrade phthalates. The broad-range degradation ability of fungi is attributed to the strong extracellular ligninolytic enzymes such as lignin peroxidase, manganese-dependent peroxidase, and laccase. For example, the cutinase-producing *F. oxysporum* showed high enzymatic activities and was able to degrade BBP (Kim et al., 2002). A treatment of BBP with fungal cutinase produced from *F. oxysporum* f. sp. *pisi* strain resulted in the formation of BMP, DMP, benzene methanol (BM), phthalic anhydride, and an unidentified compound (Kim et al., 2002). The formation of BMP and DMP was proposed to be due to the likely trans-esterification reaction products of cutinase in 0.1% methanol in the reaction medium.

9.4.3   Di-(2-ethylhexyl) phthalate (DEHP)

The industrial plasticizer DEHP is among the most abundantly used phthalate esters with an annual worldwide production estimated around 2 million tons. It is used in the manufacture of a wide variety of PVC-containing medical and consumer products to impart flexibility, strength, broad-range temperature tolerance, stability

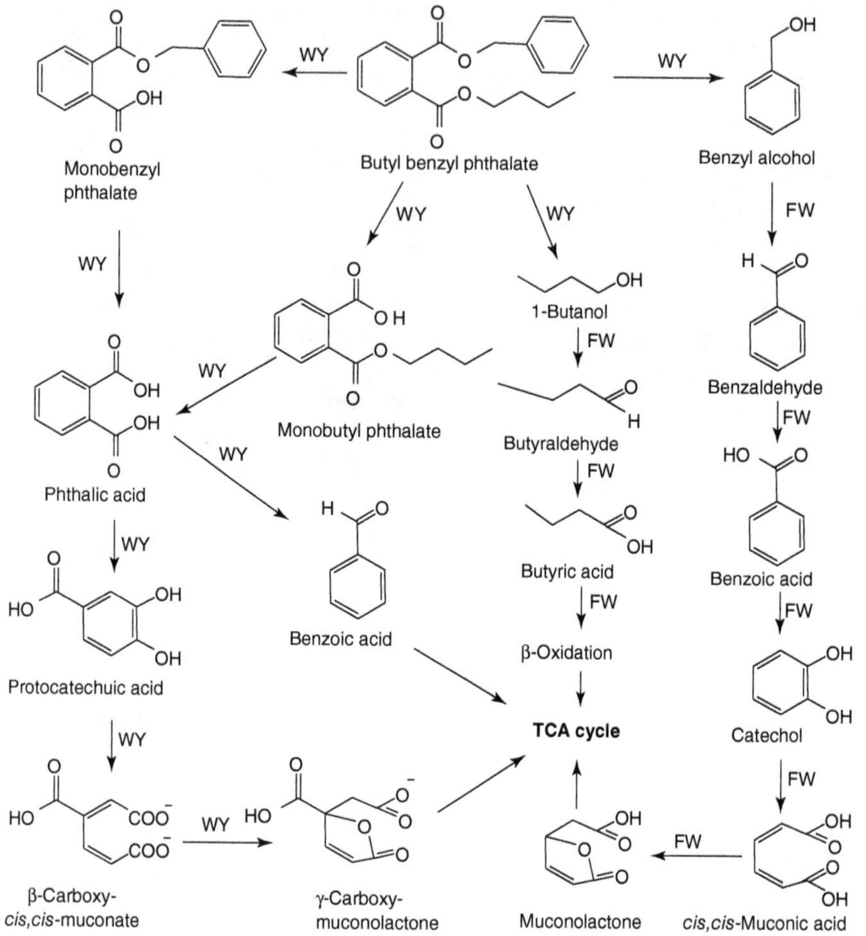

Figure 9.22 Degradation pathway of *n*-butyl benzyl phthalate by a consortium of two bacterial strains, *Arthrobacter* sp. Strain WY and *Acinetobacter* sp. Strain FW (Chatterjee and Karlovsky, 2010).

during sterilization, and optical clarity. The biological action of DEHP is very similar to that of chemicals which are collectively known as *peroxisome proliferators* (PPs). It can cross the placenta and disrupt steroid hormone synthesis. It inhibits binding to the estrogen receptor and is an anti-androgenic (Jobling et al., 1995; Harris et al., 1997; Gray et al., 1999; Moore et al., 2001).

Once DEHP enters the gastrointestinal tract, it is rapidly metabolized to mono(2-ethylhexyl) phthalate (MEHP) and 2-ethylhexanol, followed by formation of PA via pancreatic lipases (Fig. 9.23). Further metabolism occurs via oxidation by cytochrome P450 4A, yielding secondary oxidized DEHP metabolites such as mono-(2-ethyl-5-hydroxyhexyl) phthalate (5OH-MEHP), mono-(2-ethyl-5-oxohexyl)phthalate (5-oxo-MEHP), mono-(2-ethyl-5-carboxy-pentyl)phthalate

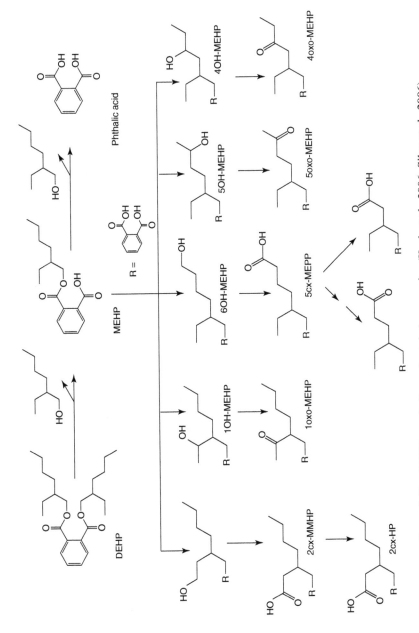

Figure 9.23 DEHP metabolic products in human urine (Koch et al., 2006; Silva et al., 2006).

(5cx-MEPP), and mono-[2-(carboxymethyl)hexyl] phthalate (2cx-MMHP), representing the major share of DEHP metabolites excreted in urine (about 70% for these four oxidized metabolites vs about 6% for MEHP) (Koch et al., 2006; Silva et al., 2006). MEHP and three oxidative metabolites of DEHP, namely 5-oxo-MEHP, 5-OH-MEHP, and 5-cx-MEPP, have been unequivocally identified using authentic standards, while others were assigned structures on the basis of their chromatographic and mass spectrometric behavior (Silva et al., 2006). There are strong indications that the secondary oxidized DEHP metabolites, not DEHP or MEHP, are the ultimate developmental toxins (Koch et al., 2006).

A bacterial strain found capable of rapidly degrading DEHP was isolated from soil and identified as *Bacillus subtilis*. The organism also utilized DBP and PA as sole carbon sources. The microorganism degraded DEHP and DBP through the intermediate formation of MEHP and MBP, respectively, which were then metabolized to PA and further by a protocatechuate pathway (Quan et al., 2005).

9.4.4   Di-*n*-octyl phthalate (DOP)

A single bacterial isolate from a municipal waste-contaminated soil, *Gordonia* sp. strain Dop5, utilized DOP as the sole energy source, completely degrading it (Sarkar et al., 2013). In the degradation process, mono-*n*-octyl phthalate, PA, protocatechuic acid, and 1-octanol were identified as the degradation products. Furthermore, PA was metabolized via protocatechuic acid involving protocatechuate 3,4-dioxygenase, while 1-octanol was metabolized by NAD^+-dependent dehydrogenases to 1-octanoic acid, which was subsequently degraded via β-oxidation, ultimately leading to TCA cycle intermediates (Fig. 9.24). The aerobic bacterium was found capable of efficiently degrading other phthalate esters of environmental concern having both shorter or longer alkyl chains (Sarkar et al., 2013). Earlier, a consortium of two bacterial strains, *Gordonia* sp. strain JDC-2 and *Anthrobacter* sp. strain JDC-32 isolated from activated sludge, was utilized to achieve complete degradation of DOP by overcoming the degradative limitations of each species alone (Wu et al., 2010). In this case, *Gordonia* sp. rapidly degraded DOP into PA, while *Arthrobacter* sp. degraded PA but not DOP (Wu et al., 2010).

9.5   INSECTICIDES

9.5.1   Methoxychlor

Incubation of methoxychlor in liver microsomes from rats and humans yields three phenolic metabolites. The metabolism of this compound is initiated by O-demethylation catalyzed by cytochrome P450 enzymes (Dehal and Kupfer, 1994). The primary metabolites were identified as mono- and bisphenol demethylated derivatives and a trihydroxy catechol involving sequential demethylations to the monohydroxy metabolite with the subsequent formation of the dihydroxy and

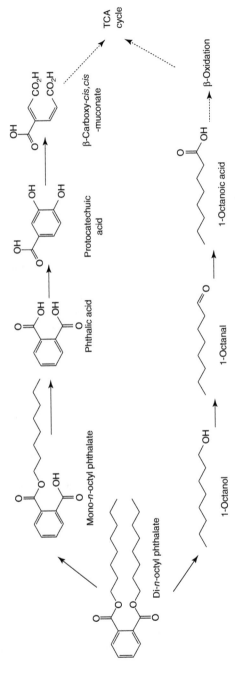

Figure 9.24 Proposed pathway for the complete degradation of di-*n*-octyl phthalate by *Gordonia* sp. strain Dop5 (Sarkar et al., 2013).

227

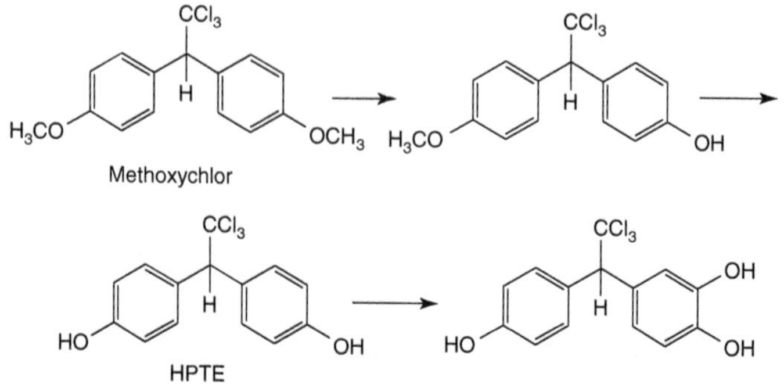

Figure 9.25   Metabolism of methoxychlor with rat liver microsomes (Kupfer et al., 1990).

trihydroxy metabolites (Fig. 9.25) (Kupfer et al., 1990). Structure–activity studies of the major metabolites of methoxychlor in rodents have shown that the mono- and bis-demethylated metabolites have the ERα agonist activity as well as the ERβ and AR antagonist activity (Gaido et al., 2000).

Metabolic transformations of methoxychlor in fungal *Cunninghamella elegans* (ATCC 36112) are catalyzed by cytochrome P450, exhibiting a strong resemblance of the xenobiotic metabolism of the mammalian system, rapidly transforming to several metabolites formed by demethylation, hydroxylation, oxidation to alkenes, and oxidative dechlorination (Fig. 9.26). Both mono- and bis-demethylated methoxychlor metabolites were found to be the most abundant products (Keum et al., 2009).

A Gram-negative bacterium isolate *Bradyrhizobium* sp. strain 17-4 from river sediment, which closely resembles *Bradyrhizobium elkanii*, mediated O-demethylation of methoxychlor to yield mono de-methylated methoxychlor as the primary degradation product. This was accompanied by the sequential O-demethylation to form the bis-demethylated derivative, oxidative dechlorination, and mono demethylated carboxylic acid, followed by multiple polar degradation products. In submerged sediment, methoxychlor degradation is proposed via initial conversion to de-Cl-methoxychlor under reductive conditions, and further degradation proceeds under oxidative conditions to phenolic derivatives and carboxylic acids leading to readily biodegradable substrates and mineralization (Fig. 9.27) (Satsuma et al., 2012).

9.6   FUNGICIDES

9.6.1   Vinclozolin

Vinclozolin produces biotransformation products *in vitro* in liver slices and *in vivo* in rats. The metabolic pathway of involves hydrolytic opening of the oxazolidine ring as the first step, forming M1 and M2 compounds, respectively, by nonenzymatic cleavage of the 3,4 and 2,3 N–C bonds. Cleavage of the 2,3 N–C bond is

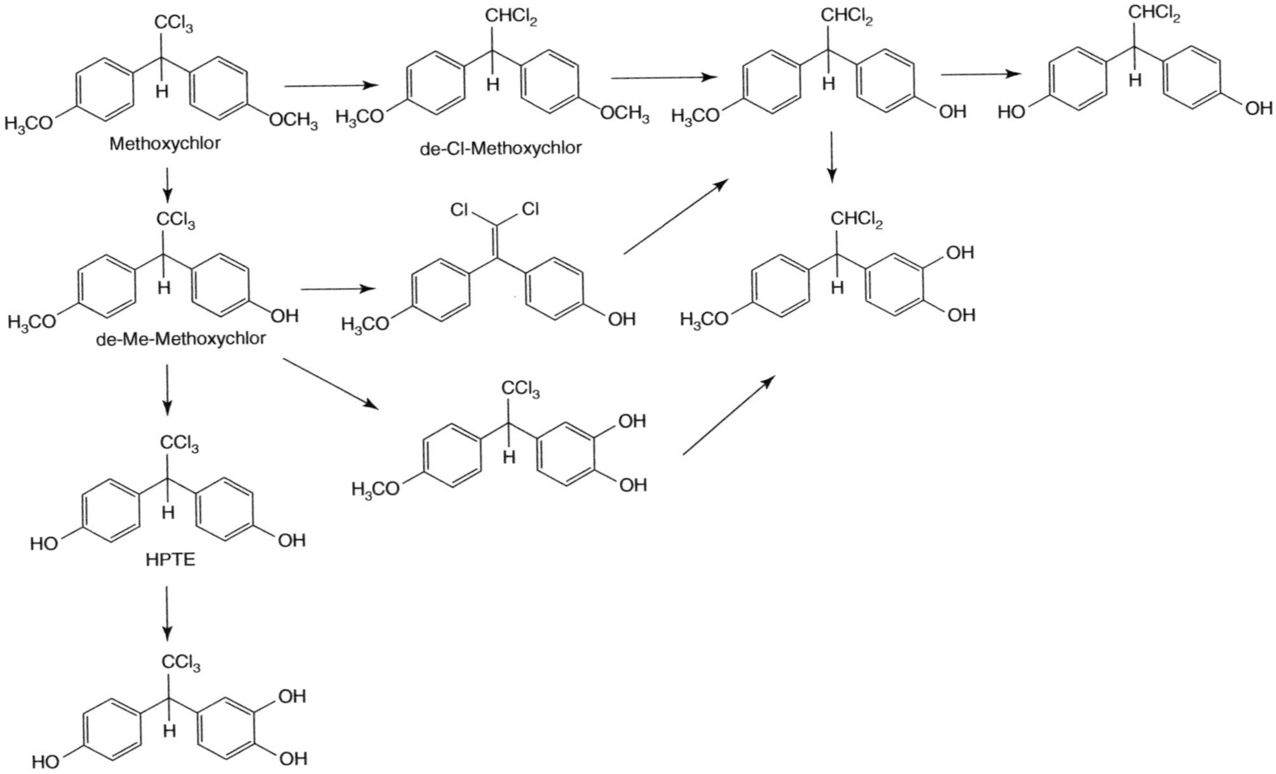

Figure 9.26 Metabolic transformation of methoxychlor by *Cunninghamella elegans* (Keum et al., 2009).

229

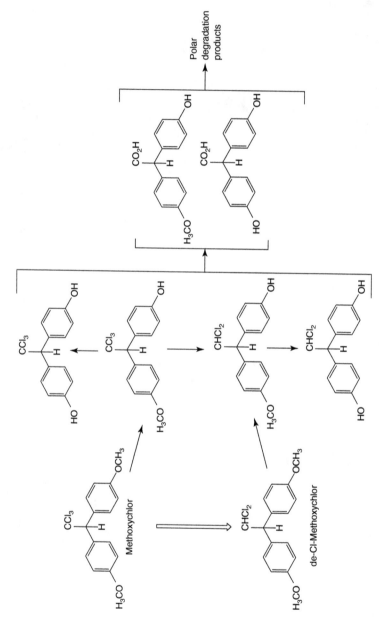

Figure 9.27 Degradation pathways of methoxychlor by *Bradyrhizobium* sp. Strain 17-4 (Satsuma et al., 2012).

followed by decarboxylation, which is not reversible, in contrast to the cleavage of the 3,4 N–C bond. The enzymatic phase I step includes the dihydroxylation of the vinyl group resulting in metabolite M4 from vinclozolin, metabolite M5 from M2, and M6 from M1 (Fig. 9.28). M5 was the major metabolite mainly present as glucurono-conjugate detected in the rat liver slices and in urine. As the end product of vinclozolin degradation, 3,5-dichloroaniline (M3) was identified in the rat liver slice, but was not detected in rat urine (Bursztyka et al., 2008).

Vinclozolin biotransformation by the fungus *C. elegans* resulted in four major metabolites (Fig. 9.29). The metabolites were identified as *N*-(2-hydroxy-2-methyl-1-oxobutene-3-yl)-3,5-dichlorophenyl-1-carbamic acid (I), the 3(*R*)- and 3(*S*)-isomers of 3′,5′-dichloro-2,3,4-trihydroxy-2-methybutyranilide (II and III), and 3′,5′-dichloro-2-hydroxy-2-methylbut-3-enanilide (IV, product identified as the metabolite M2 in Fig. 9.28) (Pothuluri et al., 2000).

9.6.2 Procymidone

Procymidone *in vivo* rat and mice metabolic pathway involves hydroxylation at the methyl group followed by oxidation to carboxylic acid and hydrolysis of the imide linkage (Fig. 9.28). The major metabolites were *N*-(3,5-dichlorophenyl)-1-carboxy-2-methylcyclopropane-1,2-dicarbo-ximide (P5) and the products (P6 and P7) yielded from P5 by hydrolysis at the imide. Small amounts of 3,5-

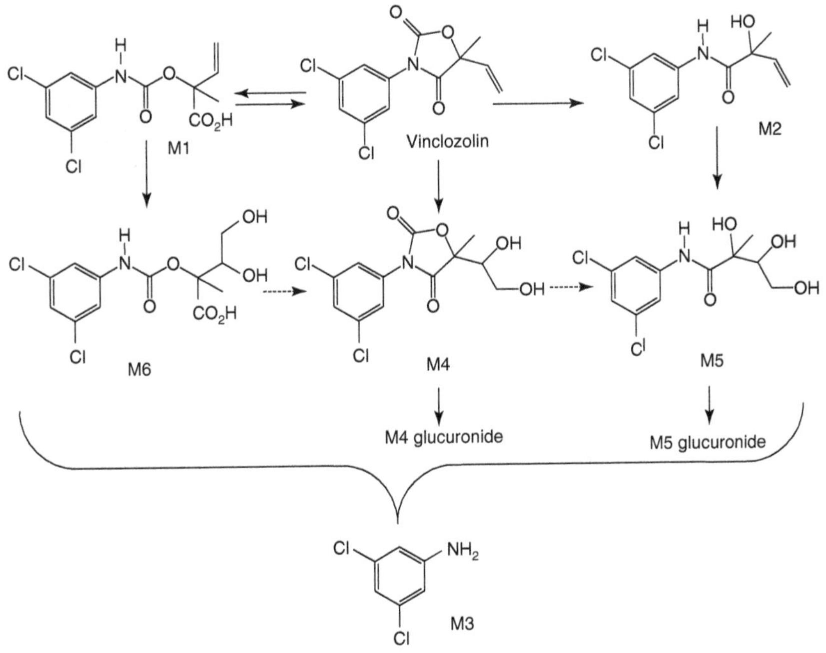

Figure 9.28 Metabolic pathways of the *in vitro* and *in vivo* biotransformations of vinclozolin. Source: Redrawn from Bursztyka et al. (2008).

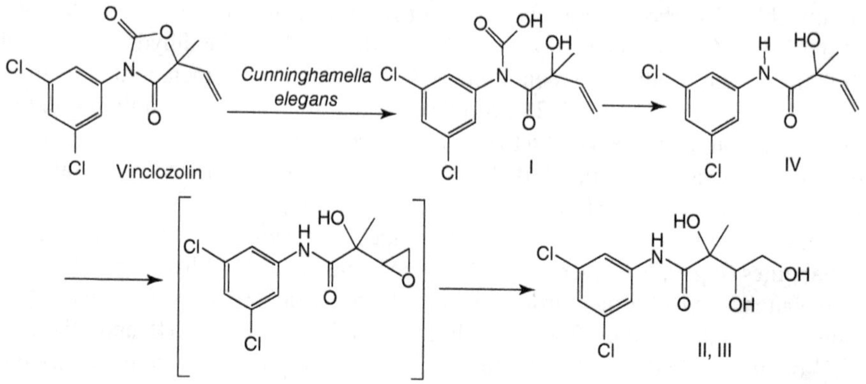

Figure 9.29 Biotransformation of vinclozolin by *Cunninghamella elegans*. Source: Redrawn from Pothuluri et al. (2000).

dichloroaniline and 2-methylcyclopropane-1,1,2-TCA were also obtained (Fig. 9.30) (Mikami et al., 1979; Shiba et al., 1991).

9.6.3   Prochloraz

Prochloraz was found to be extensively metabolized in rats. The main metabolic pathway involved opening of the imidazole ring followed by hydrolysis of the alkyl chain. A minor metabolic pathway involved aromatic hydroxylation. The main urinary metabolites identified were 2,4,6-trichlorophenoxyacetic acid (**3**) and 2-(2,4,6-trichlorophenoxy) ethanol glucuronide conjugate (**7**), accounting for 80% of the oral dose. Five other metabolites identified were 2-(2,4,6-trichloro phenoxy)ethanol (**2**), 2-(3-hydroxy-2,4,6-trichlorophenoxy)ethanol (**8**), *N*-2-(3 -hydroxy-2,4,6-trichlorophenoxy) ethyl-*N'*-propyl-urea (**6**), *N*-2-(4-hydroxy-2,6-dichlorophenoxy)ethyl-*N'*-propylurea (**5**), and *N*-2-(2,4,6-trichlorophenoxy)ethyl-urea (**4**) (Fig. 9.31) (Needham and Challis, 1991).

9.7   HERBICIDES

9.7.1   Linuron

Linuron is a systemic herbicide used to control a wide variety of annual and peren-nial broadleaf and grassy weeds. The metabolic pathway of linuron *in vivo* and *in vitro* in the rabbit and rat involved the major metabolites *N*-desmethyl linuron, *N'*-(3,4-dichlorophenyl) urea, and *N'*-(6-hydroxy-3,4-dichlorophenyl) urea (Fig. 9.32) (Anfossi et al., 1993).

The soil bacterial isolate *Variovorax* sp. strain SRS16 mineralizes linuron. The biodegradation pathway proposed initiates with hydrolysis of linuron to 3,4-dichloroaniline (DCA) and *N,O*-dimethyl- hydroxylamine, followed by conversion of DCA to Krebs cycle intermediates (Fig. 9.33) (Bers et al., 2011).

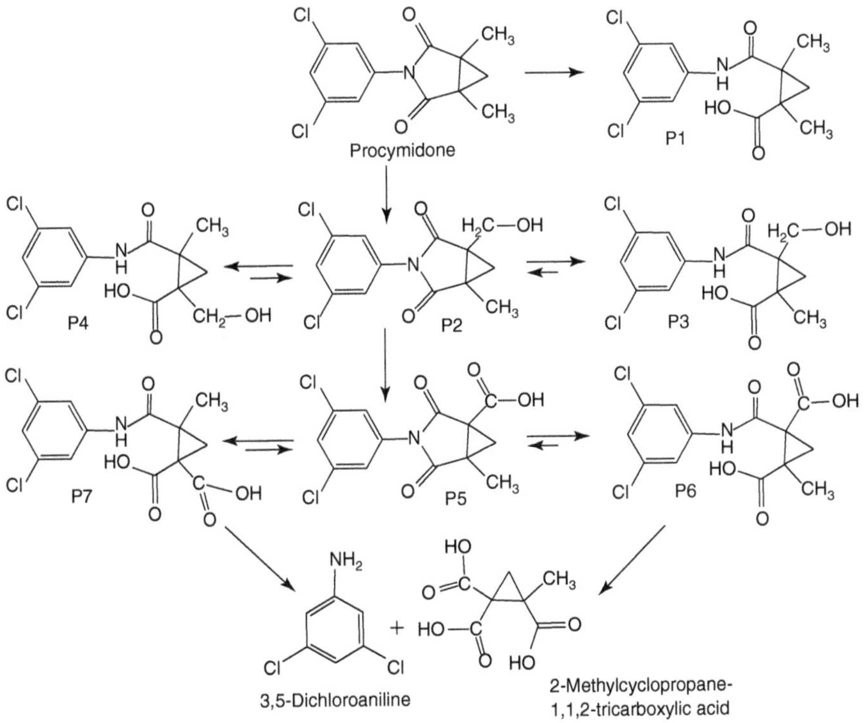

Figure 9.30 Metabolic pathway for the dicarboximide fungicide procymidone in rat and mice (Mikami et al., 1979; Shiba et al., 1991).

The soil fungus *Mortierella* sp. Gr4. degrades linuron, resulting successively in dealkylated metabolites and 3,4-dichloroaniline. Also, a new metabolite was detected as a non-aromatic diol, which remains to be fully identified (Badawi et al., 2009).

9.7.2 Atrazine

Metabolism of atrazine in mammals as well as microbes most commonly involves N-monodealkylation and hydroxylation processes. For example, atrazine undergoes biotransformation in the rodents to deisopropylatrazine (DIA), deethylatrazine (DEA), and 2-chloro-4,6-diamino-s-triazine (DACT) (Fig. 9.34) by successive rounds of oxidative N-dealkylation reactions, presumably catalyzed by P450s (Adams et al., 1990). In human microsome, three other distinct oxidation products corresponding to adding an oxygen atom into the ethyl side chain (hydroxy-ethyl atrazine, HEA) and the isopropyl side chain (hydroxy-isopropyl atrazine, HIA) and an N-oxidation product at the N-ethyl group (*N*-hydroxyatrazine, NHA) were also identified (LeBlanc and Sleno, 2011; Joo et al., 2010). Two additional metabolites

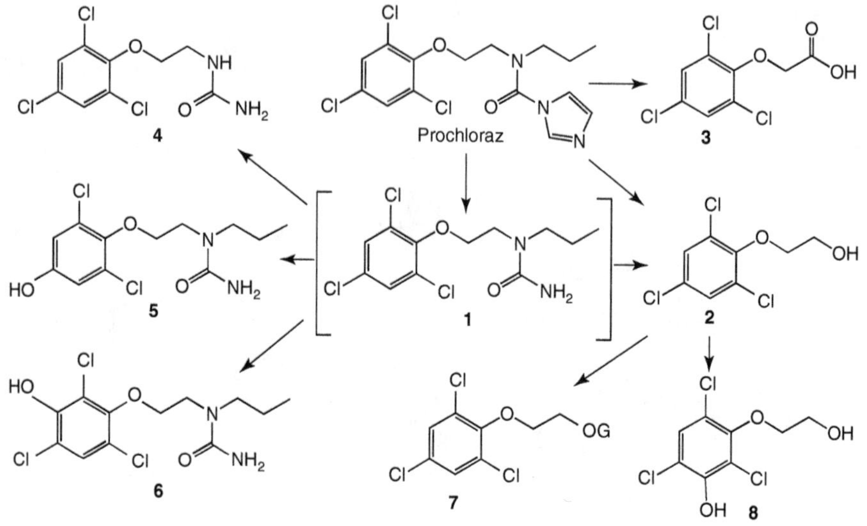

Figure 9.31 Metabolites of imidazole fungicide prochloraz in the urine of rats (Needham and Challis, 1991).

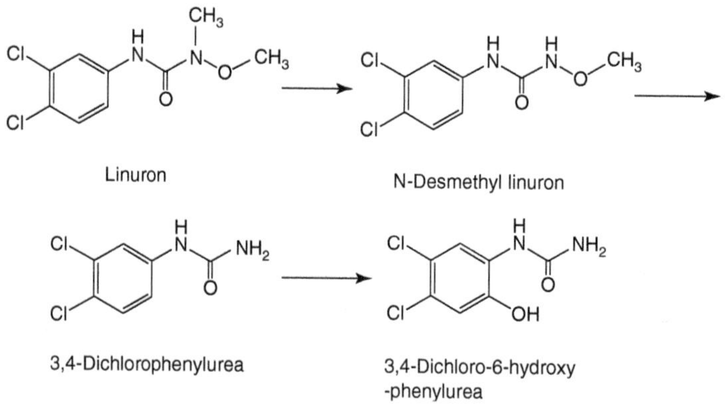

Figure 9.32 Metabolic biotransformation of the phenylurea herbicide Linuron in rabbit and rat. Source: Redrawn from Anfossi et al. (1993).

identified were dehydrogenated atrazine (DHA) and hydroxy-dehydrogenated atrazine (HDHA) (Fig. 9.34) (LeBlanc and Sleno, 2011).

Atrazine biotransformation using bacterial enrichment cultures in soil using *Pseudomonas* sp. strain ADP indicated that atrazine mineralization is initiated by the hydrolytic dechlorination reaction to produce hydroxyatrazine (Shapir et al., 2007). This undergoes two subsequent hydrolytic deamination reactions, resulting in the formation of cyanuric acid. The enzymes involved in what is constituted as the upper degradative pathway of atrazine to cyanuric acid are AtzA, AtzB, and AtzC (Fig. 9.35). The lower atrazine degradation pathway consists of ring

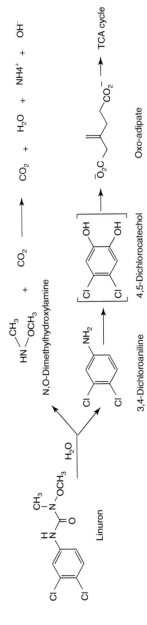

Figure 9.33 Biodegradation of linuron with the bacterial isolate *Variovorax* sp. strain SRS16 (Bers et al., 2011).

235

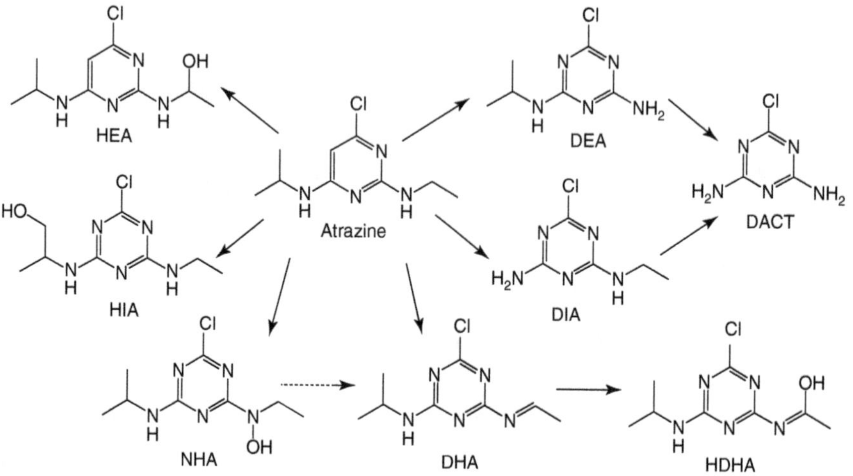

Figure 9.34 *In vitro* metabolic transformations of atrazine in human microsomes (LeBlanc and Sleno, 2011; Joo et al., 2010).

cleavage and subsequent transformation of cyanuric acid to CO_2 and NH_4 (Shapir et al., 2007).

9.8 POLYCHLORINATED BIPHENYLS (PCBs)

PCBs are a well-known class of pollutants. Given their inherent stability, PCBs are difficult to eliminate from environmental matrices. There are 209 possible PCB congeners, with their own potential for biodegradation. In general, those with fewer chlorine atoms tend to be more readily biotransformed under aerobic conditions, and the higher chlorinated congeners are more readily biotransformed under anaerobic conditions. The potential for biodegradation is a function not only of the number of chlorine atoms on a given PCB molecule but also of their placement. PCB congeners with the chlorine atom on the *ortho*-carbon tend to be more difficult to biotransform than those with the chlorine atom in the meta or para positions (Abramowicz, 1990).

Diverse aerobic bacteria capable of oxidizing PCBs have been reported (Pieper and Seeger, 2008). Bacterial strains that degrade PCBs oxidatively include various Gram-negative genera *Pseudomonas*, *Burkholderia*, *Comamonas*, *Cupriavidus*, *Sphingomonas*, *Acidovorax*, and Gram-positive genera *Rhodococcus*, *Corneybacterium*, and *Bacillus* genera (Furukawa and Fujihara, 2008). Bacterial metabolism of aromatic compounds is usually initiated by oxygenases, which catalyze the incorporation of two oxygen atoms into the aromatic ring to form arene *cis*-diols. The biphenyl 2,3-dioxygenases are of crucial importance for the successful metabolism of PCBs.

PCB congeners with three or fewer chlorines are susceptible to transformation by PCB-degrading aerobic bacteria species *Rhodococcus jostii* RHA1 and

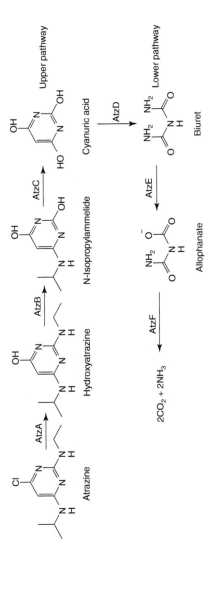

Figure 9.35 Atrazine metabolism by soilborne bacteria *Pseudomonas* sp. strain ADP (Shapir et al., 2007; de Souza et al., 1998).

Burkholderia xenovorans LB400, resulting in the accumulation of metabolites such as chlorobenzoates and 2-hydroxypenta-2,4-dienoates (Fig. 9.36) (Furukawa and Fujihara, 2008). The aerobic biotransformation of PCBs involves oxidation of the ring by a 2,3-dioxygenase, which substitutes two hydrogens with two hydroxyl groups at adjacent ortho and meta positions on the molecule, which is then dehydrogenated to a dihydroxylated PCB. The ring is then cleaved through the assistance of another dioxygenase at either of two locations. *B. xenovorans* LB400 is able to degrade a broad range of PCBs and metabolize from monochlorobiphenyls to 2,3,4,5,2′,5′-hexachlorobiphenyl congener (Field and Sierra-Alvarez, 2008).

Anaerobic biotransformation of PCBs is most effective with more highly chlorinated PCBs. Under anaerobic conditions, PCBs are transformed by reductive dehalogenation, substituting chlorine atom(s) in the molecule with hydrogen. Anaerobic PCB-dechlorinating microorganisms are expected to reduce the toxicity of PCBs and make them more aerobically degradable. The anerobic bacterium *Dehalococcoides* was demonstrated to dechlorinate 4–9 chlorines in Arochlor 1260 (Furukawa and Fujihara, 2008; Bedard et al., 2007). Such anaerobic dehalogenation generates lower chlorinated congeners, which are easily degraded aerobically (Pieper and Seeger, 2008). Typically, meta and/or para chlorines are removed to generate primarily ortho-substituted chlorobiphenyls. Stepwise dechlorination pathway of a major heptachlorobiphenyl congner in Arochlor 1260 is shown in Figure 9.37.

The yeast-like fungus *Trichosporon mucoides* and mitosporic (filamentous) fungus *Paecilomyces lilacinus* demonstrated PCB biodegradation potential of fungi, both of which are known for their biotransformation capabilities. Low chlorinated biphenyls were transformed through monohydroxylation of both the unsubstituted and the chlorinated aromatic ring of the molecules followed by the cleavage of hydroxylated ring system (Sietmann et al., 2006). Ligninolytic fungi, such as *Phanerochaete chrysosporium* and others, largely selected for the degradation of aromatic pollutants, have had little success in the degradation of PCBs. Incubation of 4-chlororobiphenyl with *T. mucoides* resulted in several transformation products with mono- and dihydroxylation of the molecule and aromatic ring cleavage products (Sietmann et al., 2006) (Fig. 9.38).

9.9   POLYBROMINATED DIPHENYL ETHERS (PBDEs)

Microbially mediated reductive dehalogenation is one of the most important routes for environmental transformation of persistent halogenated compounds. PBDEs are structurally similar to polychlorinated biphenyls and dioxins, which can be dechlorinated via reductive dehalogenation.

9.9.1   2,2′,4,4′-Tetrabromodiphenyl ether (BDE-47)

BDE-47 is an important congener in the commercial penta-BDE product and the most abundant PBDE congener found in human blood (Qiu et al., 2009).

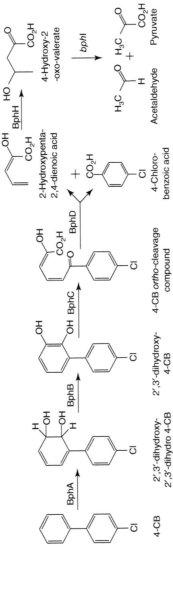

Figure 9.36 Aerobic bacterial degradation of PCBs catalyzed by bisphenyl dioxygenases (Bhps) (Furukawa and Fujihara, 2008). BphA = biphenyl 2,3-dioxygenase; BphB = *cis*-2,3-dihydro-2,3-dihydroxybiphenyl dehydrogenase; BphC = 2,3-dihydroxybiphenyl-1,2-dioxygenase; BphD = 2-hydroxy-6-phenyl-6-oxohexa-2,4-dieneoate hydrolase; BphH = 2-hydroxypenta-2,4-dieneoate hydratase; BphI = acylating acetaldehyde dehydrogenase.

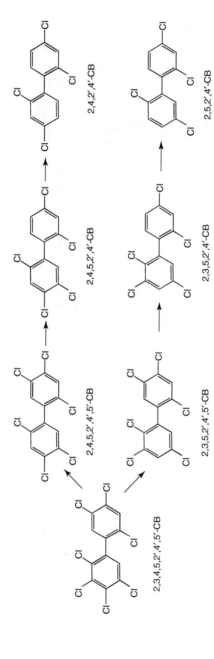

Figure 9.37 Bacterial stepwise dechlorination of 2,3,4,5,2′,4′,5′-heptachloro-biphenyl by *Dehalococcoides* bacteria (Furukawa and Fujihara, 2008).

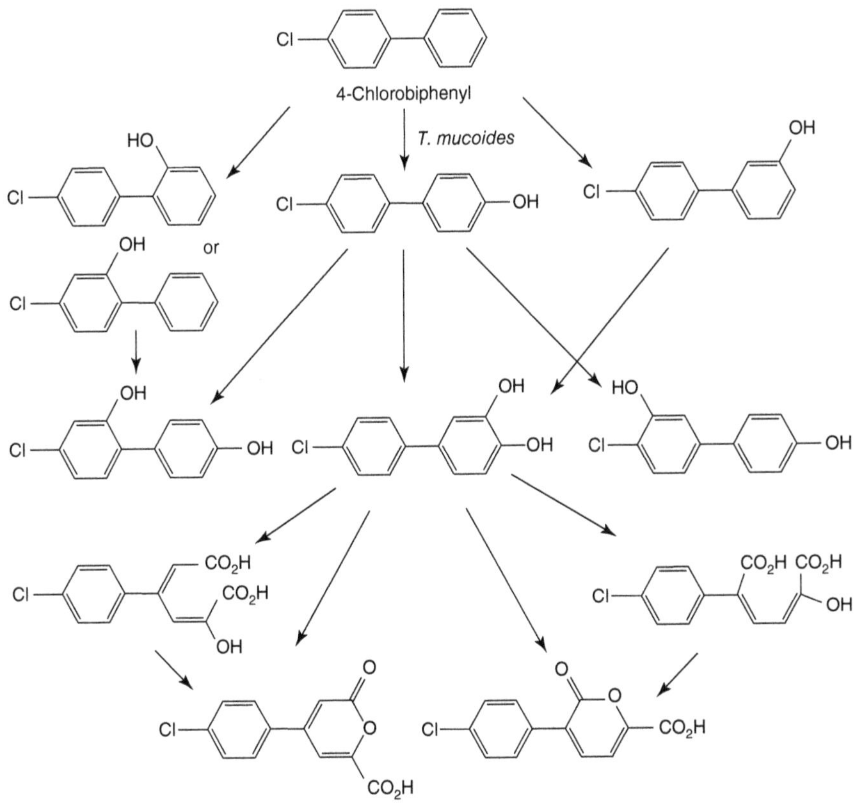

Figure 9.38 Proposed transformation pathway of 4-chlorobiphenyl by the yeast-like fungus *T. mucoides* (Sietmann et al., 2006).

Incubation of BDE-47 with phenobarbital-treated rat liver microsomes generated six hydroxylated metabolites, presumably produced by cytochrome P-450 enzymes (Qiu et al., 2007; Hamers et al., 2008). Oxidation of many aromatic xenobiotic contaminants in the liver occurs through the catalytic action of the CYP-450 isozymes of the hepatic mixed-function oxidase system. These were identified as 3-OH-BDE-47, 5-OH-BDE-47, 6-OH-BDE-47, 4-OH-BDE-42, 4′-OH-BDE-49, and 2′-OH-BDE-66 (Fig. 9.39). The last three metabolites require a bromine shift via an arene oxide during the hydroxylation process. 5-OH-BDE-47 and 6-OH-BDE-47 were the most dominant metabolites in humans and accounted for 90% of the total OH-tetra-BDE concentration (Qiu et al., 2009), while 6-OH-BDE-47 was only a minor metabolite in the rat. In addition, three bromophenols, namely 2,4,5-tribromophenol, 2,4,6-tribromophenol, and 2,4-dibromophenol, were also detected as products of the cleavage of the diphenyl ether bond. The endocrine-disrupting (ED) potencies of individual metabolites for competing with thyroxine (T4; the transport form of thyroid hormone) for binding

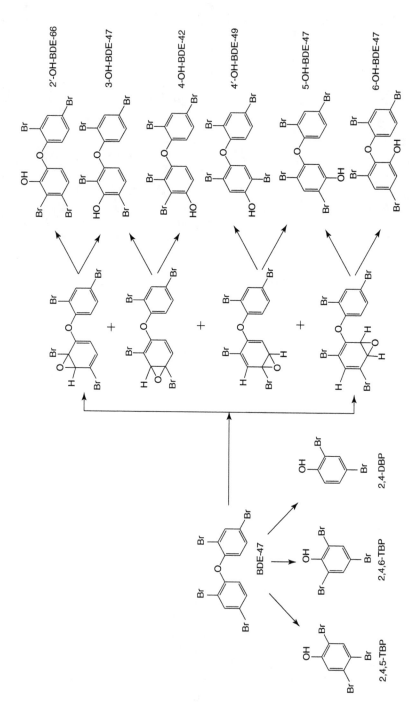

Figure 9.39 Hydroxylation pathway of BDE–47 metabolites in humans (Qiu et al., 2009).

to human transthyretin (TTR; a T4-transporting protein in plasma) were 160–1600 times higher than that of BDE-47. Similarly, individual metabolites had inhibition potencies of estradiol-sulfotransferase (E2-SULT), an enzyme responsible for sulfonation and subsequent inactivation of the endogenous hormone estradiol, 2.2–220 times higher than that of BDE-47 (Hamers et al., 2008).

9.9.2 2,2′,4,4′,5-Penta bromodiphenyl ether (BDE-99)

In another study, the metabolites of BDE-99, a major congener in the widely used commercial penta-BDE mixture, on incubation with dexamethasone-treated rat liver microsomes were identified (Erratico et al., 2011). Out of seven hydroxy metabolites of BDE-99 formed, four were identified as 2,4,5-tribromophenol, 4-OH-BDE-90, 5′-OH-BDE-99, and 6′-OH-BDE-99 (Fig. 9.40). Stapleton and colleagues examined the oxidative metabolites of BDE-99 in human tissues by exposing human liver cells *in vitro*, which resulted in the formation of 2,4,5-tribromophenol, two monohydroxylated pentabromo diphenyl ether metabolites, and an unidentified tetrabromo metabolite. BDE-99 also appeared to metabolize to a greater extent than BDE-47 (Stapleton et al., 2009).

9.9.3 3,3′,4,4′,5,5′,6,6′-Decabromodiphenyl ether (BDE-209)

The fully brominated diphenyl ether, decabromodiphenyl ether (decaBDE), is the most commonly used. Gerecke et al. (2005) reported on the microbial reductive

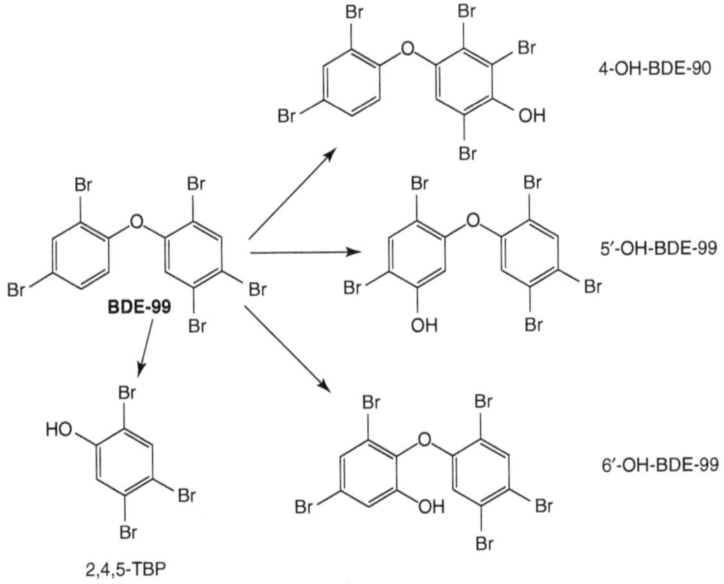

Figure 9.40 Identified metabolites of BDE-99 formed in rat liver microsomes (Erratico et al., 2011).

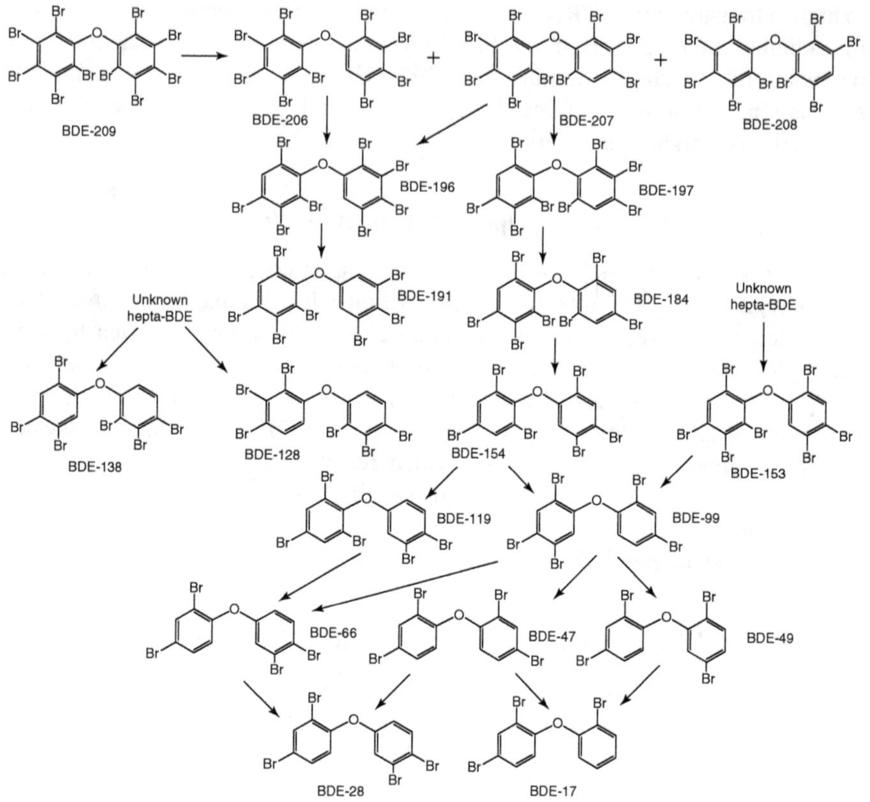

Figure 9.41 Debromination pathway of BDE-209 derived from both sediment microcosms and biomimetic system. Source: Redrawn from Tokarz et al. (2008).

debromination of *meta*- and *para*-bromines of BDE-209 to octabromodiphenyl ether congeners in anaerobic mesophilic digester sludge, which occurred over a 238-day incubation period. The product congeners were two nonabromodiphenyl ethers (BDE-207 and BDE-208) with the absence of ortho debromination to BDE-206, and six octabromodiphenyl ethers. Tokarz et al. (2008) studied reductive debromination of PBDEs in anaerobic sediment microcosms and, in parallel, in a solvent-enhanced biomimetic system. BDE-209 debrominated in sediment and biomimetic system with a corresponding increase in nona-, octa-, hepta-, and hexa-PDBEs. Reductive debromination of BDE-209 could potentially produce BDE-99 and BDE-47. A synthesis of the BDE-209 debromination sequence constructed from the combined results of both sediment microcosms and biomimetic system with BDE-209 as well as BDE-99 and BDE-47 is shown in Figure 9.41. Product congeners identified were predominantly double para-substituted (Tokarz et al., 2008).

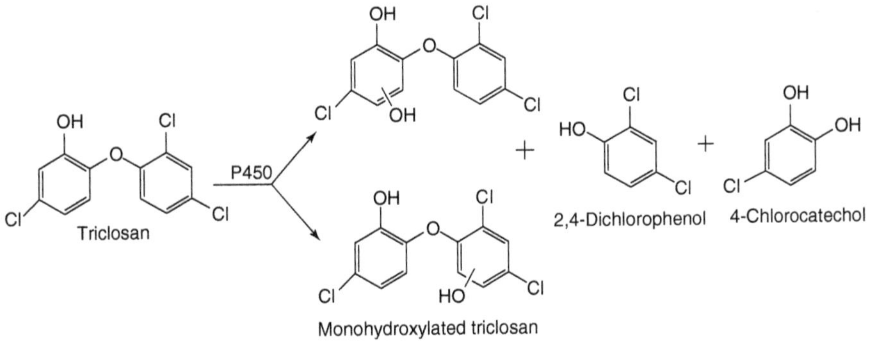

Figure 9.42   Schematic of triclosan metabolism in Wistar rats (Tulp et al., 1979).

9.10   TRICLOSAN

PCDEs are structurally and by physical properties similar to PCBs. In metabolic studies, ortho hydroxylation of the PCDEs has been found to be the dominant oxidative pathway. Triclosan, also known as Irgasan DP 300 or Irgacare MP in Europe, formed several hydroxylated metabolites as well as 2,4-dichlorophenol and 4-chlorocatechol by rats (Tulp et al., 1979). In the rat, chlorodiphenyl ethers are metabolized predominantly via aromatic hydroxylation at ortho and meta positions to the ether bond. Triclosan is hydroxylated to five different monohydroxy metabolites, which were found in urine; three of these were also present in feces. Because of the scission of the ether bond, a minor metabolic process, 2,4-dichlorophenol occurred in urine and feces, and 4-chlorocatechol in urine (Fig. 9.42) (Tulp et al., 1979; Fang et al., 2010).

Biodegradation experiments with *Sphingomonas* sp. PH-07 revealed that it was able to catabolize triclosan to intermediates which included hydroxylated compounds, monohydroxy-triclosan and dihydroxy-triclosan, and other bond cleavage products, 4-chlorophenol and 2,4-dichlotrophenol, indicating that the initial dihydroxylation occurred on both aromatic rings of triclosan (Kim et al., 2011). A microbial transformation of triclosan in fish from various lakes in Switzerland with inputs from WWTPs is reported to produce the more bioaccumulative methyltriclosan (Balmer et al., 2004).

9.11   CONCLUSIONS AND FUTURE PROSPECTS

Biotransformations of various EDCs taking place during mammalian metabolism and in microbial degradation and metabolic pathways have been compiled to appreciate the natural processes of biodegradation. Efforts to elucidate pathways for biodegradation of anthropogenic compounds began with enrichment and characterization of microbes capable of degrading pollutants from contaminated sites. In some cases, strains capable of mineralizing a pollutant could be isolated, but in other cases, degradation – often only partial – required finicky consortia. Optimization was often limited to efforts to enhance the growth of contaminant-degrading microbes. However, treatments involving biological action have several problems. The activity of the microorganisms is temperature dependent and is subject to inhibition by highly toxic pollutants.

A confluence of new technologies now offers entirely new ways of approaching the challenges of bioremediation. The fitness of microbes that express degradative enzymes can be enhanced by unbiased approaches to generate strains that have improved resistance to the toxicity of pollutants and their metabolites and the ability to survive in challenging environments. These approaches should enable the development of strains that efficiently degrade recalcitrant anthropogenic compounds in diverse contaminated environments and to thereby provide environmentally benign and relatively low-cost methods for the cleanup of contaminated sites (Copley, 2009).

Several recent studies have indicated that most pharmaceutical biotransformation products (BPs) formed under aerobic conditions have a slightly modified molecular structure featuring increased polarity, because of the introduction of hydroxyl, carboxyl, or keto moieties. On the basis of the similarity of the molecular structure to the parent compound, a significant number of BPs are expected to possess comparable biological activity as their chemical precursors. Therefore, biotransformation of compounds into metabolites that can be more or less active than the parent clearly needs to be considered in their safety evaluation. Also, the enhanced polarity improves the permeability of these compounds for several water treatment processes, such as adsorptive filtration (e.g., activated carbon), underground soil passage, or bank filtration. As a consequence, the likelihood increases that BPs are contaminating groundwater and drinking water.

REFERENCES

Abramowicz, D. A. Aerobic and anaerobic biodegradation of PCBs: a review, *Crit. Rev. Biotechnol.* **1990**, 10, 241–251.

Adams, N. H.; Levi, P.; Hodgson, E. In vitro studies of the metabolism of atrazine, simazine and terbutryn in several vertebrate species. *J. Agric. Food Chem.* **1990**, 38, 1411–1417.

Anfossi, P.; Roncada, P.; Stracciari, G. L.; Montana, M.; Pasqualucci, C.; Montesissa, C. Toxicokinetics and metabolism of linuron in rabbit: *in vivo* and *in vitro* studies, *Xenobiotica* **1993**, 23(10), 1113–1123.

Badawi, N.; Ronhede, S.; Olsson, S.; Kragelund, B. B.; Johnsen, A. H.; Jacobsen, O. S.; Aamand, J. Metabolites of the phenylurea herbicides chlorotoluron, diuron, isoproturon and linuron produced by the soil fungus *Mortierella* sp., *Environ. Pollut.* **2009**, 157(10), 2806–2812.

Baker, M. E.; Chandsawangbhuwana, C. 3D models of MBP, a biologically active metabolite of bisphenol A, in human estrogen receptor α and estrogen receptor β, *PLoS ONE* **2012**, 7(10), e46078. doi:10.1371/journal.pone.0046078

Ballou, D.; Batie, C. Phthalate oxygenase, a Rieske iron-sulfur protein from *Pseudomonas cepacia*, *Prog. Clin. Biol. Res.* **1988**, 274, 211–226.

Balmer, M. E.; Poiger, T.; Droz, C.; Romanin, K.; Bergqvist, P. A.; Muller, M. D.; Buser, H. R. Occurrence of methyl triclosan, a transformation product of the bactericide triclosan, in fish from various lakes in Switzerland, *Environ. Sci. Technol.* **2004**, 38, 390–395.

Barr, W. J. *Predicting biological degradation and toxicity of steroidal estrogens*, MS Dissertation (Civil Eng.), Univ. Pittsburgh, 2011. Available at: http://d-scholar ship.pitt.edu/10546/1/ BarrWJFall2011.pdf (accessed 02 Feb 2012).

Bedard, D. L.; Ritalahti, K. M.; Löffler, F. E. The *Dehalococcoides* population in sediment-free mixed cultures metabolically dechlorinates the commercial polychlorinated biphenyl mixture Aroclor 1260, *Appl. Environ. Microbiol.* **2007**, 73(8), 2513–2521.

Bers, K.; Leroy, B.; Breugelmans, P.; Albers, P.; Lavigne, R.; Sørensen, S. R.; Aamand, J.; De Mot, R.; Wattiez, R.; Springael, D. A novel linuron hydrolase identified by genomic-proteomic analysis of phenylurea herbicide mineralization by *Variovorax* sp. strain SRS16, *Appl. Environ. Microbiol.* **2011**, 77(24), 8754–8764.

Bursztyka, J.; Debrauwer, L.; Perdu, E.; Houanin, I.; Jaeg, J.-P.; Cravedi, J.-P. Biotransformation of vinclozolin in rat precision-cut liver slices: Comparison with *in vivo* metabolic pattern, *J. Agric. Food Chem.* **2008**, 56, 4832–4839.

Cabana, H.; Jones, J. P.; Agathos, S. N. Elimination of endocrine disrupting chemicals using white rot fungi and their lignin modifying enzymes: a review, *Eng. Life Sci.* **2007**, 7(5), 429–456.

Chatterjee, S.; Dutta, T. K. Complete degradation of butyl benzyl phthalate by a defined bacterial consortium: role of individual isolates in the assimilation pathway, *Chemosphere* **2008**, 70(5), 933–941.

Chatterjee, S.; Karlovsky, P. Removal of the endocrine disruptor butyl benzyl phthalate from the environment, *Appl. Microbiol. Biotechnol.* **2010**, 87(1), 61–73.

Coombe, R. G.; Tsong, Y. Y.; Hamilton, P. B.; Sih, C. J. Mechanisms of steroid oxidation by microorganisms: oxidative cleavage of estrone, *J. Biol. Chem.* **1966**, 241, 1587-1595.

Copley, S. D. Evolution of efficient pathways for degradation of anthropogenic chemicals, *Nature Chem. Biol.* **2009**, 5, 559–566.

Corvini, P. F. X.; Schäffer, A.; Schlosser, D. The degradation of α-quaternary nonylphenol isomers by *Sphingomonas* sp. strain TTNP3 involves a type II *ipso*-substitution mechanism, *Appl. Microbiol. Biotechnol.* **2006a**, 72, 223–243.

Corvini, P. F. X.; Schäffer, A.; Schlosser, D. Microbial degradation of nonylphenol and other alkylphenols—our evolving view, *Appl. Microbiol. Biotechnol.* **2006b**, 72(2), 223–243.

Dehal, S. S.; Kupfer, D. Metabolism of the proestrogenic pesticide methoxychlor by hepatic P450 monooxygenases in rats and humans. Dual pathways involving novel ortho ring-hydroxylation by CYP2B, *Drug Metab. Dispos.* **1994**, 22, 937–946.

Della Greca, M.; Pinto, G.; Pistillo, P.; Pollio, A.; Previtera, L.; Temussi, F. Biotransformation of ethinylestradiol by microalgae, *Chemosphere* **2008**, 70(11), 2047–2053.

Eaton, R. W. Plasmid-encoded phthalate catabolic pathway in *Arthrobacter keyseri* 12B, *J. Bacteriol.* **2001**, 183(12), 3689–3703.

Eaton, R. W.; Ribbons, D. W. Metabolism of dibutylphthalate and phthalate by *Micrococcus* sp strain 12b, *J. Bacteriol.* **1982**, 151, 48–57.

Erratico, C. A.; Moffatt, S. C.; Bandiera, S. M. Comparative oxidative metabolism of BDE-47 and BDE-99 by rat hepatic microsomes, *Toxicol. Sci.* **2011**, 123(1), 37–47.

Fang, J. L.; Stingley, R. L.; Beland, F. A.; Harrouk, W.; Lumpkins, D. L.; Howard, P. Occurrence, efficacy, metabolism, and toxicity of triclosan, *J. Environ. Sci. Health C Environ. Carcinog. Ecotoxicol. Rev.* **2010**, 28(3), 147–171.

Field, J. A.; Sierra-Alvarez, R. Microbial transformation and degradation of polychlorinated biphenyls, *Environ. Pollut.* **2008**, 155 (1), 1–12.

Furukawa, K.; Fujihara, H. Microbial degradation of polychlorinated biphenyls: biochemical and molecular features, *J. Biosci. Bioeng.* **2008**, 105, 433–449.

Gabriel, F. L.; Cyris, M.; Giger, W.; Kohler, H. P. Ipso-substitution: a general biochemical and biodegradation mechanism to cleave alpha-quaternary alkylphenols and bisphenol A, *Chem. Biodivers.*, **2007**, 4(9), 2123–2137.

Gabriel, F. L. P.; Routledge, E. J.; Heidlberger, A.; Rentsch, D.; Guenther, K.; Giger, W.; Sumpter, J. P.; Kohler, H. P. E. Isomer-specific degradation and endocrine disrupting activity of nonylphenols, *Environ. Sci. Technol.* **2008**, 42, 6399–6408.

Gabriel, F. L. P.; Mora, M. A.; Kolvenbach, B. A.; Corvini, P. F. X.; Kohler, H. P. E. Formation of toxic 2-nonyl-*p*-benzoquinones from α-tertiary 4-nonylphenol isomers during microbial metabolism of technical nonylphenol, *Environ. Sci. Technol.* **2012**, 46, 5979–5987.

Gaido, K. W.; Maness, S. C.; McDonnell, D. P.; Dehal, S. S.; Kupfer, D.; and Safe, S. Interaction of methoxychlor and related compounds with estrogen receptor alpha and beta, and androgen receptor: structure-activity studies, *Mol. Pharmacol.* **2000**, 58, 852–858.

Gerecke, A. C.; Hartmann, P. C.; Heeb, N. V.; Kohler, H. P. E.; Giger, W.; Schmid, P.; Zennegg, M.; Kohler, M., Anaerobic degradation of decabromodiphenyl ether, *Environ. Sci. Technol.* **2005**, 39(4), 1078–1083.

Gray, L. E.; Wolf, C., Jr.; Lambright, C.; Mann, P.; Price, M.; Cooper, R. L.; Ostby, J. Administration of potentially antiandrogenic pesticides (procymidone, linuron, iprodione, chlozolinate, p,p'-DDE, and ketoconazole) and toxic substances (dibutyl- and diethylhexyl phthalate, PCB 169, and ethane dimethane sulphonate) during sexual differentiation produces diverse profiles of reproductive malformations in the male rat, *Toxicol. Ind. Health* **1999**, 15(1–2), 94–118.

Haiyan, R.; Shulan, J.; Dao, W.; Ahmad, N. Degradation characteristics and metabolic pathway of 17α-ethynylestradiol by Sphingobacterium sp. JCR5, *Chemosphere* **2007**, 66(2), 340–346.

Hamers, T.; Kamstra, J. H.; Sonneveld, E.; Murk, A. J.; Visser, T. J.; Van Velzen, M. J.; Brouwer, A.; Bergman, A. Biotransformation of brominated flame retardants into potentially endocrine-disrupting metabolites, with special attention to 2,2′,4,4′-tetrabromodiphenyl ether (BDE-47), *Mol. Nutr. Food Res.* **2008**, 52(2), 284–298.

Hara, H.; Stewart, G. R.; Mohn, W. W. Involvement of a novel ABC transporter and monoalkyl phthalate ester hydrolase in phthalate ester catabolism by Rhodococcus jostii RHA1, *Appl. Environ. Microbiol.* **2010**, 76(5), 1516–1523.

Harris, C. A.; Henttu, P.; Park, M. G.; Sumpter, J. P. The estrogenic activity of phthalate esters *in vitro*, *Environ. Health Perspect.* **1997**, 105, 802–811.

Hirano, T.; Honda, Y.; Watanabe, T.; Kuwahara, M. Degradation of bisphenol A by the lignin-degrading enzyme, manganese peroxidase, produced by the white-rot basidiomycete, *Biosci. Biotechnol. Biochem.* **2000**, 64, 1958–1962.

Huang, Q.; Weber, W. J., Jr, Transformation and removal of bisphenol A from aqueous phase via peroxidase-mediated oxidative coupling reactions: efficacy, products, and pathways, *Environ. Sci. Technol.*, **2005**, 39 (16), 6029–6036.

Ike, M.; Chen, M. Y.; Jin, C. S.; Gujita, M. Acute toxicity, mutagenicity and estrogenicity of biodegradation products of bisphenol A, *Environ. Toxicol.* **2002**, 17(5), 457–461.

Isidori, M.; Lavorgna, M.; Nardelli, A.; Parrella, A. Toxicity on crustaceans and endocrine disrupting activity on Saccharomyces cerevisiae of eight alkylphenols, *Chemosphere* **2006**, 64(1), 135–143.

Jobling, S.; Reynolds, T.; White, R.; Parker, M. G.; Sumpter, J. P. A variety of environmentally persistent chemicals including some phthalate plasticizers are weakly estrogenic, *Environ. Health Perspect.* **1995**, 103, 582–587.

Joo, H.; Choi, K.; Hodgson, E. Human metabolism of atrazine, *Pest. Biochem. Physiol.* **2010**, 98, 73–79.

Junghanns, C.; Moeder, M.; Krauss, G.; Martin, C.; Schlosser, D. Degradation of xenoestrogen nonylphenol by aquatic fungi and their laccases, *Microbiology*, **2005**, 151, 45–57.

Kagle, J.; Porter, A. W.; Murdoch, R. W.; Rivera-Cancel, G.; Hay, A. G. Biodegradation of pharmaceutical and personal care products, *Adv. Appl. Microbiol.*, **2009**, 67, 65–108.

Keum, Y. S.; Lee, Y. H.; Kim, J.-H. Metabolism of methoxychlor by *Cunninghamella elegans* ATCC36112, *J. Agric. Food Chem.* **2009**, 57(17), 7931–7937.

Khunjar, W. O.; Mackintosh, S.; Skotnicka-Pitak, J.; Baik, S.; Aga, D. S.; Love, N. G. Elucidating the role of ammonia-oxidizing bacteria versus heterotrophic bacteria during the biotransformation of 17α-ethinylestradiol and trimethoprim, *Environ. Sci. Technol.* **2011**, 45 (8), 3605–3612.

Kim, Y. H.; Lee, J.; Ahn, J. Y.; Gu, M. B.; Moon, S. H. Enhanced degradation of an endocrine-disrupting chemical, butyl benzyl phthalate, by *Fusarium oxysporum* f. sp. *pisi* cutinase, *Appl. Environ. Microbiol.* **2002**, 68(9), 4684–4688.

Kim, S. J.; Kweon, O.; Jones, R. C.; Freeman, J. P.; Edmondson, R. D.; Cerniglia, C. E. Complete and integrated pyrene degradation pathway in *Mycobacterium vanbaalenii* PYR-1 based on systems biology, *J. Bacteriol.* **2007**, 189(2), 464–472.

Kim, Y. M.; Murugesan, K.; Schmidt, S.; Bokare, V.; Jeon, J. R.; Kim, E. J.; Chang, Y. S. Triclosan susceptibility and co-metabolism – a comparison for three aerobic pollutant-degrading bacteria, *Biores. Technol.* **2011**, 102(3), 2206–2212.

Koch, H. M.; Preuss, R.; Angerer, J. Di(2-ethylhexyl)phthalate (DEHP): Human metabolism and internal exposure – an update and latest results, *Int. J. Androl.* **2006**, 29, 155–165.

Kohler, H. E.; Gabriel, F. L. P.; Giger, W. ipso-substitution – a novel pathway for microbial metabolism of endocrine-disrupting 4-nonylphenols, 4-alkoxyphenols, and bisphenol A, *Chimia* **2008**, 62, 358–363.

Kolvenbach, B.; Schlaich, N.; Raoui, Z.; Prell, J.; Zuhlke, S.; Schaffer, A.; Guengerich, F. F.; Corvini, P. F. X. Degradation pathway of bisphenol A: Does *ipso* substitution apply to phenols containing α-carbon structure in the *para* position, *Appl. Environ. Microbiol.* **2007**, 73(15), 4776–4784.

Krupinski, M.; Szewczyk, R.; Długonski, J. Detoxification and elimination of xenoestrogen nonylphenol by the filamentous fungus Aspergillus versicolor, *Int. Biodeter. Biodegrad.* **2013**, 82, 59–66.

Kupfer, D.; Bulger, W. H.; Theoharides, A. D. Metabolism of methoxychlor by hepatic P-450 monooxygenases in rat and human. 1. Characterization of a novel catechol metabolite, *Chem. Res. Toxicol.* **1990**, 3(1), 8–16.

Kuramitz, H.; Natsui, J.; Sugawara, K.; Itoh, S.; Tanaka, S. Electrochemical evaluation of the interaction between endocrine disrupter chemicals and estrogen receptor using 17 β-estradiol labeled with daunomycin, *Anal. Chem.* **2002**, 74, 533–538.

Kurisu, F.; Ogura, M.; Saitoh, S.; Yamazoe, A.; Yagi, O. Degradation of natural estrogen and identification of the metabolites produced by soil isolates of Rhodococcus sp and Sphingomonas sp., *J. Biosci. Bioeng.* **2010**, 109(6), 576–582.

LeBlanc A.; Sleno, L. Atrazine metabolite screening in human microsomes: detection of novel reactive metabolites and glutathione adducts by LC-MS, *Chem. Res. Toxicol.* **2011**, 24, 329–339.

Lee, H. B.; Liu, D. Degradation of 17β-estradiol and its metabolites by sewage bacteria, *Water Air Soil Poll.* **2002**, 134, 353–368.

Lee, S. M.; Lee, J. W.; Koo, B. W.; Kim, M. K.; Choi, D. H.; Choi, I. G. Dibutyl phthalate biodegradation by the white rot fungus, *Polyporus brumalis, Biotechnol. Bioeng.* **2007**, 97, 1516–1522.

Liang, D. W.; Zhang, T.; Fang, H. H. P. Phthalates biodegradation in the environment, *Appl. Microbiol. Biotechnol.* **2008**, 80, 183–198.

Lloret, L.; Eibes, G.; Moreira, M. T.; Feijoo, G.; Lema, J. M. Removal of estrogenic compounds from filtered secondary wastewater effluent in a continuous enzymatic membrane reactor. Identification of biotransformation products, *Environ. Sci. Technol.* **2013**, doi:10.1021/es304783k

Mao, L.; Lu, J.; Habteselassie, M.; Luo, Q.; Gao, S.; Cabrera, M.; Huang, Q. Ligninase-mediated removal of natural and synthetic estrogens from water: II. Reactions of 17β-estradiol, *Environ. Sci. Technol.* **2010**, 44 (7), 2599–2604.

Masuda, M.; Yamasaki, Y.; Ueno, S.; Inoue, A. Isolation of bisphenol A-tolerant/degrading *Pseudomonas monteilii* strain N-502, *Extremophiles* **2007**, 11, 355–362.

Mikami, N.; Satogami, H.; Miyamoto, J. Metabolism of procymidone in rats, *J. Pestic. Sci.* **1979**, 4(2), 165–174.

Moore, R. W.; Rudy, T. A.; Lin, T. M.; Ko, K.; Peterson, R. E. Abnormalities of sexual development in male rats with in utero and lactational exposure to the antiandrogenic plasticizer di(2-ethylhexyl) phthalate, *Environ. Health Perspect.* **2001**, 109(3), 229–237.

Nakamura, S.; Tezuka, Y.; Ushiyama, A.; Kawashima, C.; Kitagawara, Y.; Takahashi, K.; Ohta, S.; Mashino, T. *Ipso* substitution of bisphenol A catalyzed by microsomal cytochrome P450 and enhancement of estrogenic activity, *Toxicol. Lett.* **2011**, 203(1), 92–95.

Nativelle, C.; Picard, K.; Valentin, I.; Lhuguenot, J. C.; Chagnon, M. C. Metabolism of N-butyl benzyl phthalate in the female Wistar rat. Identification of new metabolites, *Food Chem. Toxicol.* **1999**, 37, 905–917.

Needham, D.; Challis, I. R. The metabolism and excretion of prochloraz, an imidazole-based fungicide, in the rat, *Xenobiotica* **1991**, 21, 1473–1482.

Nicotra, S.; Intra, A.; Ottolina, G.; Riva, S.; Danieli, B. Laccase-mediated oxidation of the steroid hormone 17β-estradiol in organic solvents, *Tetrahedron: Asymmetry* **2004**, 15(18), 2927–2931.

Nomura, S.; Daidoji, T.; Inoue, H.; Yokota, H. Differential metabolism of 4-n- and 4-*tert*-octylphenols in perfused rat liver, *Life Sci.* **2008**, 83(5–6), 223–228.

Pieper, D. H.; Seeger, M. Bacterial metabolism of polychlorinated biphenyls, *J. Mol. Microbiol. Biotechnol.* **2008**, 15(2–3), 121–138.

Porter, A. W.; Hay, A. G. Identification of *opdA*, a gene involved in biodegradation of the endocrine disrupter octylphenol, *Appl. Environ. Microbiol.* **2007**, 73(22), 7373–7379.

Pothuluri, J. V.; Freeman, J. P.; Heinze, T. M.; Beger, R. D.; Cerniglia, C. E. Biotransformation of vinclozolin by the fungus *Cunninghamella elegans*, *J. Agric. Food Chem.* **2000**, 48(12), 6138–6148.

Qiu, X.; Mercado-Feliciano, M.; Bigsby, R. M.; Hites, R. A. Measurement of polybrominated diphenyl ethers and metabolites in mouse plasma after exposure to a commercial pentabromo diphenyl ether mixture, *Environ. Health Perspect.* **2007**, 115, 1052–1058.

Qiu, X.; Bigsby, R. M.; Hites, R. A. Hydroxylated metabolites of polybrominated diphenyl ethers in human blood Samples from the United States, *Environ. Health Perspect.* **2009**, 117(1), 93–98.

Quan, C. S.; Liu, Q.; Tian, W. J.; Kikuchi, J.; Fan. S. D. Biodegradation of an endocrine-disrupting chemical, di-2-ethylhexyl phthalate, by *Bacillus subtilis* no. 66, *Appl. Microbiol. Biotechnol.* **2005**, 66, 702–710.

Richardson, S. D.; Ternes, T. A. Water analysis: emerging contaminants and current issues, *Anal. Chem.* **2011**, 83, 4614–4648.

Rozalska, S.; Szewczyk, R.; Długonski, J. Biodegradation of 4-n-nonylphenol by the non-ligninolytic filamentous fungus *Gliocephalotrichum simplex*: a proposal of a metabolic pathway, *J. Hazard. Mat.* **2010**, 180(1–3), 323–331.

Russ, A. S.; Vinken, R.; Schuphan, I.; Schmidt, B. Synthesis of branched para-nonylphenol isomers: occurrence and quantification in two commercial mixtures, *Chemosphere* **2005**, 60, 1624–1635.

Sakai, K.; Yamanaka, H.; Moriyoshi, K.; Ohmoto, T.; Ohe, T. Biodegradation of bisphenol A and related compounds by *Sphingomonas* sp. strain BP-7 isolated from seawater, *Biosci. Biotechnol. Biochem.* **2007**, 71, 51–57.

Sakuyama, H.; Endo, Y.; Fujimoto, K.; Hatano, Y. Oxidative degradation of alkylphenols by Horseradish peroxidase, *J. Biosci. Bioeng.*, **2003**, 96(3), 227–231.

Sarkar, J.; Chowdhury, P. P.; Dutta, T. K. Complete degradation of di-*n*-octyl phthalate by *Gordonia* sp. strain Dop5, *Chemosphere* **2013**, 90, 2571–2577.

Sasaki, M.; Maki, J.; Oshiman, K.; Matsumura, Y.; Tsuchido, T. Biodegradation of bisphenol A by cells and cell lysate from Sphingomonas sp. strain AO1, *Biodegradation* **2005**, 16(5), 449–459.

Satsuma, K.; Masuda, M.; Sato, K. O-Demethylation and successive oxidative dechlorination of methoxychlor by *Bradyrhizobium* sp. Strain 17-4, isolated from river sediment, *Appl. Environ. Microbiol.* **2012**, 78(15), 5313–5319.

Shapir, N.; Mongodin, E. F.; Sadowsky, M. J.; Daugherty, S. C.; Nelson, K. E.; Wackett, L. P. Evolution of catabolic pathways: genomic insights into microbial s-triazine metabolism, *J. Bacteriol.* **2007**, 189, 674–682.

Shiba, K.; Kaneko, H.; Yoshino, H.; Kakuta, N.; Iba, K.; Nakatsuka, I.; Yoshitake, A.; Yamada, H.; Miyamoto, J. Comparative metabolism of procymidone in rats and mice, *J. Pestic. Sci.* **1991**, 16, 27–33.

Sietmann, R.; Gesell, M.; Hammer, E.; Schauer, F. Oxidative ring cleavage of low chlorinated biphenyl derivatives by fungi leads to the formation of chlorinated lactone derivatives, *Chemosphere* **2006**, 64, 672–685.

Silva, M. J.; Samandar, E.; Preau, J. L., Jr.; Needham, L. L.; Calafat, A. M. Urinary oxidative metabolites of di (2-ethylhexyl) phthalate in humans, *Toxicology.* **2006**, 219(1–3), 22–32.

Silva, M. J.; Samandar, E.; Reidy, J. A.; Hauser, R.; Needham, L. L.; Calafat, A. M. Metabolite profiles of di-n-butyl phthalate in humans and rats, *Environ. Sci. Technol.* **2007**, 41(21), 7576–7580.

Skotnicka-Pitak, J.; Khunjar, W. O.; Love, N. G.; Aga, D. S. Characterization of metabolites formed during the biotransformation of 17α-ethinylestradiol by *Nitrosomonas europaea* in batch and continuous flow bioreactors, *Environ. Sci. Technol.* **2009**, 43, 3549–3555.

de Souza, M. L.; Newcombe, D.; Alvey, S.; Crowley, D. E.; Hay, A.; Sadowsky, M. J.; Wackett, L. P. Molecular basis of a bacterial consortium: Interspecies catabolism of atrazine, *Appl. Environ. Microbiol.* **1998**, 64, 178–218.

Spivack, J., Leib, T. K.; Lobos, J. H. Novel pathway for bacterial metabolism of bisphenol A. Rearrangements and stilbene cleavage in bisphenol A metabolism, *J. Biol. Chem.* **1994**, 269,7323–7329.

Staples, C. A.; Peterson, D. R.; Parkerton, T. F.; Adams, W. J. The environmental fate of phthalate esters: a literature review, *Chemosphere* **1997**, 35, 667–749.

Stapleton, H. M.; Kelly, S. M.; Pei, R.; Letcher, R. J.; Gunsch, C. Metabolism of polybrominated diphenyl ethers (PBDEs) by human hepatocytes in vitro, *Environ. Health Perspect.* **2009**, 117 (2), 197–202.

Stolz, A. Molecular characteristics of xenobiotic-degrading sphingomonads, *Appl. Microbiol. Biotechnol.* **2009**, 81(5), 793–811.

Suzuki, T.; Nakagawa, Y.; Takano, I.; Yasuda, K. Environmental fate of bisphenol A and its biological metabolites in river water and their xeno-estrogenic activity, *Environ. Sci. Technol.* **2004**, 38, 2389–2396.

Tanaka, T.; Tamura, T.; Ishizaki, Y.; Kawasaki, A.; Kawase, T.; Teraguchi, M.; Taniguchi, M. Enzymatic treatment of estrogens and estrogen glucoronide, *J. Environ. Sci.* **2009**, 21(6), 731–735.

Tanghe, T.; Dhooge, W.; Verstraete, W. Formation of the metabolic intermediate 2,4,4-trimethyl-2-pentanol during incubation of a *Sphingomonas* sp. strain with the xeno-estrogenic octylphenol, *Biodegradation* **2000**, 11, 1–19.

Ternes, T. A.; Kreckel, P.; Mueller, J. Behavior and occurrence of estrogens in municipal sewage treatment plants. II. Aerobic batch experiments with activated sludge, *Sci. Total Environ.* **1999**, 225, 91–99.

Testa, B.; Soine, W. Principles of drug metabolism, in *Burger's Medicinal Chemistry and Drug Discovery*, Abraham, D. J., ed., 6th ed., Vol. 2, Hoboken, NJ: Wiley-Interscience, **2003**, pp. 431–498.

Tezuka, Y.; Takahashi, K.; Suzuki, T.; Kitamura, S.; Ohta, S.; Nakamura, S.; Mashin, T. Novel metabolic pathways of *p*-n-nonylphenol catalyzed by cytochrome P450 and estrogen receptor binding activity of new metabolites, *J. Health Sci.* **2007**, 53(5), 552–561.

Thibaut, R.; Jumel, A.; Debrauwer, L.; Rathahao, E.; Lagadic, L.; Cravedi, J.-P. Identification of 4-*n* nonylphenol metabolic pathways and residues in aquatic organisms by HPLC and LC-MS analyses, *Analusis* **2000**, 28(9), 793–801.

Tokarz, J. A., 3rd; Ahn, M. Y.; Leng, J.; Filley, T. R.; Nies, L. Reductive debromination of polybrominated diphenyl ethers in anaerobic sediment and a biomimetic system, *Environ. Sci. Technol.* **2008**, 42, 1157–1164.

Tulp, M. T.; Sundstrom, G.; Martron, L. B.; Hutzinger, O. Metabolism of chlorodiphenyl ethers and Irgasan DP 300, *Xenobiotica* **1979**, 9(2), 65–77.

Uchida, H.; Fukuda, T.; Miyamoto, H.; Kawabata, T.; Suzuli, M.; Uwajima, T. Polymerization of bisphenol A by purified laccase from *Trametes villosa, Biochem. Biophys. Res. Commun.* **2001**, 287, 355–358.

Vallini, G.; Grassinetti, S.; Andrea, F. D.; Catelani, G; Agnolucci, M. Biodegradation of 4-(1-nonyl)phenol by axenic cultures of the yeast Candida aquaetextoris: identification of microbial breakdown products and proposal of a possible metabolic pathway, *Int. Biodeterior. Biodegrad.* **2001**, 47, 133–140.

Van Zelm, R.; Huijbregts, M. A. J.; Van De Meent, D., Transformation products in the life cycle impact assessment of chemicals, *Environ. Sci. Technol.* **2010**, 44, 1004–1009.

Wagner, M.; Nicell, J. A. Evaluation of horseradish peroxidase for the treatment of estrogenic alkylphenols, *Water Quality Res. J. Can.*, **2005**, 40(2), 145–154.

Wu, X.; Liang, R.; Dai, Q.; Jin, D.; Wang, Y.; Chao, W. Complete degradation of di-n-octyl phthalate by biochemical cooperation between *Gordonia* sp. strain JDC-2 and *Arthrobacter* sp. strain JDC-32 isolated from activated sludge, *J. Hazard. Mat.* **2010**, 176(1–3), 262–268.

Xu, X. R.; Li, H. B.; Gu, J. D. Elucidation of n-butyl benzyl phthalate biodegradation using high performance liquid chromatography and gas chromatography–mass spectrometry, *Anal. Bioanal. Chem.* **2006**, 386, 370–375.

Ye, X.; Bishop, A. M.; Needham, L. L.; Calafat, A. M. Identification of metabolites of 4-nonylphenol isomer 4-(3', 6'-dimethyl-3'-heptyl) phenol by rat and human liver microsomes, *Drug. Metabol. Dispos.* **2007**, 35(8), 1269–1274.

Yi, T.; Harper, W. F., Jr., The link between nitrification and biotransformation of 17α-ethinylestradiol, *Environ. Sci. Technol.* **2007**, 41, 4311–4316.

Yoshihara, S.; Mizutare, T.; Makishima, M.; Suzuki, N.; Fujimoto, N.; Igarashi, K.; Ohta, S. Potent estrogenic metabolites of bisphenol A and bisphenol B formed by rat liver S9 fraction: their structures and estrogenic potency, *Toxicol. Sci.* **2004**, 78(1), 50–59.

Yoshimoto, T.; Nagai, F.; Fujimoto, J.; Watanabe, K.; Mizukoshi, H.; Makino, T.; Kimura, K.; Saino, H.; Sawada, H.; Omura, H. Degradation of estrogens by *Rhodococcus zopfii* and *Rhodococcus equi* isolates from activated sludge in wastewater treatment plants, *Appl. Environ. Microbiol.* **2004**, 70, 5283-5289.

Zalco, D.; Costagliola, R.; Dorio, C.; Rathahao, E.; Cravedi, J. P. In vivo metabolic fate of the xeno-estrogen 4-*n*-nonylphenol in Wistar rats, *Drug Metabol. Dispos.* **2003**, 31(2), 168–178.

Zhang, C.; Zeng, G.; Yuan, L.; Yu, J.; Li, J.; Huang, G.; Xi, B.; Liu, H. Aerobic degradation of bisphenol A by *Achromobacter xylosoxidans* strain B-16 isolated from compost leachate of municipal solid waste, *Chemosphere* **2007**, 68, 181–190.

10

ABIOTIC DEGRADATIONS/ TRANSFORMATIONS OF EDCs THROUGH OXIDATION PROCESSES

10.1 INTRODUCTION

Endocrine disrupting chemicals (EDCs) are ubiquitous in the environment, especially in aquatic ecosystems. Therefore, these contaminants are emerging as a major concern for water quality, as multiple EDCs have been detected in wastewater effluents and surface waters. Studies have shown that many EDCs are not completely degraded or removed with conventional wastewater treatment plant (WWTP) processes, allowing the micro contaminants to enter the environment via treated wastewater effluents. Most water and wastewater treatments plants currently in operation have not been specifically designed to remove exotic bioactive xenobiotics (Daughton, 2007). There are no federal or state standards for such contaminants – so these compounds are becoming more and more prevalent, especially in surface waters. Surface water is widely used as water resource for drinking water. Therefore, the widespread occurrence of EDCs in surface waters may pose a problem to water utilities.

The U.S. Geological survey (USGS) reported that some of most prevalent organic wastewater contaminants in impacted US streams were detergent metabolites, plasticizers, and pharmaceuticals including potent synthetic hormones (Kolpin et al., 2002). In the samples of rivers surveyed, the contaminants present were nonylphenol (NP) (in 50%), bisphenol A (BPA) (in 41%), 17α-ethinyl estradiol (EE2, in 16%), and 17β-estradiol (E2, in 11%) (Kolpin et al., 2002). BPA is released into the aquatic environment from industrial discharges, landfill leachate, and water streams containing plastic debris. Alkyphenols, such as NP, enters the environment through wastewater streams with nonylphenol polyethoxylates

Endocrine Disruptors in the Environment, First Edition. Sushil K. Khetan.
© 2014 John Wiley & Sons, Inc. Published 2014 by John Wiley & Sons, Inc.

(NPEOs), the nonionic surfactants. Raw textile mill effluents have very high levels of NP and NPEOs (Neamtu and Frimmel, 2006a). Under anaerobic conditions, such as those found in sewers, and biotreatment operations at WWTPs, NPEO is oxidized to NP. Phthalates are easily transported to the environment during manufacture, disposal, and leaching from plastic materials, in which they are bonded noncovalently to allow the required degree of flexibility.

The growing environmental problem requires the development of processes capable of efficiently eliminating these EDCs and the associated hormonal disruptions. Conventional treatment techniques, including coagulation, precipitation, and activated sludge processes, may not be highly effective in removing EDCs, while the advanced treatment options, such as granular activated carbon (GAC), membrane, as well as chemical and advanced oxidation processes (AOPs), have shown satisfactory results. Chemical oxidation has been widely applied for disinfection of drinking water and wastewaters and for the elimination of undesired micropollutants from drinking water. Ozone, chlorine, and chlorine dioxide are the currently widely used oxidants in water treatment. Photolysis by UV irradiation also is a common practice in disinfecting drinking water. AOPs, including photochemical and nonphotochemical processes such as UV, ozonation, Fenton's reagent, and combinations thereof, are the processes involving *in situ* generation of highly reactive hydroxyl radicals with an oxidation potential of 2.8 V, which nonselectively attack a large group of organic chemicals.

Electron density effects of functional groups and the degree of protonation affect the potential reactivity of organic compounds with oxidants. Electron-donating (e.g., hydroxyl, amine) or electron-withdrawing (e.g., carboxyl) functional groups lead to increasing and decreasing reactivity, respectively, for substituted aromatic rings. For example, free chlorine reacts rapidly with phenolic compounds, mainly through the reaction between HOCl and the deprotonated phenolate anion. This results in sequential chlorine addition to the aromatic ring, followed by ring cleavage. The reactivity of the phenolic functional group likely explains the rapid transformation during chlorination of some estrogenic hormones (estradiol, ethynylestradiol, estriol, estrone), which contain phenolic moieties (Westerhoff et al., 2005).

Although HOCl is assumed to be the active oxidant when chlorine is used in aqueous environment, evidence has shown that a little-known chlorine monoxide (Cl_2O) species is the predominant chlorinating agent during the chlorination of the herbicide dimethenamid (Sivey et al., 2010). It is quite likely that it could have been the active reactant species in other reactions but has not been considered (Richardson and Ternes, 2011).

Ozone (O_3) is a powerful oxidant and can oxidize pollutants either directly or by generating ˙OH radicals which then react with other species. These two pathways compete for the substrates to be oxidized. Molecular O_3 and ˙OH radical have high oxidation potentials, 2.07 and 2.80 V, respectively. Lower pH (pH < 4) favors the oxidation via molecular ozone which is more selective and reacts with specific groups. The production of hydroxyl radicals mainly occurs at high pH, which is considered an AOP. Thus, the radical oxidation pathway dominates under alkaline conditions, while direct oxidation with molecular ozone predominates under acidic ones.

Photocatalysis and photolytic degradation of EDCs in an aqueous matrix were also investigated, although the former is more effective than UV light alone. The heterogeneous photocatalytic process photo-excites a semiconductor catalyst, such as TiO_2, in contact with water. Many AOPs use H_2O_2, the oxidizing strength of which is relatively weak. However, UV irradiation combined with H_2O_2 increases the rate and potency of oxidation through the generation of ˙OH radicals and has been effective in degrading several EDCs in water (Rosenfeldt and Linden, 2004; Chen et al., 2006). The synergistic use of ozone with H_2O_2 or in association with UV irradiation, such as UV/H_2O_2 and O_3/H_2O_2, is justified to reduce the selectivity of action in the hope of amplifying the destruction of trace organics. At sufficient contact time and proper operating conditions, it leads to the total degradation and mineralization of target pollutants. Gultekin and Ince (2007) have comprehensively reviewed the degradation of BPA, alkylphenols, and phthalates by direct and indirect photolysis by UV and photocatalysis with TiO_2.

Many of the AOP-driven degradation of EDCs in oxygenated solutions are focused mainly on the degradation kinetics, but have not dealt with degradation pathway or identified the oxidation by-products or end products. Here, we focus on the degradation reactions of EDCs, where degradation products are well identified and/or the mechanism of degradation is delineated.

10.2 NATURAL AND SYNTHETIC ESTROGENS

10.2.1 17β-Estradiol (E2) and Estrone (E1)

Natural estrogens of 17β-estradiol (E2) and estrone (E1) are basic female sex hormones and are well known to exhibit estrogenic activities potently, even at very low concentrations (in the ng/l range). They are reported to be important EDCs in the aquatic environment, and may be associated with increased incidences of hermaphrodite carp and trout in British rivers that receive significant inputs of domestic effluents. These EDCs have been detected at low levels in wastewaters and surface waters in both the United States and European countries and must be treated before entering the public drinking water supply.

10.2.1.1 Chlorination with HOCl Treatment of E2 with sodium hypochlorite results in three chlorine-substituted E2 and E1 products, namely 2,4-dichloro-E2, monochloro-E1, 2,4-dichloro-E1, and four by-products such as 4-[2-(2,6-dichloro-3-hydroxyphenyl)ethyl]-7α-methyloctahydroinden-5-one (molecular weight 356) which were identified in chlorinated E2 solution (Fig. 10.1) (Hu et al., 2003).

The estrogenic activity of the aqueous chlorinated solution of E2, as assessed by yeast two-hybrid assay, was found similar to or slightly lower than before chlorination up to 60 min of contact time. The activity was found to be reduced to 40% of that before chlorination after 120–180 min contact time (Hu et al., 2003).

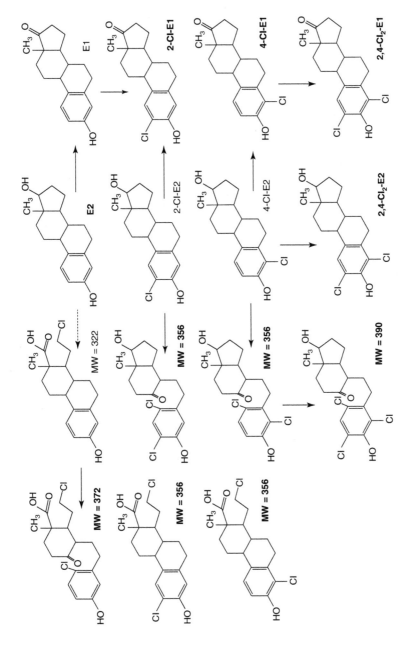

Figure 10.1 Aqueous chlorination pathway of 17β-estradiol (E2) with HOCl. Boldface captioned compounds were detected in the experiment (Hu et al., 2003).

10.2.1.2 Oxidation with KMnO₄ Oxidation of E2 by potassium permanganate in water led to 10 oxidation products detected by liquid chromatography-tandem mass spectrometry (LC-MS/MS) (Jiang et al., 2012). The proposed structures (Fig 10.2) reveal that Mn^{VII} initially attacks the hydroxyl group in the aromatic ring, leading to the formation of a series of quinone-like and aromatic-ring-opening products, while the alcohol and group at position C17 remain intact.

10.2.1.3 Ozonation Ozone oxidized steroids (estradiol, or estrone) containing phenolic moieties more efficiently. The oxidation products formed during the ozonation of the natural hormones E2 and E1 were identified as the same two major products 1 and 2 (Fig. 10.3) (Huber et al., 2004). Product 2 is a decomposition product of the cyclohexadione intermediate.

Treatment of E2 and E1 in water with ozone was further investigated, and the products formed identified with ultra-performance (UP) LC-MS/MS with a triple-quadrupole and a quadrupole time-of-flight instrument (Pereira et al., 2011). Two similar products were formed with both E2 and E1. In the case of E2, the product 1 with molecular ion (m/z of 288) was identified as 10ε-17β-dihydroxy-1,4-estradieno-3-one (Fig. 10.4), also identified in the photocatalytic reactions of E2 (Ohko et al., 2002; Mai et al., 2008; Zhao et al., 2008). Product 2 with m/z of 278 was proposed on the basis of the ozonolysis of the phenolic moiety (Fig. 10.4). The

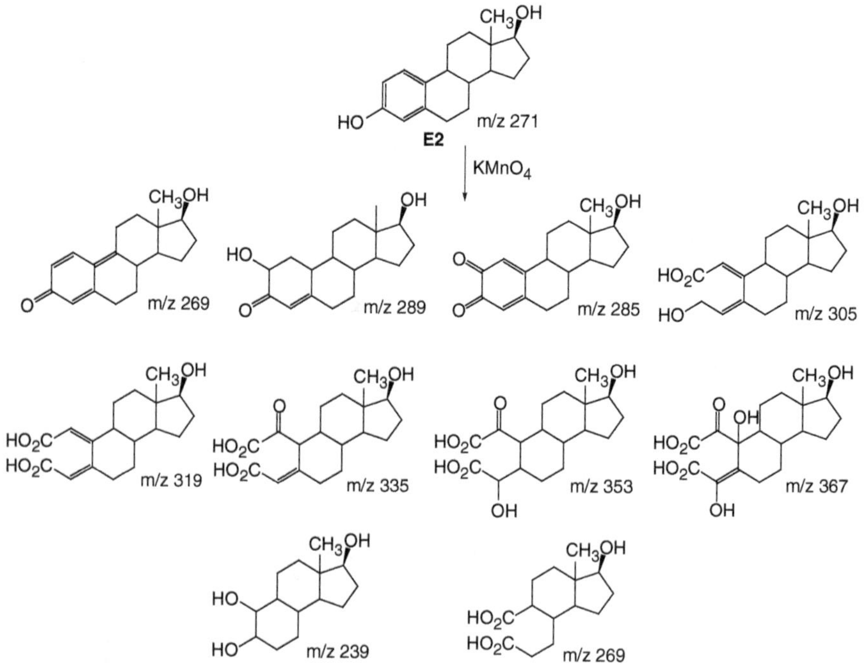

Figure 10.2 Structures of oxidation products formed by the reaction of E2 with KMnO₄. Source: Redrawn from Jiang et al. (2012).

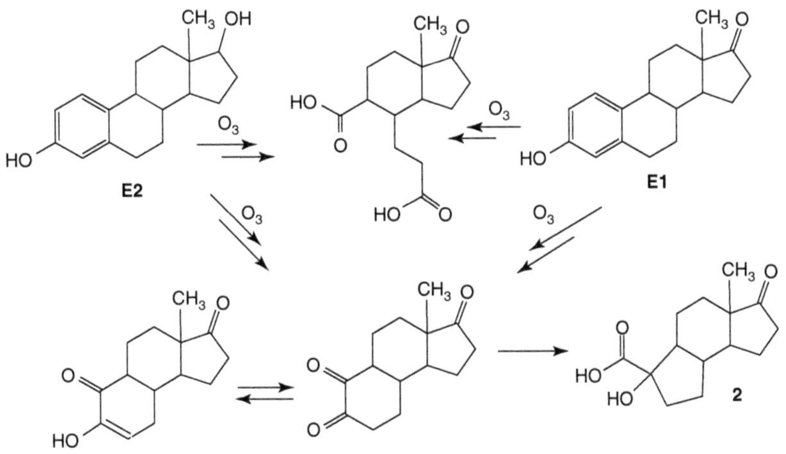

Figure 10.3 Oxidation products formed by the reaction of O_3 with E2 and E1 (Huber et al., 2004).

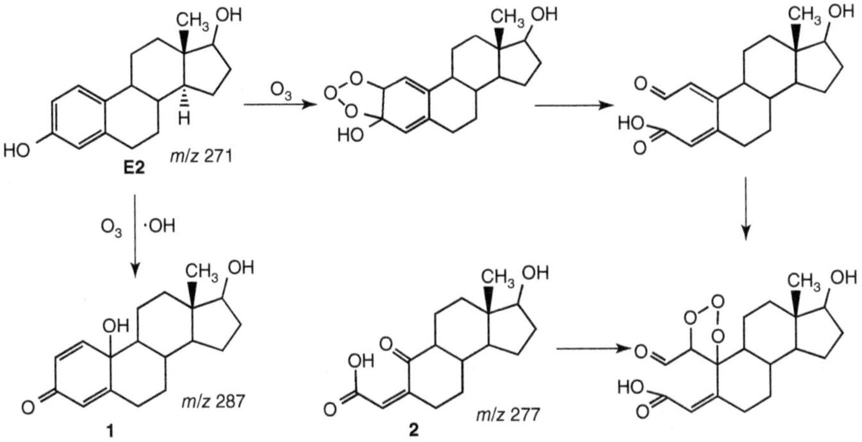

Figure 10.4 Ozonation of E2 in water (Pereira et al., 2011).

corresponding two products of ozone treatment of E1 were found with 2 mass units less (Pereira et al., 2011).

It was observed that estrogenic activity remained in the disinfected waters containing E2 after water ozonation, probably because of the newly formed oxidation by-products (Alum et al., 2004; Kim et al., 2004; Bila et al., 2007; Maniero et al., 2008) even at doses of 10 mg/l (Bila et al., 2007).

10.2.1.4 Photocatalytic degradation A photocatalysis of E2 in TiO_2 suspension under UV irradiation resulted in a gradual increase of CO_2 until it reached a constant value when E2 totally degraded in 3 h (Ohko et al., 2002; Mai et al., 2008). The degradation pathway mainly involved the OH radical attack producing 2-hydroxyestradiol (**1**), and subsequent ring opening leading to dicarboxylic acids. Another pathway involved the rearrangement of phenol moiety and reaction with OH and OOH radicals forming 10ε-17β-dihydroxy-1,4-estradien-3-one (**2**) and 10ε-hydroperoxide-17β-hydroxy-1,4-estradien-3-one (**3**), respectively (Fig. 10.5). The intermediates produced during the photocatalytic reaction did not exhibit any potent estrogenic activity in the treated water.

The reaction of E2 in the presence of a photo-Fenton catalyst α-FeOOH/H_2O_2 and UV led to several identifiable intermediates and, eventually, total degradation. The YES bioassay revealed removal of estrogenicity originating from E2, its degradation products. The products identified with the help of LC-MS/MS and gas chromatography–mass spectrometry (GC-MS) are shown in Figure 10.6 (Zhao et al., 2008).

10.2.2   17α-Ethinylestradiol (EE2)

10.2.2.1   Chlorination   Primary products of aqueous chlorination of EE2 were identified as 2-Cl-EE2 with about 20% yield and 4-Cl-EE2 with 80% yield. Further chlorination of these two products resulted in the formation of 2,4-Cl2-EE2 as a secondary intermediate (Fig. 10.7) (Lee et al., 2008). The monochloro-EE2s still exhibited approximately 13% relative potency (RP) of EE2 as calculated from estrogenic activity by *in vitro* yeast estrogen (YES) assay. 4-Chloro-EE2 showed similar estrogen receptor binding activity as the parent compound, whereas 2,4-dichloro-EE2 was about 10 times less potent than EE2 (Moriyama et al., 2004). Further rapid chlorination of monochloro-EE2s efficiently removed estrogenic activity (Lee et al., 2008).

10.2.2.2   Oxidation with Ozone   Ozone attacks the phenolic moiety of EE2 in the primary step. On the basis of studies on the ozonation of two model compounds bearing the characteristic functional groups, namely, the phenol and acetylene moiety attached to a cyclohexane ring, and of the experimental results, the initial oxidation products were proposed as 2-OH EE2 (**1**), 4-OH EE2 (**2**), 2,3-quinone EE2 (**3**), 3,4-quinone EE2 (**6**), and muconic-EE2 (**4**) (Fig. 10.8) (Huber et al., 2004), resulting in greater than 87% reduction in estrogenic activity as measured by a yeast *in vitro* assay (Lee et al., 2008). The reduced estrogenicity is attributed to the cleavage of the phenolic moiety of EE2 because the 3-hydroxy group and the aromatic ring of the phenolic moiety are of particular importance for the binding of estrogens to the estrogen receptor (Larcher et al., 2012; Lee et al., 2008).

10.3   BISPHENOL A

BPA is ubiquitous in the aquatic environment. Several chemical degradation processes including advanced oxidation processes for the removal of aqueous BPA reported in the literature are reviewed here.

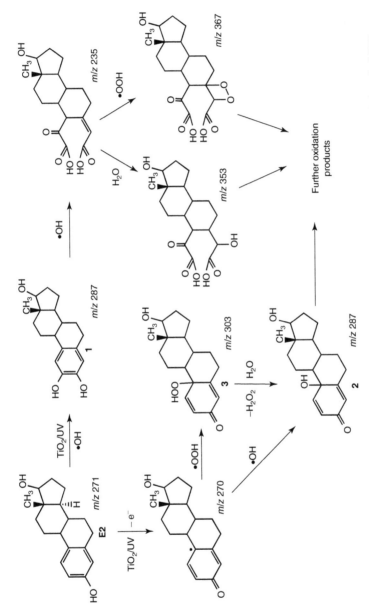

Figure 10.5 E2 degradation pathway proposed with TiO$_2$ photocatalysis (Ohko et al., 2002; Mai et al., 2008).

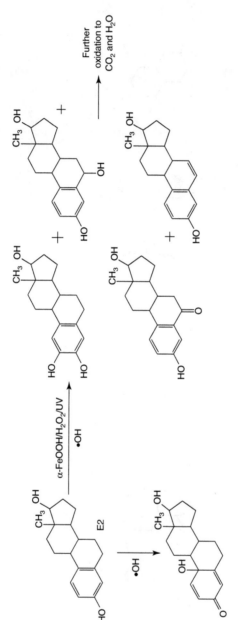

Figure 10.6 Photo-Fenton degradation of E2 in presence of α-FeOOH/H₂O₂ and UV (Zhao et al., 2008).

262

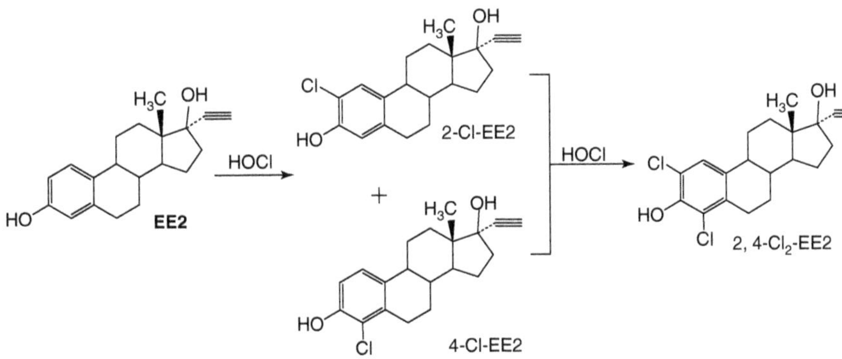

Figure 10.7 Products of aqueous chlorination of EE2 (Moriyama et al., 2004; Lee et al., 2008).

10.3.1 Chlorination with HOCl

Disinfection by chlorination is an essential treatment of water supply systems, and phenolic compounds are known to be reactive to hypochlorite. BPA reacts very efficiently with chlorine to form chlorinated BPA in the early stages of the reaction. The chlorinated BPA solution was found to contain 13 products including 4-chloro-BPA, 2,6′-dichloro-BPA; 2,6-dichloro-BPA; 2,2′,6′-trichloro-BPA; 2,2′,6,6′-tetrachloro-BPA; trichlorophenol; 4-isopropyl-2′-hydroxylphenol, and six kinds of polychlorinated phenoxyphenols (PCPPs) (Fig. 10.9) (Hu et al., 2002a). The products of aqueous chlorination of BPA exerted greater estrogenic activity (~24 times) than the parent BPA itself, as evaluated by YES assay (Hu et al., 2002a, 2002b; Alum et al., 2004).

Lee et al. (2004), on the other hand, used yeast two-hybrid and estrogen receptor competition assays, finding that the estrogenicity of the water samples declined but was not eliminated by chlorination. They suggested that there was a trade-off between the benefits accrued in removing BPA by chlorination and the disadvantages of accumulating chlorinated BPA by-products (Lee et al., 2004).

10.3.2 Catalytic Oxidation with H_2O_2

High substrate selectivity, high reaction rates, and high stoichiometric efficiencies of catalytic reactions allow efficient treatment at low pollution concentrations. BPA oxidation by iron-tetrasulfophthalocyanine (FeTsPc) (Fig. 10.10) and H_2O_2 reaction in water resulted in the formation of 4-isopropyl phenol and BPA-*o*-quinone, identified as reaction intermediates. After BPA was significantly degraded, the concentration of 4-isopropyl phenol and BPA-*o*-quinone reached their maxima and then gradually decreased, indicating that these intermediates underwent further oxidation to the final reaction products, namely, acetic, oxalic, and maleic acids, etc. (Kim et al., 2008). Immobilizing FeTsPc onto Amberlite (Amb), an ion exchange resin, accelerated complete removal of BPA in the presence of H_2O_2 at pH 7.5. BPA removal was caused by adsorption

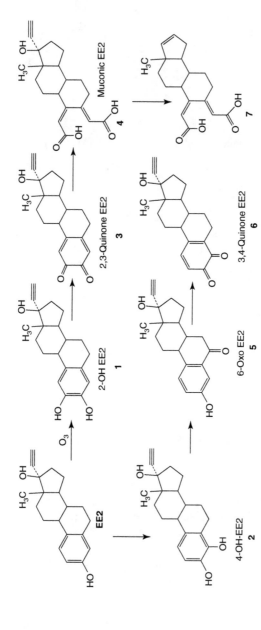

Figure 10.8 Initial transformation products during the reaction of EE2 with ozone (Huber et al., 2004; Lee et al., 2008; Vieira et al., 2010; Larcher et al., 2012).

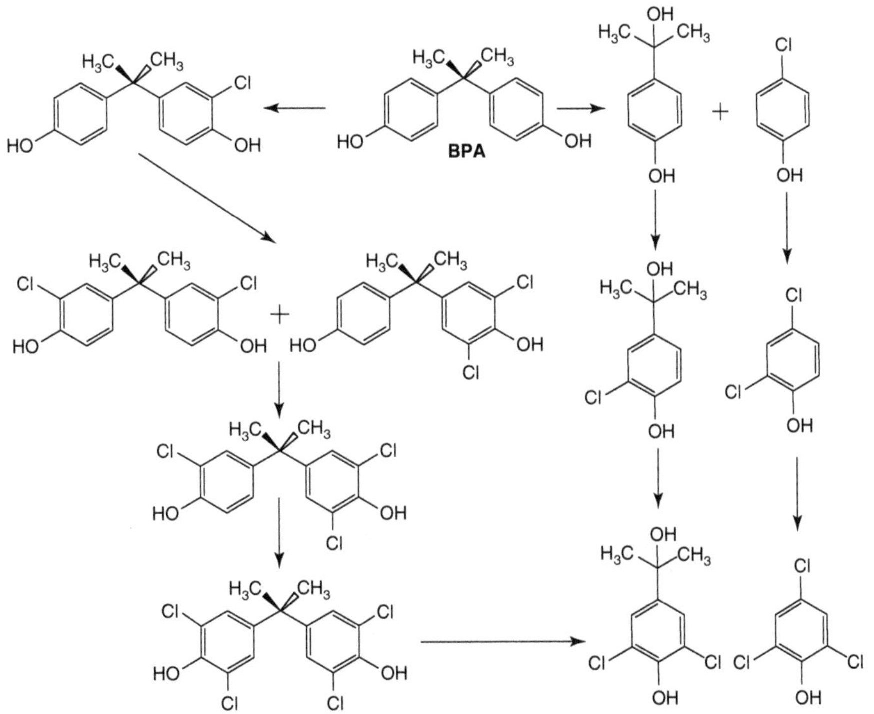

Figure 10.9 Pathways of chlorination of BPA by HOCl (Hu et al., 2002a).

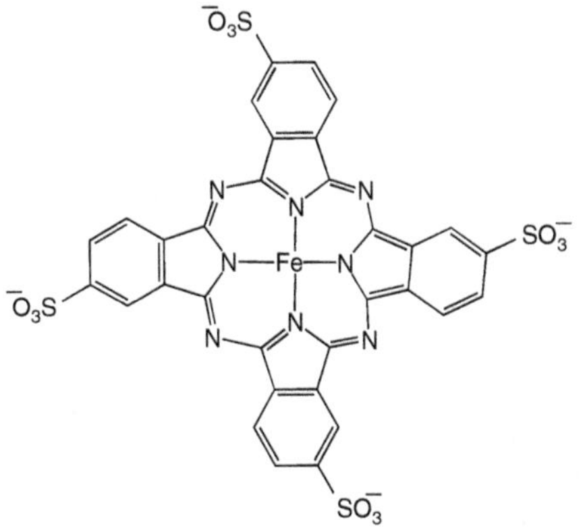

Figure 10.10 Iron (III)-2,9,16,23-tetrasulfophthalo-cyanine (FeTsPc).

by Amb and catalytic oxidation when H_2O_2 was incorporated. At least 35% of total BPA removal was attributed to catalytic oxidation via a mechanism analogous to the homogeneous $FeTsPc/H_2O_2$ (Kim et al., 2009). The FeTsPc–Amb system maintained most of its initial BPA removal efficiency even after several injections of BPA and H_2O_2, while the homogeneous FeTsPc system gradually decreased to approximately 10% of its initial efficiency by deactivation (Kim et al., 2009).

10.3.3   Oxidation with $KMnO_4$

The permanganate ion (Mn^{VII}; $KMnO_4$) is a strong oxidizing agent that has been widely used for *in situ* chemical oxidation in remediating groundwater, and is a preoxidant. $KMnO_4$-led oxidative degradation reactions of BPA, tetrachloro-bisphenol A (TCBPA), and tetrabromo-bisphenol A (TBBPA) in water using the $BaHPO_4$ buffer have been reported. Oxidation of BPA and tetra-halogenated derivatives proceeded similarly, although rate constant for BPA was one-third that of TCBPA and TBBPA, and half-life was nearly three times longer (Bastos et al., 2008).

Recently, in an aqueous permanganate-led oxidation of BPA, 11 degradation intermediates were detected by LC-MS/MS, eight of which were found to be common with other oxidation processes. Three intermediates with *m/z* 248, 246, and 196 were assigned to the tentative structures in the proposed BPA degradation pathway (Fig. 10.11) (Zhang et al., 2013).

TBBPA, a major flame retardant with uses in high-impact polystyrene, phenolic resins, and adhesives and has a large production volume, was investigated

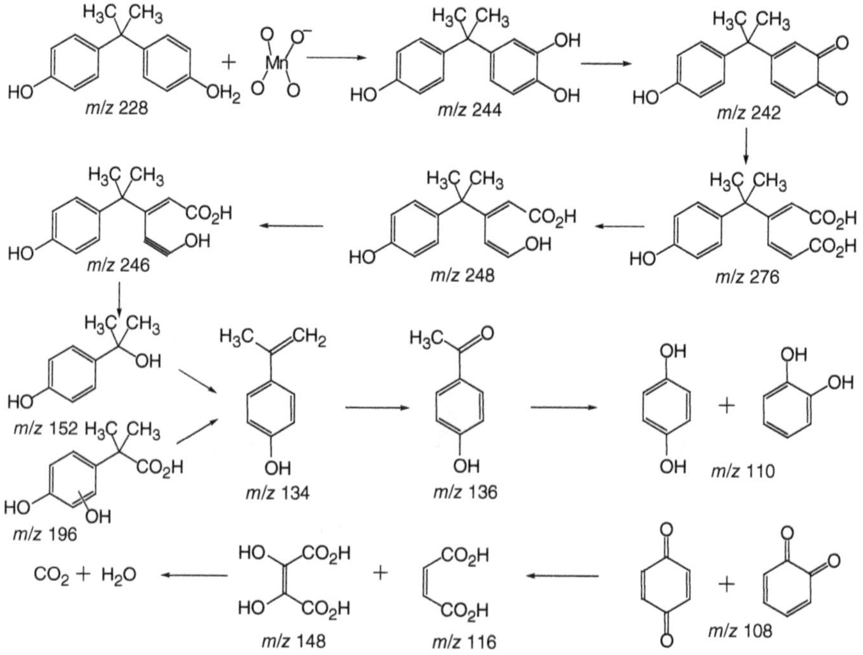

Figure 10.11 Proposed degradation pathway of BPA oxidation by aqueous permanganate (Zhang et al., 2013).

for $KMnO_4$ oxidation in water. The products identified included 2,6-dibromo-4-isopropenyl phenol, 2-(3,5-dibromo-4-hydroxy-phenyl)-2-propanol, and 4-hydroxy-2,6-dibromophenol (Bastos et al., 2008).

10.3.4 Oxidation with MnO_2

The mineral birnessite (δ-MnO_2), which occurs naturally in soils and sediments, was demonstrated to be very efficient toward the oxidation of organic compounds containing phenolic and/or aniline moieties, via formation of an intermediate radical triggering a series of radical reactions. BPA (4.4 µM) treatment with δ-MnO_2 (800 µM) in a pH 4.5 solution was found to eliminate nearly all (>99%) BPA in 6 min (Lin et al., 2009). A total of 11 products or intermediates (Fig. 10.12) were identified triggered by the BPA radical formed through electron transfers to MnO_2, representing reactions of radical coupling, fragmentation, substitution, and elimination. However, most of the products identified are phenolic in nature and may still have estrogenic properties (Lin et al., 2009).

10.3.5 Treatment with Zero-Valent Aluminum

Zero-valent iron (ZVI) has been successfully investigated on the activation of oxygen for oxidative degradation of aquatic organic contaminants (Noradoun et al., 2003). Similarly, zero-valent aluminum (ZVAl) in acidic pH (<4) has also been demonstrated to oxidatively degrade several organic compounds (Bokare and Choi, 2009). However, aluminum metal generates Al^{3+} and OH^- ions during the course of the reaction, which leads to an increase in pH, resulting in complete inhibition of the oxidation process (Bokare and Choi, 2009).

Recently, BPA degradation has been investigated by ZVAl in acidic aqueous solution containing 2 mg/l BPA and 4 g/l aluminum at pH 1.5, removing 75% BPA in 12 h (Liu et al., 2011). Addition of Fe^{2+} accelerated the reaction, presumably because of enhanced formation of ·OH via the reaction in which greater than 99% BPA was removed in 12 h with 1.0 µM Fe^{2+} and in 8 h with 10 µM Fe^{2+}. The primary products identified include mono-hydroxy BPA, hydroquinone, 2-(4-hydroxyphenyl)propane, and 4-isopropenyl phenol (Fig. 10.13). The peak areas of the primary products reduced in the GC-MS analysis after 24 h, suggesting further oxidation to short-chain carboxylic acids. Formic and acetic acids were detected by ion chromatography (Liu et al., 2011).

10.3.6 Ozonation

Ozone (O_3) has been shown to be an effective disinfectant and powerful oxidizer. Ozonation is one of the most widely investigated techniques owing to the fact that it is commonly used for water treatment as a clarifying and disinfecting agent. The mechanism of organic matter removal in ozonated waters is either direct oxidation by molecular ozone or indirect oxidation by ·OH radicals formed by the decomposition of ozone in alkaline conditions. Molecular ozone is a selective electrophile that reacts with amines, phenols, and double bonds, whereas ·OH reacts less selectively with organic compounds.

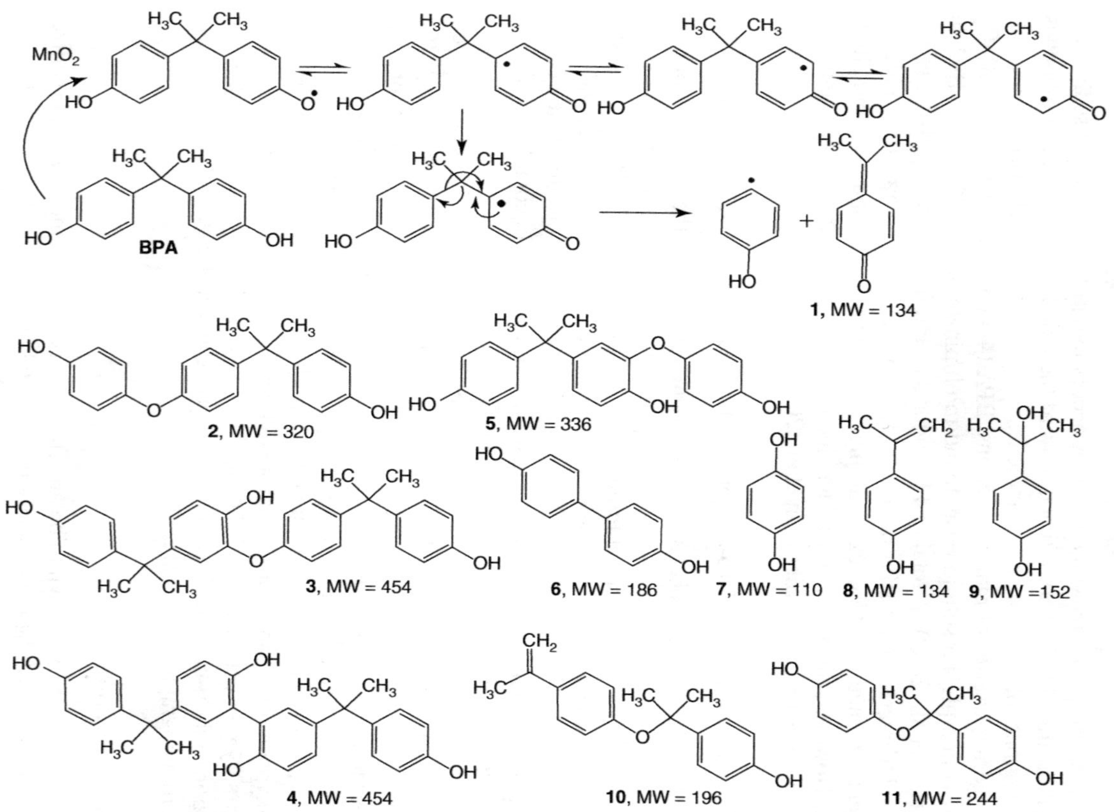

Figure 10.12 Oxidation products of BPA with MnO_2 in an aqueous solution (Lin et al., 2009).

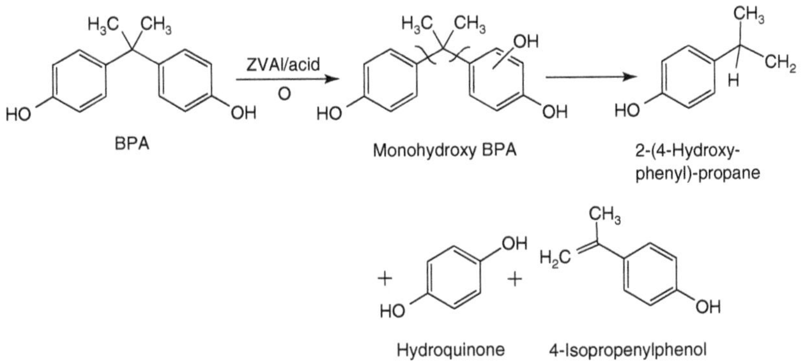

Figure 10.13 Oxidation of BPA by zero-valent aluminum (Liu et al., 2011).

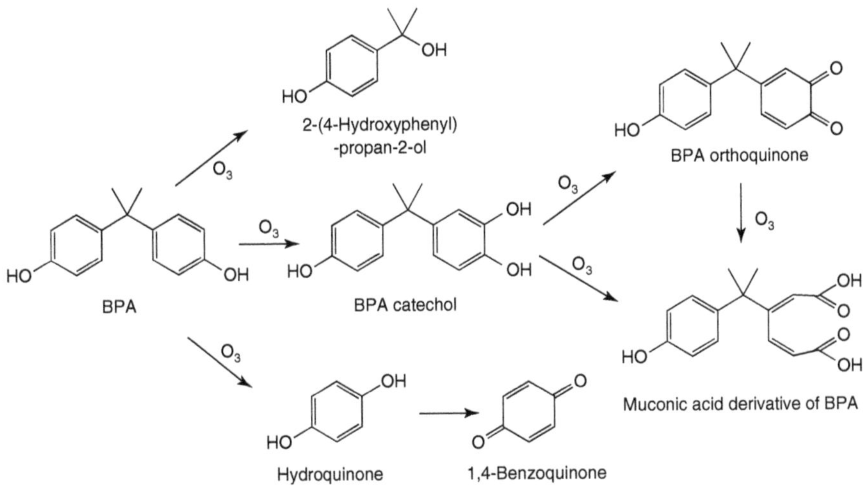

Figure 10.14 Ozonation of bisphenol A in aqueous solution (Deborde et al., 2008).

Ozonation of BPA in aqueous solution resulted in five major transformation products, in addition to three minor products. The identified products include catechol, orthoquinone, and muconic acid derivative of BPA, and benzoquinone and 2-(4-hydroxyphenyl)-propan-2-ol (Fig. 10.14) (Deborde et al., 2008). These compounds further degraded to smaller and more polar compounds, such as acids, under the reaction conditions, as formation of each of the products increased initially and then progressively decreased before complete BPA removal (Deborde et al., 2008).

Lenz et al. (2004) reported 1.4 mg/l ozone and 5 min of contact time as the optimum conditions for complete destruction of both parent BPA (0.002 µM; 0.5 µg/l) and estrogenic activity.

10.3.7   Fenton Reaction

BPA degradation employing the Fenton process using ferrous sulfate and H_2O_2 in deionized and natural waters resulted in BPA elimination and seven primary intermediates involving reactive $\cdot OH$ radicals. These are monohydroxylated-4-isopropenylphenol, 4-isopropenyl phenol, 4-hydroxyacetophenone, dihydroxylated bisphenol A, quinone of dihydroxylated bisphenol A, monohydroxylated bisphenol A, and quinone of monohydroxylated bisphenol A (Torres et al., 2007) (Fig. 10.15). Ultrasonic treatment of BPA at 300 kHz and 80 W, which also generates OH radicals, gave similar primary intermediates (Torres et al., 2007).

An earlier investigation of BPA degradation in water employing electrochemically generated Fenton reagent had also identified these intermediates except monohydroxylated-4-isopropenylphenol (Gozmen et al., 2003). In another study with BPA conducted with sub-stoichiometric amounts of H_2O_2 in the Fenton reaction, a wide array of aromatic intermediates were identified including the earlier identified products and several products formed from oxidative coupling reactions (Poerschmann et al., 2010). In addition, a number of ring-opened

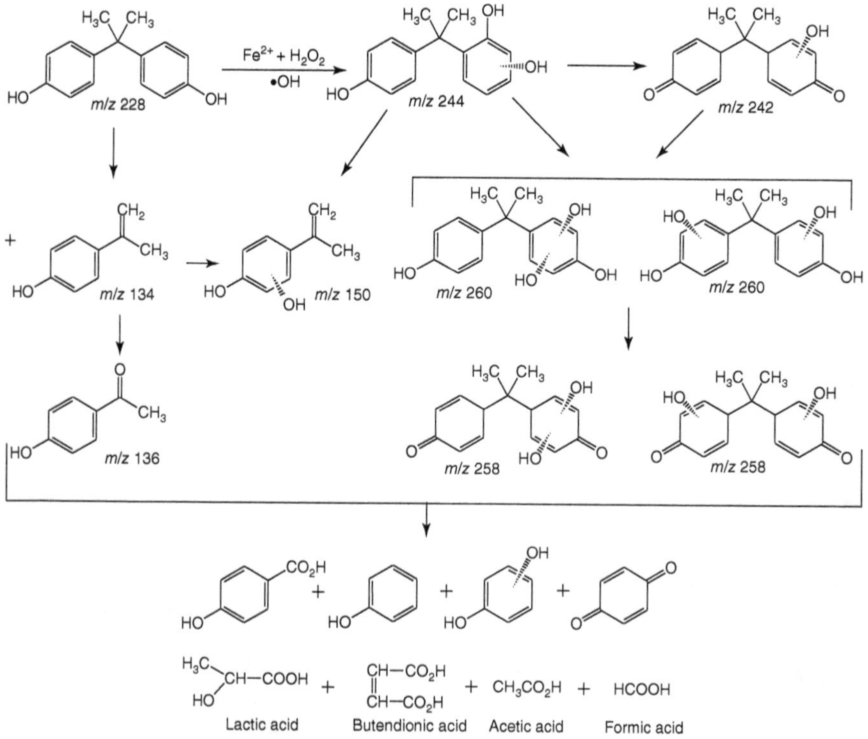

Figure 10.15   BPA degradation employing Fenton reaction or ultrasound (Torres et al., 2007; Poerschmann et al., 2010; Gozmen et al., 2003).

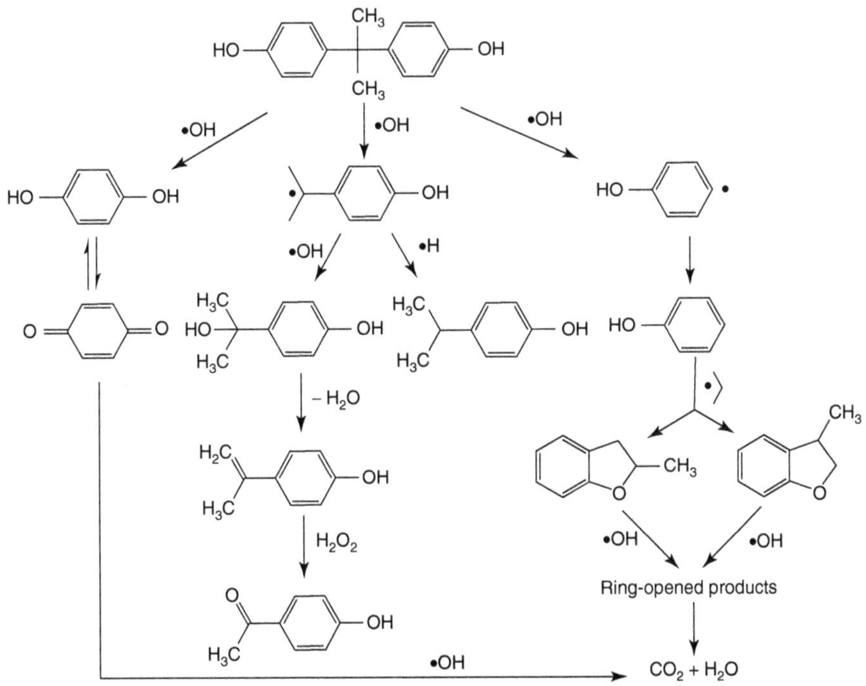

Figure 10.16   BPA degradation pathway by photo-Fenton process (Katsumata et al., 2004).

products such as lactic and acetic acids and dicarboxylic acids were also detected as intermediates (Fig. 10.15).

Treatment of BPA with the Fenton reagent in water under UV irradiation resulted in greater than 90% mineralization after 36 h. The decomposition of BPA produced six intermediates, namely, phenol, *p*-hydroquinone, 4-isopropylphenol, 4-isopropenyl-phenol, 4-hydroxyacetophenone, and methyl benzofurans. Some oxidative ring-opened products identified include formic and acetic acids and acetaldehyde, and finally CO_2 (Fig. 10.16) (Katsumata et al., 2004). It was observed that the estrogenic activity of BPA decreased with irradiation time (Neamtu and Frimmel, 2006b).

Advanced oxidation processes, such as the Fenton and photo-Fenton processes, lead to similar BPA half-lives of 1–2 min, but the Fenton system is able to generate ·OH radicals:

$$Fe(II) + H_2O_2 \rightarrow Fe(III) + HO^{\cdot} + HO^- \tag{10.1}$$

In the photo-Fenton process, the presence of UV light contributes to the formation of ·OH as well as to maintaining Fe(II) in solution:

$$Fe(OH)^{2+} \xrightarrow{h\nu} Fe(II) + HO^{\cdot} \tag{10.2}$$

The photo-Fenton process was found to be most effective in terms of mineralization and reduction in toxicity, likely because of the formation of ·OH radicals as well as to the maintenance of Fe(II) in solution, which reacts with H_2O_2 generating ·OH (Reaction 10.1). Once H_2O_2 is depleted in the presence of UV light, Reaction 10.2 is the main source of radicals. On the contrary, in absence of light, Fe(II) is oxidized almost completely to Fe(III) (Rodríguez et al., 2010).

10.3.8 Photolytic and Photocatalytic Degradation

Exposure of an aqueous solution of BPA to UV/H_2O_2 at a fluence rate of 1000 mJ/cm^2 (typical of irradiation rate in water treatment plants) led to greater than 90% degradation of BPA and nearly total removal of estrogenic activity (Rosenfeldt and Linden, 2004). A similar study employing a low-pressure UV lamp operated at 5000 mJ/cm^2 in presence of 10 and 25 mg/l H_2O_2 reported 80% and 97% removal of BPA, respectively, and significantly reduced aqueous estrogenic activity *in vitro* and *in vivo* (Chen et al., 2006). The concentration of H_2O_2 was found to be critical in ensuring sufficient OH radicals in solution. The photolysis of BPA in presence of O_3 (18.7×10^{-3} mmol/min) using a low-pressure Hg UV lamp led to complete conversion (Irmak et al., 2005).

Photocatalysis is a chemical oxidation process in which a metal oxide semiconductor immersed in water irradiated by near-UV light ($\lambda < 385$ nm) results in the formation of free ·OH radicals. Among several semiconductors, TiO_2 is the most widely used catalyst owing to its excellent UV-light photocatalytic activity, photostability, nontoxicity, and water insolubility under most environmental conditions.

The photocatalytic degradation of BPA using TiO_2-loaded mesoporous silica MCM-41 under UV irradiation ($\lambda = 365-366$ nm) resulted in the isolation of intermediates identified as 2-methyl-2,3-dihydrobenzofuran, 4-hydroxyacetophenone,1,1-diethoxyethane, isobutanol, and 3-methylbutanol (Tao et al., 2011). BPA photodecomposition intermediates were also identified earlier, using composite TiO_2–zeolite sheets (Fukahori et al., 2003) and TiO_2 (Ohko et al., 2001). A degradation mechanism was proposed by the initial formation of 4-hydroxyphenyl-dimethylmethanol and phenol via the photocleavage of the phenyl groups by ·OH radicals attack (Tao et al., 2011). The aromatic intermediates were further oxidized through ring cleavage, which were mineralized into CO_2 and H_2O. The degradation pathway of BPA is shown in Figure 10.17.

Similarly, solar photocatalytic degradation using TiO_2 resulted in complete mineralization of aqueous BPA forming stoichiometric amounts of CO_2 (Kaneco et al., 2004).

10.4   4-OCTYLPHENOL AND 4-NONYLPHENOL

10.4.1   Chlorination

In drinking water, the chlorination of 4-nonylphenol (4-NP) resulted in seven reaction products, identified as 2-chloro-4-NP, 2,6-dichloro-4-NP, trichlorophenol, and

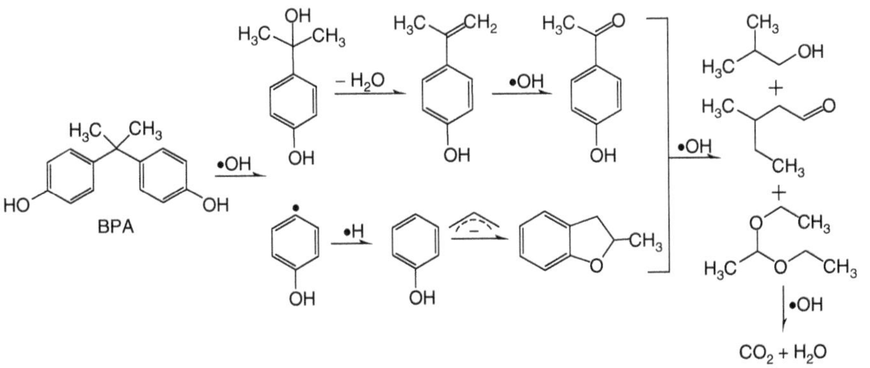

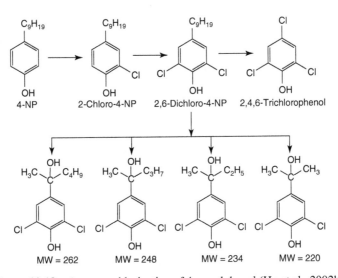

Figure 10.17 Photocatalytic degradation pathway of BPA using TiO_2/MCM-41 (Tao et al., 2011).

2,6-dichloro derivatives of 4-propyl-2'-hydroxyphenol, 4-isobutyl-2'-hydroxyphenol, 4-isoamyl-2'-hydroxyphenol, and 4- isopentyl-2'-hydroxyphenol by GC-MS (Fig. 10.18) (Hu et al., 2002b). It was found that 4-NP rapidly reacted with sodium hypochlorite, and mono and dichlorinated products were predominant in 1 h reaction time. When the reaction time was extended to 2 h, trichlorophenol and four degradation products derived from 2,6-dichloro-4-NP were obtained (Fig. 10.18). The aqueous chlorinated 4-NP solution elicited anti-estrogenic activity (Hu et al., 2002b).

Figure 10.18 Aqueous chlorination of 4-nonylphenol (Hu et al., 2002b).

10.4.2 Ozonation

NP degradation by molecular ozone was found to have the kinetic rate constant $3.90 \pm 0.10 \times 10^4$ M^{-1} s^{-1} (Ning et al., 2007; Deborde et al., 2005). The initial reaction product of ozone was identified as 2-hydroxy 4-nonylphenol (Ning et al., 2007). In a separate study, ozonation of 4-nonylphenol yielded a mixture of a 4-nonylbenzoquinone homolog, 4-nonylcatechol homolog, and carboxylic compounds (Sun et al., 2008). Using a recombinant yeast bioassay, 4-nonylcatechol homologs were found to have higher and 4-nonylbenzoquinone homologs lower estrogenic activity than 4-nonylphenol (Sun et al., 2008).

The reactivity of octylphenol (OP) degradation by ozone was found to be similar to NP degradation, as the ozone attack was not on the alkyl chain but at the aromatic ring structure. The kinetic rate constant of OP degradation by molecular ozone was $4.33 \pm 0.18 \times 10^4$ (Ning et al., 2007).

10.4.3 Photocatalytic Degradation

The degradation rate of both 4-OP and 4-NP in aqueous solution using UV-solar simulation light was found to be slow. The direct photolytic degradation rate constant for OP in pure water was calculated to be 1.70×10^{-2} h^{-1}. The results indicated that the oxidation rate increased in the presence of H_2O_2 and nitrate. The dominant intermediate products of photodegradation of both 4-NP and 4-OP were phenol, 1,4-dihydroxylbenzene, and 1,4-benzoquinine. The estrogenic activity of OP and NP (using the YES test), which remained unaffected using a UV-solar simulator in the presence of carbonate ions, decreased in natural waters and nearly disappeared on the addition of 50 mM H_2O_2 to the initial solution (Neamtu et al., 2009; Neamtu and Frimmel, 2006a).

Similarly, the UV (253.7 nm) photolysis of 4-*tert*-octylphenol in aqueous solution yielded 4-*tert*-octylcatechol and a dimeric product (Fig. 10.19). In comparison, the UV/H_2O_2 photoinduced degradation yielded 4-*tert*-octylcatechol and a quinonic compound, which was also obtained by the oxidation of 4-*tert*-octylcatechol by H_2O_2. The structure of the quinonic compound has been proposed to be 2-hydroxy-5-*tert*-octylbenzoquinone (Fig. 10.19) (Mazellier and Leverd, 2003).

The photolysis of 4-*tert*-octylphenol photoinduced by iron (III) aqua complexes resulted in the formation of 4-*tert*-octylcatechol as one of the main degradation products and by-products from hydrogen abstraction from the alkyl group, benzoquinone, and 4-hydroxyacetophenone (Brand et al., 1998).

10.5 PARABENS

Parabens, commonly used antimicrobial preservatives in cosmetics, food, pharmaceutical products, and personal care products, have been reported to have estrogenic- and antiandrogenic-like properties.

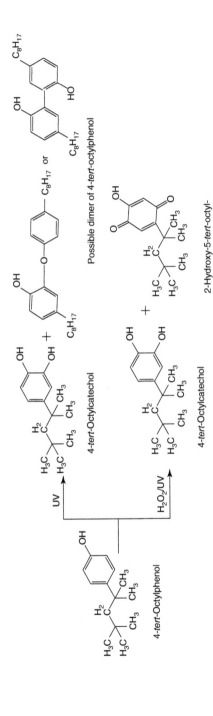

Figure 10.19 Transformation of 4-*tert*-octylphenol by UV irradiation and by a UV/H$_2$O$_2$ process in aqueous solution (Mazellier and Leverd, 2003).

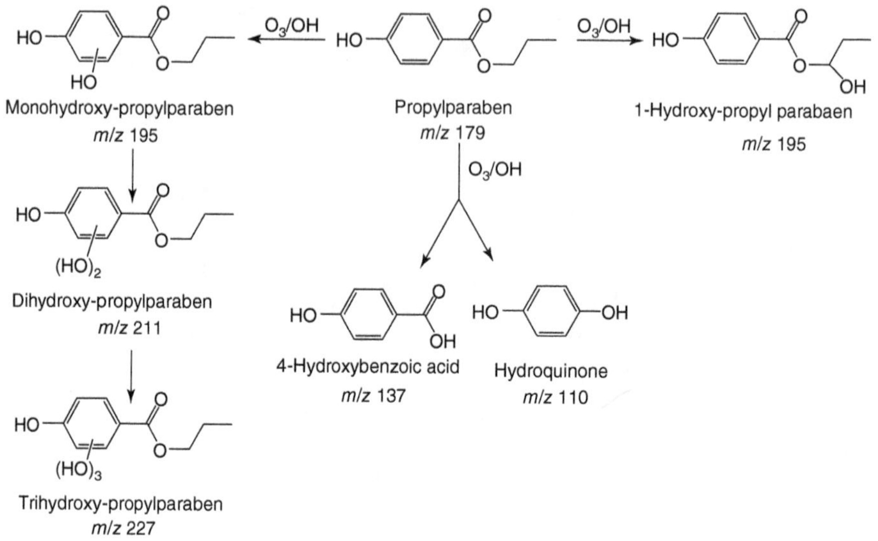

Figure 10.20 Oxidation of propylparaben with ozone (Tay et al., 2010).

10.5.1 Ozonation

Ozone treatment of a homologous series of four parabens resulted in similar transformation and degradation products. For example, propylparaben formed mono-, di-, and trihydroxy ring products, monohydroxylation on the side chain, and 4-hydroxybenzoic acid and hydroquinone (Fig 10.20) (Tay et al., 2010).

10.5.2 Photocatalytic Degradation

Photocatalytic degradation of propylparaben with TiO_2 using a high-pressure mercury lamp (max. emission at 365 nm) as a light source employed ˙OH as oxidative species. Eleven products were identified, including four monohydroxylated products (*m/z* 179), three dihydroxylated products (*m/z* 211), one product (*m/z* 195) with a carbonyl group, 4-hydroxybenzoic acid, and two dihydroxybenzenes (*m/z* 110) (Fig 10.21). In addition, two unidentified products with *m/z* 97 and 165 were also obtained in the reaction (Fang et al., 2013). The estrogenic activity of propylparaben was completely removed after a reaction time of 90 min.

10.6 PHTHALATES – PHOTOCATALYTIC DEGRADATION

Phthalates are recalcitrant to biodegradation and photolytic degradation in the natural environment, with their hydrolysis half-life estimated to be about 20 years (Bajt et al., 2001). This recalcitrance is due to the presence of benzene carboxylic groups and lack of light response at wavelengths greater than 300 nm.

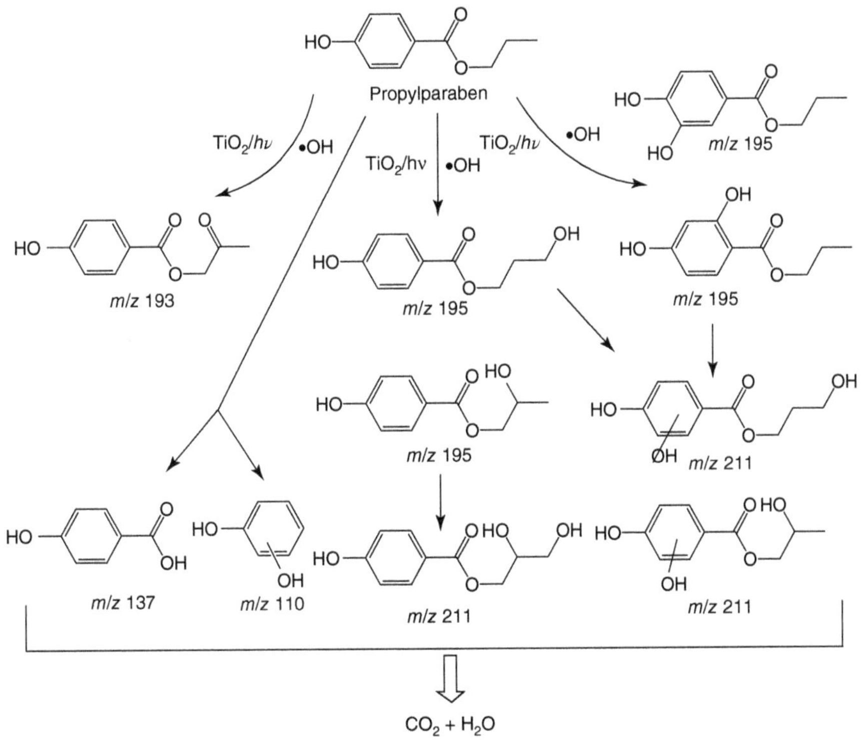

Figure 10.21   Photocatalytic degradation of propylparaben (Fang et al., 2013).

10.6.1   Dibutyl Phthalate (DBP)

Photocatalytic degradation of DBP catalyzed by porous polyoxotungstate/TiO_2 nanocomposites of less than 10 nm particle size under simulated sunlight irradiation (λ = 320–680 nm) achieved 98% conversion (Xu et al., 2010). It was found that the photocatalytic activity of TiO_2 was enhanced by a synergistic effect between POM ($H_3PW_{12}O_{40}$) molecules and the TiO_2 matrix. The ·OH radicals produced in the reaction were visualized to attack the aliphatic chain and the aromatic ring, forming hydroxylated isomer intermediates, which on further oxidation lost the butoxy groups. On the basis of the identified intermediates and small aliphatic acids, a degradation pathway of DBP has been proposed (Fig. 10.22) (Xu et al., 2010).

10.6.2   *n*-Butyl Benzylphthalate

A photocatalytic degradation of butyl benzyl phthalate (BBP) was achieved using UV light in the presence of the photocatalyst TiO_2. Irradiation (at 350 nm for 2 h) of an aqueous solution containing TiO_2 (2 g/l) degraded nearly 0.8 mg/l of BBP, and the process followed a pseudo-first-order kinetics. On the basis of the identified

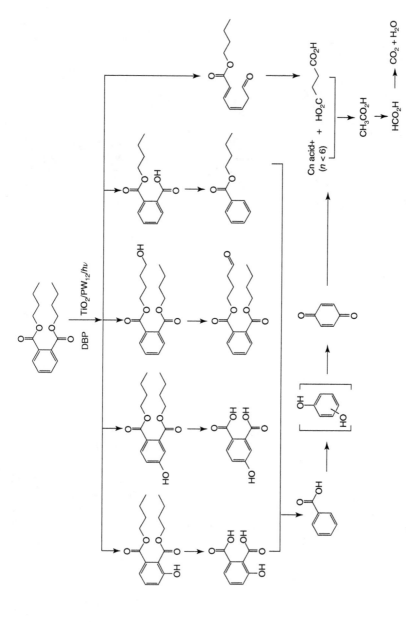

Figure 10.22 Photocatalytic degradation pathway of aqueous DBP in the PW₁₂/TiO₂/simulated sunlight system (Xu et al., 2010).

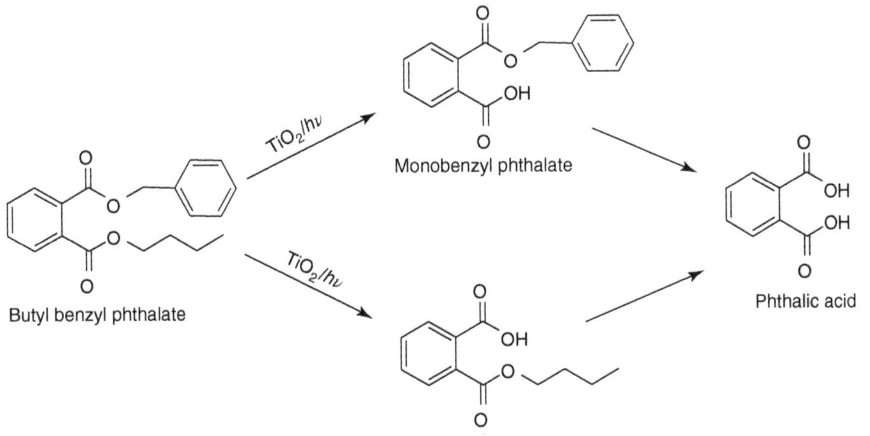

Figure 10.23 Proposed pathways for the photocatalytic degradation of BBP (Xu et al., 2009).

intermediate products, the degradation pathway proposed the conversion of BBP into a radical anion and then the formation of an anionic species with the addition of a hydroxyl radical in the corresponding carbon atom. This species then becomes protonated and loses a butanol or benzyl alcohol from the BBP moiety, forming MBuP and MBzP. Monoesters are then transformed to produce phthalic acid by the action of electrons and hydroxyl radicals (Fig. 10.23). Phthalic acid is finally mineralized to CO_2 and water (Xu et al., 2009).

10.6.3 Di(2-Ethylhexyl)phthalate (DEHP)

The photocatalytic oxidation of di(2-ethylhexyl)phthalate (DEHP) in solution using TiO_2 completely removed the former in 150 min of irradiation time. The proposed degradation pathway involves the cleavage of aliphatic chain, with aromatic ring remaining intact. The degradation pathway proposed initial ·OH and ·H radicals attacking the aliphatic chain of DEHP producing intermediates such as mono(2-ethylhexyl)phthalate (MEHP), p-hydroxy-(2-ethylhexyl)benzoate, 2-ethylhexylbenzoate, monobutylphthalate (MBP), and phthalic and benzoic acids (Chung and Chen, 2009). Subsequently, the aromatic ring cleaved, leading mineralization to CO_2 and H_2O (Chung and Chen, 2009). The intermediates formed during the photocatalytic degradation of DEHP are shown in Figure 10.24.

10.7 LINURON

10.7.1 Treatment with O_3, UV, and UV/O_3

Degradation of the phenyl urea herbicide linuron has been reported employing ozonation, photolysis, and combined UV/O_3. In the ozonation of linuron, N-terminus demethoxylation, dechlorination, and hydroxylation on the benzene

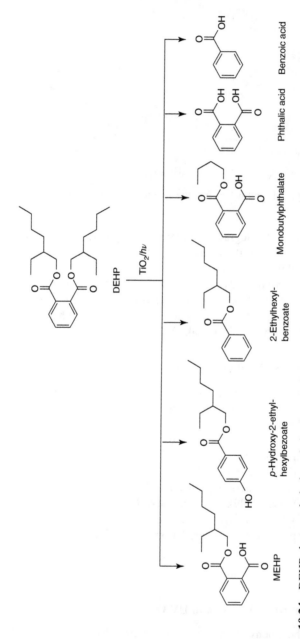

Figure 10.24 DEHP photocatalytic degradation intermediates. Source: Modified from Chung and Chen, 2009; the products identified by GC-MS were incorrectly assigned as open-chain di-*n*-octyl-phthalate products instead of 2-ethylhexyl phthalate esters.

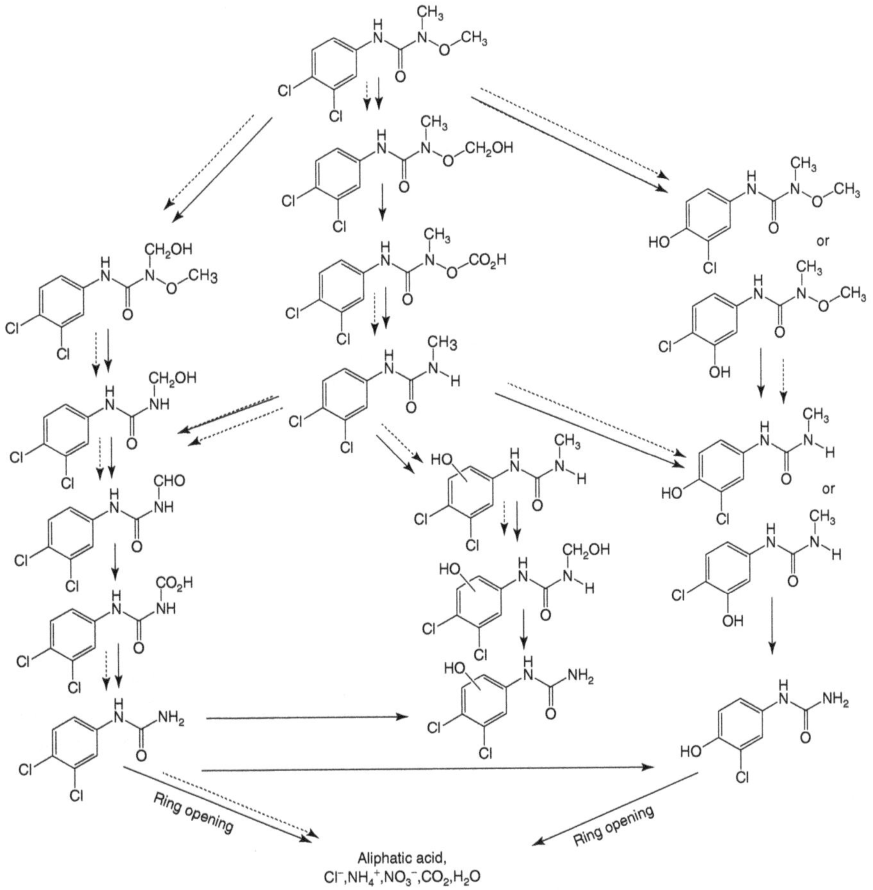

Figure 10.25 Degradation pathways of linuron by ozonation and UV/O$_3$ processes (Rao and Chu, 2010). Solid arrows indicate UV/O$_3$ process, while dashed arrows indicate ozonation.

ring were found to be involved. The major mechanism for linuron decay in the photolysis under the irradiation of UV at 254 nm was found to be N-terminus demethoxylation, photohydrolysis with or without dechlorination, and N-terminus demethylation (Fig 10.25) (Rao and Chu, 2010). The UV/O$_3$ process was found to give best performance in terms of linuron decay and mineralization.

10.8 ATRAZINE

10.8.1 Fenton Reaction

Fenton reaction treatment of atrazine resulted in its total degradation, forming oxalic acid, urea, formic acid, acetic acid, and acetone, identified as stable final small molecules (Mackul'ak et al., 2011).

10.8.2   Reaction with Ozone, Ozone/H$_2$O$_2$, and Ozone/OH Radicals

Combined treatment of atrazine with ozone and H$_2$O$_2$ resulted in the retention of the triazine ring and oxidative dealkylation with or without replacement of the 2-chloro group by hydroxyl group, ammeline being the final degradation product (Nelieu et al., 2000). Reaction with ozone and ozone/hydroxyl radicals formed analogous products with the additional formation of the acetamido group from one of the N-alkylated groups (Acero et al., 2000).

10.8.3   Treatment with δ-MnO$_2$

A treatment of atrazine with synthetic birnessite (δ-MnO$_2$) in the aqueous phase resulted in abiotic dealkylation and hydrolysis, possibly via nonoxidative mechanisms. The major products were hydroxylated mono- and didealkylatrazine. Ammeline and cyanuric acid also were detected (Shin and Cheney, 2005). The proposed abiotic pathway for the transformation of atrazine on δ-MnO2 was found to be identical to the biotic pathway (Fig. 9.34).

10.8.4   Reductive Dechlorination

Cobalt or nickel porphyrins in aqueous solutions selectively transformed atrazine involving dechlorination and migration of a methyl group to yield a symmetric product 2,4-bis(ethylamine)-6-methyl-s-triazine. Nickel 5,10,15,20 tetrakis(1-methyl-4-pyridinio)porphyrin tetra(p-toluene-sulfonate) (TMPyP) was activated by nanosized zero-valent iron (nZVI). Cobalt porphyrins were activated by titanium (III) citrate as the electron donor (Nelkenbaum et al., 2009).

10.8.5   Photocatalytic Degradation

Exposure of an aqueous solution of atrazine containing TiO$_2$ and oxygen under simulated sunlight resulted in the mineralization of ring substituents, with several intermediates identified, and cyanuric acid as the final product of the degradation process (Fig. 10.26) (Parra et al., 2004; Pelizzetti et al., 1990). Cyanuric acid, which is known to be in equilibrium with its tautomeric form isocyanuric acid, remained resistant to further degradation (Tetzlaff and Jenks, 1999).

10.9   POLYBROMINATED DIPHENYL ETHER (PBDE) FLAME RETARDANTS

10.9.1   Photochemical Degradation

The widespread use of PBDEs as flame retardants in consumer products world-wide has caused these to be regarded as pervasive environmental contaminants. Decabromo diphenylether (BDE-209) is a widely used flame retardant, and

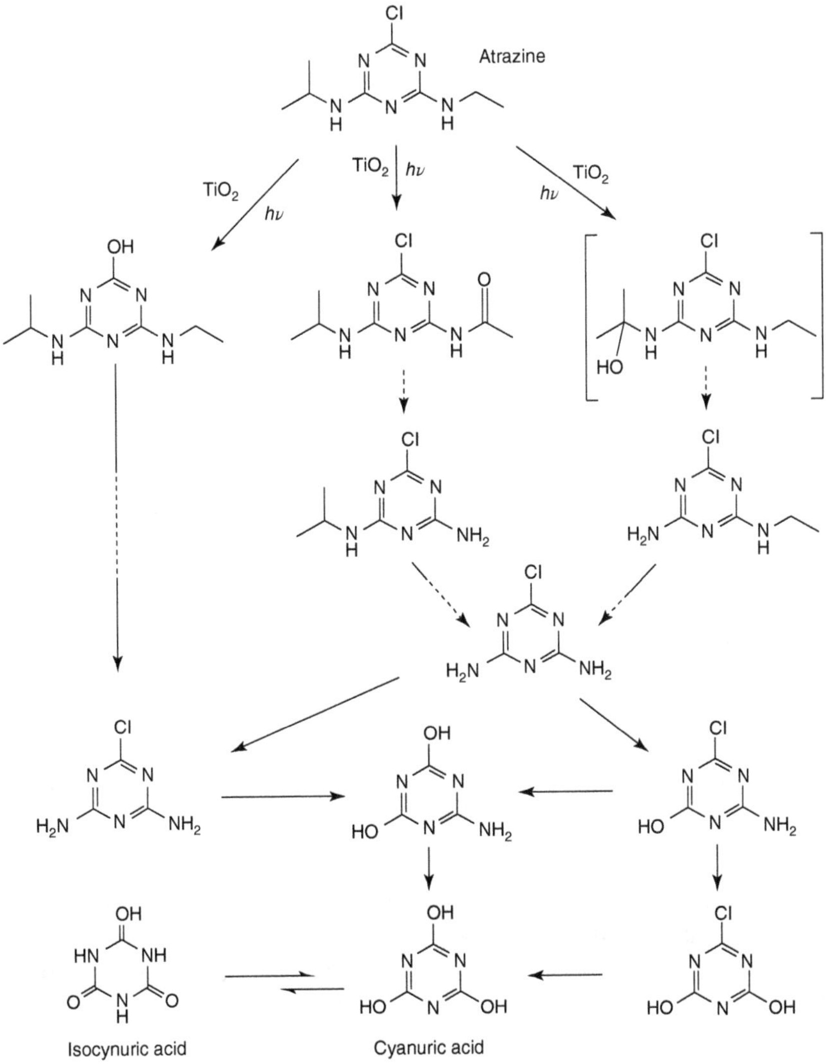

Figure 10.26 Photocatalytic degradation of atrazine (Pelizzetti et al., 1990).

photochemical transformation is considered to be an important fate process in the environment.

BDE-209 is rapidly photolyzed under UV-B and UV-C irradiation (Soderstrom et al., 2004). Photolysis of BDE-209 in methanol/water (80 : 20) after 100 min irradiation in natural sunlight produced several debrominated products consisting of all three nona-BDEs and at least seven octa-BDEs, five of which were major products. Products included eight hepta-BDEs, two of which were major products, and small amounts of hexa-BDEs (Fig. 10.27) (Eriksson et al., 2004). In another

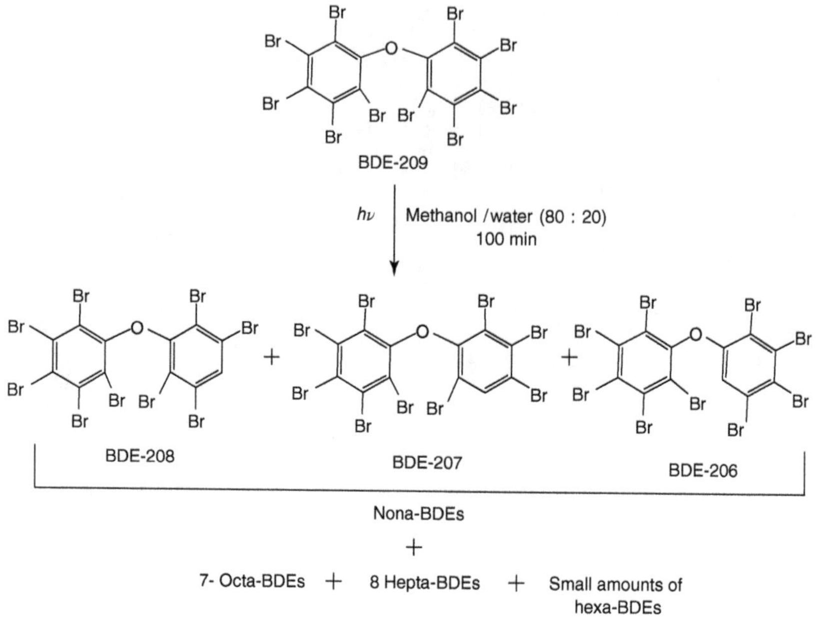

Figure 10.27 Photochemical degradation of Deca-BDE (BDE-209) (Eriksson et al., 2004).

study, solar irradiation of BDE-209 in hexane after 34 h reductively debrominated to 43 PBDE congeners detected having 3–9 bromine atoms. Out of these, 21 congeners were identified by GC retention times and mass spectral fragmentation patterns, including the congeners 2,2′,4,4′,5-pentabromodiphenyl ether and 2,2′,4,4′-tetrabromo diphenyl ether (Bezares-Cruz et al., 2004). Exposure of nonabrominated diphenyl ethers (BDE-206, 207, and 208) independently to natural sunlight resulted in rapid photodegradation to octa- and hepta-brominated PBDEs. BDE-207 experienced the most rapid photodegradation while BDE-206 was found to be the slowest (Davis and Stapleton, 2009).

10.9.2   TiO$_2$-Mediated Photocatalytic Debromination

The TiO$_2$-mediated photocatalytic debromination of BDE-209 in CH$_3$CN resulted in 90% removal principally in the formation of the nona-bromo (BDE-206), octa-bromo (BDE-203 + BDE-196), hepta-bromo (BDE-183), hexa-bromo (BDE-153), penta-bromo (BDE-99) congners, and, finally, 1,1′,3,3′-tetrabromodiphenyl ether (BDE-47) (Sun et al., 2009). When photocatalytic oxidation of BDE-209 was conducted in aqueous TiO$_2$ dispersions, 95.6% debromination resulted under 12 h UV irradiation. The reaction generated brominated dienoic acids intermediates which were further degraded on prolonged UV irradiation (Huang et al., 2013).

10.9.3   Zero-Valent Iron Reductive Debromination

ZVI is known to be a reducing agent for many organic compounds under anaerobic conditions. BDE-209 in an acetone–water mixture was also reductively debrominated by immobilized nanoscale zero-valent iron (n-ZVI) particles on a cation-exchange resin, with less brominated congeners being produced with increasing retention time (Li et al., 2007).

10.10   TRICLOSAN

In surface waters, triclosan is one of the two most commonly found chemicals in the United States (Carr et al., 2011). In addition, triclosan is reported to transform to highly toxic polychlorinated dioxins when exposed to sunlight (Latch et al., 2003). Various chemical oxidation processes can be applied to remove or restrict the presence of triclosan in drinking water and wastewater treatment.

10.10.1   Clorination with HOCl

Upon treatment with chlorine, triclosan is transformed by chlorination at the ortho and para positions of its phenol ring to form three chlorinated ticlosan derivatives – two tetrachlorinated (1 and 2) and one pentachlorinated hydroxylated diphenyl ether (3), as well as 2,4-dichlorophenol (4) (Fig. 10.28) (Canosa et al., 2005). In the experiments with excess free chlorine, formation of

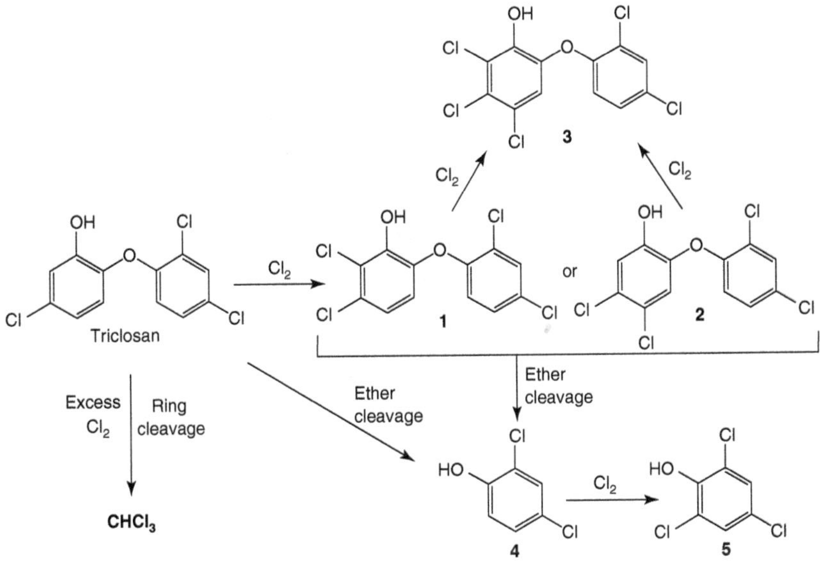

Figure 10.28   Free-chlorine-mediated oxidation of triclosan (Rule et al., 2005).

2,4,6-trichlorophenol (**5**) and chloroform was observed. A reaction pathway proposed involves ring cleavage reactions releasing chloroform and formation of other chlorinated organics by ring chlorination (Fig. 10.28) (Rule et al., 2005; Fiss et al., 2007).

10.10.2   Oxidation with $KMnO_4/MnO_2$

Oxidative removal of triclosan in water using $KMnO_4$ as an oxidant has been reported (Jiang et al., 2009). Mn(VII) could readily oxidize triclosan, and a phosphate buffer significantly enhanced the oxidation. The reactions displayed autocatalysis under slightly acidic pH, suggesting the catalytic role of the formed MnO_2. This contention was supported by the promoting effects of the addition of preformed MnO_2 colloids on Mn(VII) oxidations of triclosan (Jiang et al., 2009). However, no reaction products were identified in this study.

In another study, oxidative transformation of triclosan by manganese dioxide yielded primarily coupling and p-hydroquinone products (Fig. 10.29). Formation of trace amount of 2,4-dichlorophenol was also reported (Zhang and Huang, 2003).

10.10.3   Ozonation

Triclosan treatment with ozone in aqueous solution resulted in transformation products identified as 2,4-dichlorophenol, chloro-catecol, mono-hydroxy-triclosan, and di-hydroxy-triclosan (Chen et al., 2012).

10.10.4   Photochemical Transformation

Use of large amounts of triclosan in consumer products is routinely observed in WWTP influents. Direct photolysis has been found to be an important loss process for triclosan in the environment. The four major photoproducts identified were 2,8-dichlorodibenzodioxin (2,8-DCDD), 4,5′-dichloro-[1,1′-biphenyl]-2,2′-diol ($(OH)_2PCB$-13), 5-chloro-2-(4-chloro-phenoxy)phenol, and 2,4-dichlorophenol (Latch et al., 2005; Ferrer et al., 2004; Kliegman et al., 2013). In addition, the formation of polymerization products has been reported at high triclosan concentrations (100 µM) (Chen et al., 2008) (Fig. 10.30). Experimental and computational results indicate a likely biradical intermediate in dioxin, biphenyl, and phenoxyphenol product formation (Kliegman et al., 2013).

In surface waters downstream, where wastewater is disinfected with chlorine, the ring-chlorinated triclosan derivatives have been found to undergo photochemical transformation to form di-, tri-, and tetrachlorinated dioxins (Fig. 10.31) which accumulate in downstream sediments (Buthet et al., 2010). The dioxin products from the chlorinated triclosan derivatives are potentially of greater concern than 2,8-DCDD, because dioxin receptor binding/toxicity increases with chlorine substitution in the lateral positions (Safe, 1986). The toxicity implications of this dioxin pool composition are difficult to assess, as the specific dioxin congeners derived

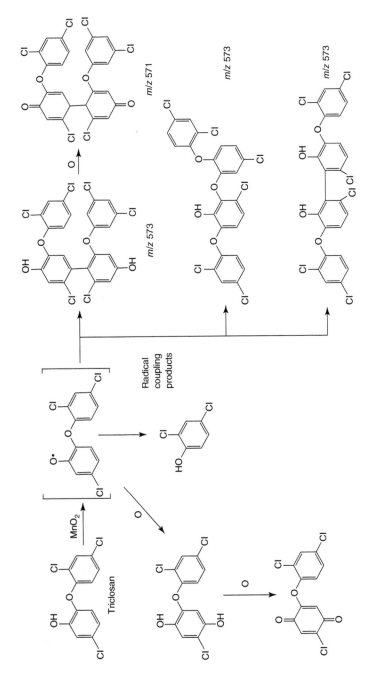

Figure 10.29 Oxidative transformation of triclosan with MnO$_2$. Source: Adapted from Zhang and Huang, (2003).

287

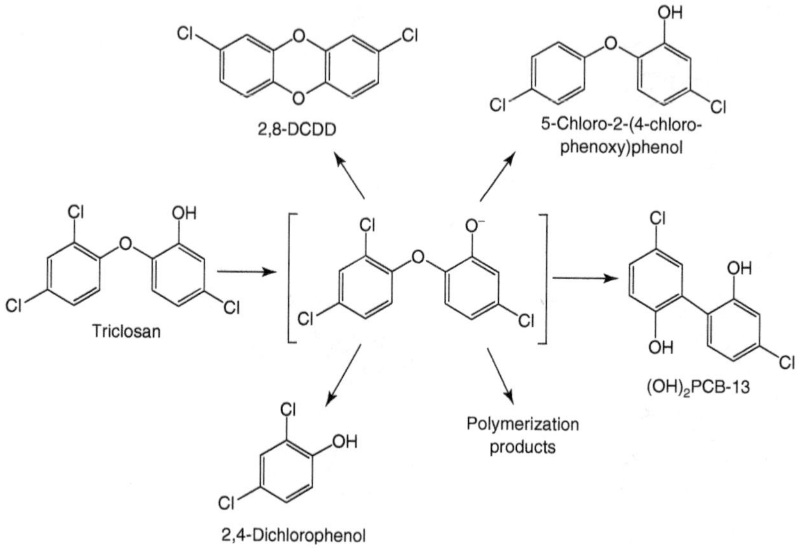

Figure 10.30 Photochemical degradation products of triclosan (Kliegman et al. 2013).

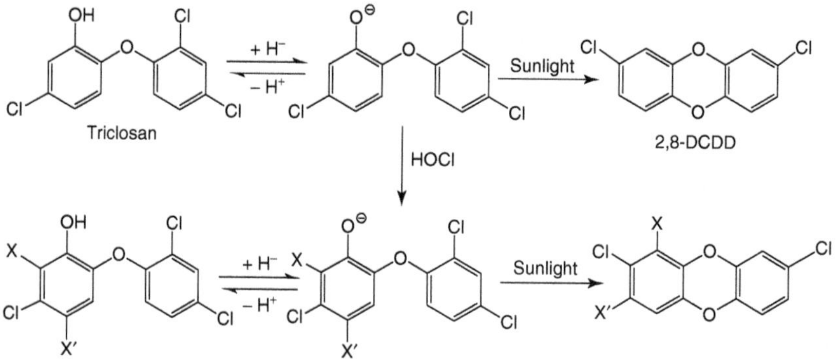

Figure 10.31 Photochemical transformations of triclosan and its chlorinated analogs to polychlorinated dibenzo-*p*-dioxins (Buthet et al., 2010).

from triclosan have not been assigned toxic equivalency factors. Nevertheless, the available data indicate that the toxicity and receptor binding of these congeners are much weaker than those of 2,3,7,8-tetrachlorodibenzodioxin (2,3,7,8-TCDD) (Buthet et al., 2010).

Photocatalysis of triclosan mediated by TiO_2 was more effective, producing no detectable 2,8-DCDD. Addition of a radical scavenger in the reaction produced the dioxin intermediate, indicating that the formation of radicals was able to degrade the dioxin intermediate during the reaction (Son et al., 2009).

10.11   PFOA AND PFOS

Perfluorooctane sulfonate (PFOS) and perfluorooctanoic acid (PFOA) are widely used in a variety of applications, including polymer additives, lubricants, fire retardants and suppressants, and surfactants. These compounds are oxidatively recalcitrant, photochemically inert, and resistant to both biotic and abiotic degradation (Key et al., 1998).

10.11.1   Modified Fenton Reaction

PFOA is nearly inert to the reaction with hydroxyl radicals produced during the Fenton reaction (Moriwaki et al., 2005). A modified Fenton's reagent using high concentrations of H_2O_2 and initiators such as soluble iron(III), characterized as *catalyzed hydrogen peroxide propagation* (CHP), generated reactive oxygen species in addition to hydroxyl radical, including perhydroxyl radical ($HO_2\cdot$), superoxide radical anion ($O_2\cdot-$), and hydroperoxide anion (HO_2-). Superoxide and hydroperoxide have high nucleophilic reactivity in aqueous systems. Reactions with 1 M H_2O_2 and 0.5 mM iron(III) at pH 3.5 degraded PFOA to mineralization by 89% over 150 min, with generation of near stoichiometric equivalents of fluoride. However, in the presence of a hydroxyl radical scavenger 2-propanol (1 M), only 24% of the PFOA was lost over 150 min, compared to 89% in the system without 2-propanol, suggesting that presence of hydroxyl radicals was important for efficient decomposition (Mitchell et al., 2014).

10.11.2   Sonochemical Degradation

The sonochemical treatment of PFOS and PFOA resulted in 99% degradation in 60 min. The decomposition products were formed by shortening of the perfluorocarbon chain and resulted in lowering of the toxicity (Moriwaki et al., 2005).

10.11.3   Photocatalytic Reaction

TiO_2-based photocatalysis is strong enough to decompose most organics, but it has not been found effective for PFOA decomposition. In comparison, indium oxide (In_2O_3) possesses significantly higher activity under UV irradiation, with the rate constant about 8.4 times higher than that by TiO_2. A photocatalysis reaction based on In_2O_3 led to PFOA decomposition forming C_2-C_7 shorter chain perfluorocarboxylic acids as major intermediates of PFOA (Li et al., 2012).

10.12   CONCLUSIONS

The oxidations of numerous EDCs with various oxidant systems have been investigated in the field of water treatment processes and environmental remediation. However, the reaction products and the mechanisms of oxidation of certain EDCs are not yet available. Hence, further study of the oxidation of these EDCs by oxidants is necessary. Some of the intermediates and products identified in the degradation of EDCs are potentially toxic and recalcitrant to further oxidation. These need be carefully considered when designing and optimizing various remediation systems.

REFERENCES

Acero, J. L.; Stemmler, K.; Gunten, U. V. Degradation kinetics of atrazine and its degradation products with ozone and OH radicals: a predictive tool for drinking water treatment, *Environ. Sci. Technol.* **2000**, 34, 591–597.

Alum, A.; Yoon, Y.; Westerhoff, P.; Abbaszadegan, M. Oxidation of bisphenol A, 17β-estradiol, and 17α-ethynyl estradiol and by-product estrogenicity, *Environ. Toxicol.* **2004**, 19, 257–264.

Bajt, O.; Mailhot, G.; Bolte, M. Degradation of dibutyl phthalate by homogeneous photocatalysis with Fe(III) in aqueous solution, *Appl. Catal. B* **2001**, 33(3), 239–248.

Bastos, P. M.; Eriksson, J.; Green, N.; Bergman, Å. A standardized method for assessment of oxidative transformations of brominated phenols in water, *Chemosphere* **2008**, 70(7), 1196-1202.

Bezares-Cruz, J.; Jafvert, C. T., Hua, I. Solar photodecomposition of decabromodiphenyl ether: products and quantum yield, *Environ. Sci. Technol.* **2004**, 38(15), 4149–4156.

Bila, D.; Montalva, A. F.; Azevedo, D. A.; Dezotti, M. Estrogenic activity removal of 17-estradiol by ozonation and identification of by-products, *Chemosphere* **2007**, 69, 736–746.

Bokare, A. D.; Choi, W. Zero-valent aluminum for oxidative degradation of aqueous organic pollutants, *Environ. Sci. Technol.*, **2009**, 43(18), 7130–7135.

Brand, N.; Mailhot, G.; Le Bolte, M. Degradation photoinduced by Fe(III): method of alkylphenol ethoxylates removal in water, *Environ. Sci. Technol.* **1998**, 32, 2715–2720.

Buthet, J. M.; Steen, P. O.; Sueper, C.; Blumentritt, D.; Vikesland, P. J.; Arnold, W. A.; McNeill, K. Dioxin photoproducts of triclosan and its chlorinated derivatives in sediment cores, *Environ. Sci. Technol.* **2010**, 44, 4545.

Canosa, P.; Morales, S.; Rodriguez, I., et al. Aquatic degradation of triclosan and formation of toxic chlorophenols in presence of low concentrations of free chlorine, *Anal. Bioanal. Chem.* **2005**, 383, 1119–1126.

Carr, D.L., Morse, A.N., Zak, J.C., and Anderson, T.A. Microbially mediated degradation of common pharmaceuticals and personal care products in soil under aerobic and reduced oxygen conditions, *Water Air Soil Pollut.* **2011**, 216, 633–642.

Chen, P. J.; Linden, K. G.; Hinton, D. E.; Kashiwada, S.; Rosenfeldt, E. J.; Kullman, S. W. Biological assessments of bisphenol A degradation in water following direct photolysis and UV advanced oxidation, *Chemosphere* **2006**, 65(7), 1094–110.

Chen, Z.; Cao, G.; Song, Q. Photo-polymerization of triclosan in aqueous solution induced by ultraviolet radiation, *Environ. Chem. Lett.* **2008**, 8 (1), 33–37.

Chen, X.; Richard, J.; Liu, Y.; Dopp, E.; Tuerk, J.; Bester, K. Ozonation products of triclosan in advanced wastewater treatment, *Water Res.* **2012**, 46(7), 2247–2256.

Chung, Y. C.; Chen, C. Y. Degradation of di-(2-ethylhexyl) phthalate (DEHP) by TiO_2 photocatalysis, *Water Air Soil Pollut.* **2009**, 200(1–4), 191–198.

Daughton, C. G. Pharmaceuticals in the environment: sources and their management, In *Analysis, Fate and Removal of Pharmaceuticals in the Water Cycle*, Petrovic, M.; Barcelo, D., eds., Comprehensive Analytical Chemistry Series, Volume 50, Amsterdam: Elsevier, **2007**, pp. 1–58, Chapter 1.

Davis, E. F.; Stapleton, H. M. Photodegradation pathways of nonabrominated diphenyl ethers, 2-ethylhexyl-tetrabromobenzoate and di(2-ethylhexyl)tetrabromophthalate: identifying potential markers of photodegradation, *Environ. Sci. Technol.* **2009**, 43(15), 5739–5746.

Deborde, M.; Rabouan, S.; Duguet, J. P.; Legube, B. Kinetics of aqueous ozone-induced oxidation of some endocrine disruptors, *Environ. Sci. Technol.* **2005**, 39, 6086–6092.

Deborde, M.; Rabouan, S.; Mazellier, P.; Duguet, J. P.; Legube, B. Oxidation of bisphenol A by ozone in aqueous solution, *Water Res.* **2008**, 42, 4299–4308.

Eriksson, J.; Green, N.; Marsh, G.; Bergman, A., Photochemical decomposition of 15 polybrominated diphenyl ether congeners in methanol/water, *Environ. Sci. Technol.* **2004**, 38(11), 3119–3125.

Fang, H.; Gao, Y.; Li, G.; An, J.; Wong, P. K.; Fu, H.; Yao, S.; Nie, X.; An, T. Advanced oxidation kinetics and mechanism of preservative propylparaben degradation in aqueous suspension of TiO$_2$ and risk assessment of its degradation products, *Environ. Sci. Technol.*, **2013**, 47 (6), 2704–2712.

Ferrer, I.; Mezcua, M.; Goez, M. J.; Thurman, E. M.; Agüera, A.; Hernando, M. D.; Fernańdez-Alba, A. R. Liquid chromatography/ time-of-flight mass spectrometric analyses for the elucidation of the photodegradation products of triclosan in wastewater samples, *Rapid Commun. Mass Spectrom.* **2004**, 18(4), 443–450.

Fiss, E. M.; Rule, K. L.; Vikesland, P. J. Formation of chloroform and other chlorinated by-products by chlorination of triclosan-containing antibacterial products, *Environ. Sci. Technol.* **2007**, 41(7), 2387–2394.

Fukahori, S.; Ichiura, H.; Kitaoka, T.; Tanaka, H. Capturing of bisphenol A photodecomposition intermediates by composite TiO$_2$–zeolite sheets, *Appl. Catal. B* **2003**, 46 (3), 453-462.

Gozmen, B.; Oturan, M. A.; Oturan, N.; Erbatur, O. Indirect electrochemical treatment of bisphenol A in water via electrochemically generated Fenton's reagent, *Environ. Sci. Technol.* **2003**, 37, 3716–3723.

Gultekin, I.; Ince, N. H. Synthetic endocrine disruptors in the environment and water remediation by advanced oxidation processes, *J. Environ. Manage.* **2007**, 85, 816–832.

Hu, J. Y.; Aizawa, T.; Ookubo, S. Products of aqueous chlorination of bisphenol A and their estrogenic activity, *Environ. Sci. Technol.* **2002a**, 36, 1980–1987.

Hu, J. Y.; Xie, G. H.; Aizawa, T. Products of aqueous chlorination of 4-nonylphenol and their estrogenic activity, *Environ. Toxicol. Chem.* **2002b**, 21(10), 2034–2039.

Hu, J.; Cheng, S.; Aizawa, T.; Terao, Y.; Kunikane, S. Products of aqueous chlorination of 17β-estradiol and their estrogenic activities, *Environ. Sci. Technol.* **2003**, 37 (24), 5665–5670.

Huang, A.; Wang, N.; Lei, M.; Zhu, L.; Zhang, Y.; Lin, Z.; Yin, D.; Tang, H. Efficient oxidative debromination of decabromodiphenyl ether by TiO$_2$-mediated photocatalysis in aqueous environment, *Environ. Sci. Technol.* **2013**, 47(1), 518–525.

Huber, M. M.; Ternes, T. A.; von Gunten, U. Removal of estrogenic activity and formation of oxidation products during ozonation of 17α-ethinylestradiol, *Environ. Sci. Technol.* **2004**, 38, 5177–5186.

Irmak, S.; Erbatur, O.; Akgerman, A. Degradation of 17β-estradiol and BPA in aqueous medium by ozone and ozone/UV techniques, *J. Hazard. Mater.* **2005**, 126, 54–62.

Jiang, J.; Pang, S.Y.; Ma, J. Oxidation of triclosan by permanganate (Mn(VII)): importance of ligands and in situ formed manganese oxides, *Environ. Sci. Technol.* **2009**, 43(21), 8326–8331.

Jiang, J.; Pang, S. Y.; Ma, J.; Liu, H. Oxidation of phenolic endocrine disrupting chemicals by potassium permanganate in synthetic and real waters, *Environ. Sci. Technol.* **2012**, 46(3), 1774–1781.

Kaneco, S.; Rahman, M. A.; Suziki, T.; Katsumata, H.; Ohta, K. Optimization of solar photocatalytic degradation conditions of bisphenol A in water using titanium dioxide, *J. Photochem. Photobiol. A Chem.* **2004**, 163, 419–424.

Katsumata, H.; Kawabe, S.; Kaneco, S.; Suzuki, T.; Ohta, K. Degradation of bisphenol A in water by the photo-Fenton reaction, *J. Photochem. Photobiol. A Chem.* **2004**, 162(2–3), 297–305.

Key, B. D.; Howell, R. D.; Criddle, C. S. Deflourination of organofluorine sulfur compounds by *Pseudomonas sp.* strain D2, *Environ. Sci. Technol.* **1998**, 32(15), 2283–2287.

Kim, S. E.; Yamada, H.; Tsuno, H. Evaluation of estrogenicity for 17β-estradiol decomposition during ozonation, *Ozone Sci. Eng.*, **2004**, 26(6), 563–571.

Kim, J. H.; Park, P. K.; Kwon, H.; Lee, S.; Lee, C. H. A Novel hybrid system for the removal of endocrine disrupting chemicals: Nanofiltration and homogeneous catalytic oxidation. *J. Membr. Sci.* **2008**, 312, 66.

Kim, J. H.; Kim, S. J.; Lee, C. H.; Kwon, H. H. Removal of toxic organic micropollutants with FeTsPc-immobilized amberlite/H_2O_2: effect of physicochemical properties of toxic chemicals, *Ind. Eng. Chem. Res.* **2009**, 48, 1586–1592.

Kliegman, S.; Eustis, S. N.; Arnold, W. A.; McNeill, K. Experimental and theoretical insights into the involvement of radicals in triclosan phototransformation, *Environ. Sci. Technol.* **2013**, 47(13), 6756–6763.

Kolpin, D. W.; Furlong, E. T.; Meyer, M. T.; Thurman, E. M.; Zaugg, S. D.; Barber, L. B.; Buxton, H. T. Pharmaceuticals, hormones, and other organic wastewater contaminants in U.S. streams, 1999–2000: a national reconnaissance. *Environ. Sci. Technol.* **2002**, 36(6), 1202–1211.

Larcher, S.; Delbes, G.; Robaire, B.; Yargeau, V. Degradation of 17α-ethinylestradiol by ozonation – identification of the by-products and assessment of their estrogenicity and toxicity, *Environ. Int.* **2012**, 39(1), 66–72.

Latch, D. E.; Packer, J. L.; Arnold, W. A.; McNeill, K. Photochemical conversion of triclosan to 2,8-dichlorodibenzo-p-dioxin in aqueous solution, *J. Photochem. Photobiol. A: Chem.* **2003**, 158(1), 63–66.

Latch, D. E.; Packer, J. L.; Stender, B. L.; VanOverbeke, J.; Arnold, W. A.; McNeill, K. Aqueous photochemistry of triclosan: formation of 2,4-dichlorophenol, 2,8-dichlorodibenzo-*p*-dioxin, and oligomerization products, *Environ. Toxicol. Chem.* **2005**, 24(3), 517–525.

Lee, B. C.; Kamata, M.; Akatsuka, Y.; Takeda, M.; Ohno, K.; Kamei, T.; Magara, Y. Effects of chlorine on the decrease of estrogenic chemicals, *Water Res.* **2004**, 38 (3), 733-739.

Lee, Y.; Escher, B. I.; von Gunten, U. Efficient removal of estrogenic activity during oxidative treatment of waters containing steroid estrogens, *Environ. Sci. Technol.* **2008**, 42, 6333–633.

Lenz, K.; Beck, V.; Fuerhacker, M. Behaviour of bisphenol A (BPA), 4-nonylphenol (4-NP) and 4-nonylphenol ethoxylates (4-NP1EO, 4-NP2EO) in oxidative water treatment processes, *Water Sci. Technol.*, **2004**, 50(5), 141-147.

Li, A.; Chao Tai, C.; Zhao, Z.; Wang, Y.; Zhang, Q.; Jiang, G.; Hu, J. Debromination of decabrominated diphenyl ether by resin-bound iron nanoparticles, *Environ. Sci. Technol.* **2007**, 41(19), 6841–6846.

Li, X.; Zhang, P.; Jin, L.; Shao, T.; Li, Z; Cao, J. Efficient photocatalytic decomposition of perfluorooctanoic acid by indium oxide and its mechanism, *Environ. Sci. Technol.* **2012**, 46(10), 5528–5534.

Lin, K.; Liu, W.; Gant, J. Oxidative removal of bisphenol A by manganese dioxide: efficacy, products, and pathways, *Environ. Sci. Technol.* **2009**, 43(10), 3860–3864.

Liu, W.; Zhang, H.; Cao, B.; Lin, K.; Gan, J. Oxidative removal of bisphenol A using zero valent aluminum–acid system, *Water Res.* **2011**, 45(4) 1872–1878.

Mackul'ak, T.; Prousek, J.; Švorc, L. Degradation of atrazine by Fenton and modified Fenton reactions, *Monatsh. Chem.* **2011**, 142(6), 561–567.

Mai, J.; Sun, W.; Xiong, L.; Liu, Y.; Ni, J. Titanium dioxide mediated photocatalytic degradation of 17β-estradiol in aqueous solution, *Chemosphere* **2008**, 73, 600–606.

Maniero, M.G.; Bila, D.M.; Dezotti, M. Degradation and estrogenic activity removal of 17β-estradiol and 17α-ethinylestradiol by ozonation and O_3/H_2O_2, *Sci. Total Environ.* **2008**, 407, 105–115

Mazellier, P.; Leverd, J. Transformation of 4-*tert*-octylphenol by UV irradiation and by an H_2O_2/UV process in aqueous solution, *Photochem. Photobiol. Sci.* **2003**, 2, 946–953.

Mitchell, S. M.; Ahmad, M.; Teel, A. L.; Watts, R. J. Degradation of perfluorooctanoic acid by reactive species generated through catalyzed H_2O_2 propagation reactions, *Environ. Sci. Technol. Lett.* **2014**, 1(1), 117–121.

Moriwaki, H.; Takagi, Y.; Tanaka, M.; Tsuruho, K.; Okitsu, K.; Maeda, Y. Sonochemical decomposition of perfluorooctane sulfonate and perfluorooctanoic acid, *Environ. Sci. Technol.* **2005**, 39(9), 3388–3392.

Moriyama, K.; Matsufuji, H.; Chino, M.; Takeda, M. Identification and behavior of reaction products formed by chlorination of ethynylestradiol, *Chemosphere* **2004**, 55, 839–847.

Neamtu, M.; Frimmel, F.H. Photodegradation of endocrine disrupting chemical nonylphenol by simulated solar UV-irradiation, *Sci. Total Environ.* **2006a**, 369 (1–3), 295-306.

Neamtu, M.; Frimmel, F.H. Degradation of endocrine disrupting bisphenol A by 254nm irradiation in different water matrices and effect on yeast cells, *Water Res.* **2006b**, 40(20), 3745-3750.

Neamtu, M.; Popa, D. M.; Frimmel, F. H. Simulated solar UV-irradiation of endocrine disrupting chemical octylphenol, *J. Hazard. Mater.* **2009**, 164 (2-3), 1561–1567.

Nelieu, S.; Kerhoas, L.; Einhorn, J. Degradation of atrazine into ammeline by combined ozone/hydrogen peroxide treatment in water, *Environ. Sci. Technol.* **2000**, 34, 430–437.

Nelkenbaum, E.; Dror, I.; Berkowitz, B. Reductive dechlorination of atrazine catalyzed by metalloporphyrins, *Chemosphere* **2009**, 75(1), 48–55.

Ning, B.; Graham, N.; Zhang, Y. Degradation of octylphenol and nonylphenol by ozone – Part I: direct reaction, *Chemosphere* **2007**, 68, 1163–1172.

Noradoun, C.; Engelmann, M. D.; McLaughlin, M.; Hutcheson, R.; Breen, K.; Paszczynski, A.; Cheng, I. F. Destruction of chlorinated phenols by dioxygen activation under aqueous room temperature and pressure conditions. *Ind. Eng. Chem. Res.* **2003**, 42, 5024–5030.

Ohko, Y.; Ando, I.; Niwa, C.; Tatsuma, T.; Yamamura, T.; Nakashima, T.; Kubota, Y.; Fujishima, A. Degradation of bisphenol A in water by TiO$_2$ photocatalyst, *Environ. Sci. Technol.* **2001**, 35(11), 2365–2368.

Ohko, Y.; Iuchi, K.; Niwa, C.; Tatsuma, T.; Nakashima, T.; Iguchi, T.; Kubota, Y.; Fujishima, A. 17β-estradiol degradation by TiO$_2$ photocatalysis as a means of reducing estrogenic activity, *Environ. Sci. Technol.* **2002**, 36(19), 4175–4181.

Parra, S.; Stanca, S. E.; Guasaquillo, I.; Thampi, K. R. Photocatalytic degradation of atrazine using suspended and supported TiO$_2$, *Appl. Catal. B* **2004**, 51, 107-116

Pelizzetti, E.; Maurino, V.; Minero, C.; Carlin, V.; Pramauro, E.; Zerbinati, O.; Tosato, M. L. Photocatalytics degradation of atrazine and other s-triazine herbicides, *Environ. Sci. Technol.* **1990**, 24, 1559–1565.

Pereira, R. de O.; de Alda, M. L.; Joglar, J.; Daniel, L. A.; Barceló, D. Identification of new ozonation disinfection byproducts of 17β-estradiol and estrone in water, *Chemosphere* **2011**, 84(11), 1535-1541.

Poerschmann, J.; Trommler, U.; Górecki, T. Aromatic intermediate formation during oxidative degradation of Bisphenol A by homogeneous sub-stoichiometric Fenton reaction, *Chemosphere* **2010**, 79(10), 975–986.

Rao, Y. F.; Chu, W. Degradation of linuron by UV, ozonation and UV/O$_3$ processes – effect of anions and reaction mechanism, *J. Hazard. Mater.* **2010**, 180, 514–523.

Richardson, S. D.; Ternes, T. A. Water analysis: emerging contaminants and current Issues, *Anal. Chem.* **2011**, 83, 4614–4648.

Rodríguez, E. M.; Fernández, G.; Klamerth, N.; Maldonado, M. I.; Álvarez, P. M.; Malato, S. Efficiency of different solar advanced oxidation processes on the oxidation of bisphenol A in water, *Appl. Catal. B* **2010**, 95(3–6), 228–237.

Rosenfeldt, E. J.; Linden, K.G. Degradation of endocrine disrupting chemicals bisphenol A, ethinylestradiol, and estradiol during UV photolysis and advanced oxidation processes, *Environ. Sci. Technol.* **2004**, 38(20), 5476–5483.

Rule, K. L.; Ebbett, V. R.; Vikesland, P. J. Formation of chloroform and chlorinated organics by free-chlorine-mediated oxidation of triclosan, *Environ. Sci. Technol.* **2005**, 39, 3176-3185.

Safe, S. H. Comparative toxicology and mechanism of polychlorinated dibenzo-*p*-dioxins and dibenzofurans, *Annu. Rev. Pharmacol. Toxicol.* **1986**, 26, 371–399.

Shin, J. Y.; Cheney, M. A. Abiotic dealkylation and hydrolysis of atrazine by birnessite, *Environ. Toxicol. Chem.* **2005**, 24(6), 1353–1360.

Sivey, J. D.; McCullough, C. E.; Roberts, A. L. Chlorine monoxide (Cl$_2$O) and molecular chlorine (Cl$_2$) as active chlorinating agents in reaction of dimethenamid with aqueous free chlorine, *Environ. Sci. Technol.* **2010**, 44, 3357–3362.

Soderstrom, G.; Sellstrom, U.; De Wit, C. A.; Tysklind, M., Photolytic debromination of decabromo-diphenyl ether (BDE 209), *Environ. Sci. Technol.* **2004**, 38(1), 127-132.

Son, H. S.; Ko, G.; Zoh, K. D. Kinetics and mechanism of photolysis and TiO$_2$ photocatalysis of triclosan, *J. Hazard. Mater.* **2009**, 166(2–3), 954–960.

Sun, Q.; Deng, S.; Huang, J.; Yu, G. Relationship between oxidation products and estrogenic activity during ozonation of 4-nonylphenol, *Ozone Sci. Eng.* **2008**, 30, 120–126.

Sun, C.; Zhao, D.; Chen, C.; Ma, W.; Zhao, J. TiO$_2$-mediated photocatalytic debromination of decabromodiphenyl ether: kinetics and intermediates, *Environ. Sci. Technol.* **2009**, 43, 157–162.

Tao, H.; Hao, S.; Chang, F., et al. Photodegradation of bisphenol A by titana nanoparticles in mesoporous MCM-41, *Water Air Soil Pollut.* **2011**, 214(1–4), 491–498.

Tay, K. S.; Rahman, N. A.; Bin Abas, M. R. Ozonation of parabens in aqueous solution: kinetics and mechanism of degradation, *Chemosphere* **2010**, 81 (11), 1446–1453.

Tetzlaff, T. A.; Jenks, W. S. Stability of cyanuric acid to photocatalytic degradation, *Org. Lett.* **1999**, 1(3), 463–465.

Torres, R. A.; Abdelmalek, F.; Combet, E.; Pétrier, C.; Pulgarin, C. A comparative study of ultrasonic cavitation and Fenton's reagent for bisphenol A degradation in deionised and natural waters, *J. Hazard. Mater.* **2007**, 146(3), 546–551.

Vieira, K. M.; Nascentes, C. C.; Augusti, R. Ozonation of ethinylestradiol in aqueous-methanolic solution: direct monitoring by electrospray ionization mass spectrometry, *J. Braz. Chem. Soc.* **2010**, 21(5), 787–794.

Westerhoff, P.; Yoon, Y.; Snyder, S.; Wert, E. Fate of endocrine-disruptor, pharmaceutical, and personal care product chemicals during simulated drinking water treatment processes, *Environ. Sci. Technol.* **2005**, 39(17), 6649–6663.

Xu, X. R.; Li, S. X.; Li, X. Y.; Gu, J. D.; Chen, F.; Li, X. Z.; Li, H. B. Degradation of n-butyl benzyl phthalate by UV/TiO$_2$, *J. Hazard. Mater.* **2009**, 164, 527–532.

Xu, L.; Yang, X.; Guo, Y., et al., Simulated sunlight photodegradation of aqueous phthalate esters catalyzed by the polyoxotungstate/titania nanocomposite, *J. Hazard. Mater.* **2010**, 178(1–3), 1070–1077.

Zhang, H.; Huang, C. H. Oxidative transformation of triclosan and chlorophene by manganese oxides, *Environ. Sci. Technol.* **2003**, 37, 2421–2430.

Zhang, J.; Sun, B.; Guan, X. Oxidative removal of bisphenol A by permanganate: Kinetics, pathways and influences of co-existing chemicals, *Sep. Purif. Technol.* **2013**, 107, 48–53.

Zhao, Y.; Hu, J.; Jin, W. Transformation of oxidation products and reduction of estrogenic activity of 17β-estradiol by a heterogeneous photo-Fenton reaction, *Environ. Sci. Technol.* **2008**, 42, 5277–5284.

PART III

SCREENING AND TESTING FOR POTENTIAL EDCs, IMPLICATIONS FOR WATER QUALITY SUSTAINABILITY, POLICY AND REGULATORY ISSUES, AND GREEN CHEMISTRY PRINCIPLES IN THE DESIGN OF SAFE CHEMICALS AND REMEDIATION OF EDCs

11

SCREENING AND TESTING PROGRAMS FOR EDCs

11.1 INTRODUCTION

Testing the responses to a chemical at the cellular level in an *in vitro* system in the laboratory provides a tool to screen a large number of chemicals in a short time. *In vitro* assays are often cell based but also include isolated tissue (e.g., metabolically active liver homogenate) and cells transfected with a human receptor system. These are only approximations, as they lack the complexity of an organism with its feedback loops, crosstalk between different biological pathways, metabolism, etc. because these are typically performed in a controlled environment of a test tube or microtiter plate. *In vivo* assays are exposure tests used to determine the toxicity of a chemical(s) to a target organism and/or tissues/organs/cells of the organism. *In vivo* animal models offer direct evidence of chemical toxicity in a living organism, but this strength is offset by the weaknesses of low throughput and excessive demand of resources.

There remains a great deal of uncertainty regarding the use of *in vitro* tests as a replacement of *in vivo* assays for toxicity testing of endocrine disruptor chemicals (EDCs), requiring validation and/or calibration with regard to their predictive power and relevance for living organisms (Hecker and Hollert, 2011). The *in vitro* assays have limited ability to metabolize substances and if a metabolite is an EDC, it may not be detected by these assays. However, it is recognized that *in vitro* methods are more appropriate than *in vivo* tests in terms of cost effectiveness and screening efficiency for identifying a chemical as a potential EDC from among a large number of compounds. The identified compound can be prioritized for assessing its *in vivo* toxicological effects, which clearly are the most appropriate for determining endocrine disrupting activity.

Endocrine Disruptors in the Environment, First Edition. Sushil K. Khetan.
© 2014 John Wiley & Sons, Inc. Published 2014 by John Wiley & Sons, Inc.

TABLE 11.1   OCED Conceptual Framework for Tiered EDC Toxicity Assessment (OECD, 2002)

Level	Objective	Examples
1	Sorting/prioritization (existing information)	Physical and chemical properties; exposure; available toxicological data
2	*In vitro* assays (Mechanistic data)	Receptor binding; transcriptional activation; steroidogenesis *invitro*; QSAR
3	*In vivo* assays (single endocrine effect)	Uterotrophic assay; Hershberger assay/fish vitellogenin assay
4	*In vivo* assays (multiple endocrine effects)	Enhanced OECD 407; rat pubertal assay/fish gonadal histopathology assay
5	*In vivo* assays (endocrine and other effects)	First/second-generation mammalian assay/partial or full life cycle assays (fish, birds)

Abbreviation: QSAR, quantitative structure–activity relationship.

The US Environmental Protection Agency (USEPA) and the Organization for Economic Cooperation and Development (OECD) have developed conceptual frameworks for screening and testing EDCs (Gelbke et al., 2004). The primary focus of the USEPA's Endocrine Disruptor Screening Program (EDSP) has been to evaluate endocrine effects that may affect reproduction and development. It concentrates on screening for three major endocrine disruption (ED) end points, namely estrogenic, androgenic, and thyroidal, by biologically based assays, with several orthogonal mechanisms.

The OECD Conceptual Framework for Testing and Assessment of potential EDCs (2002) and its revised version (2011) comprises five levels corresponding to different levels of biological complexity (OECD, 2002, 2012). This conceptual framework, unlike EDSP, does not represent a testing strategy, but rather a flexible tool box in which the information the various tests provide can be categorized at the different hierarchical levels, such as informing endocrine toxicity outcome pathways and moving from *in silico* to *in vitro* and *in vivo*. The information on mechanisms/pathways can contribute to the detection of the hazards of ED and allows assays and tests to be added as deemed necessary on the basis of new insights or developments (see, e.g., Table 11.1).

11.2   ENDOCRINE DISRUPTOR SCREENING PROGRAM (EDSP)

The US Congress enacted in 1996 Section 408(p) of the Food Quality Protection Act (FQPA). This directed the USEPA to develop and implement a screening program using "validated test systems" to investigate the potential of chemicals to induce adverse health effects through endocrine pathways. In 1998, the USEPA created the EDSP to regulate EDCs as mandated in the FQPA and the Safe Drinking Water Amendments Act of 1996. The program established a framework for priority setting, screening, and testing more than 87,000 chemicals in commerce. The underlying concept behind the program is that prioritization will be based on existing information about chemical uses, production volume, structure–activity, and toxicity. A two-tier testing approach was developed, which included a screening battery of relatively short-term *in vitro* and *in vivo* assays in Tier 1 to identify chemicals with the potential to interfere with the endocrine system. The initial tests aim to complement one another to screen chemicals for potential ED activity to enable the identification of specific endocrine mechanisms of chemicals, and to relate this to a biological response in a whole organism. Chemicals flagged in the first tier of testing are then subject to Tier 2 testing intended to determine the specific effect and the lowest dose at which it occurs.

11.2.1　EDSP Tier 1

In 2009, the USEPA issued test guidelines for 11 screening assays, including competitive binding, reporter gene, and enzyme inhibition assays, to be conducted as part of the Tier 1 Screening Program. The goal of the Tier 1 EDSP was to detect alterations of hypothalamic–pituitary–gonadal (HPG) axis function and identify substances that have the potential to interact with the estrogen (E), androgen (A), or thyroid (T) hormone system in mammals and other taxa, for further testing in Tier 2. Tier 2 is proposed to consist of multigenerational *in vivo* reproductive and developmental toxicity tests in several species and is intended to determine whether a chemical can cause adverse effects resulting from E, A, or T modulation. These three hormone systems appear to have the broadest range of potential effects as well as the greatest number of ligands with which they interact. It is designed to work as a whole to allow detection of estrogen- and androgen-mediated effects by various modes of action, including receptor binding (agonist and antagonist), transcriptional activation, steroidogenesis, and HPG feedback. In addition, rodent and amphibian *in vivo* assays were selected on the basis of their capacity to detect direct and indirect effects on thyroid function (hypothalamic–pituitary–thyroidal, HPT) feedback (Hecker and Hollert, 2011). The assays included in EDSP Tier 1 (Fig. 11.1) are given in Table 11.2.

One issue with the *in vitro* EDSP assays is that the assays have limited ability to metabolize substances and if a metabolite is the EDC, these assays may not detect it. In some known cases, such as vinclozolin and methoxychlor, it is the metabolites that are the most active agents and an *in vitro* system may not identify the parent compound as having the potential to interact with the endocrine system when taken in by a complete organism (Stoker and Zorrilla, 2010).

The *in vivo* assays, in general, use the traditional approach in toxicology of starting with a very high initial dose (reference) and other doses that are very high by endocrine standards. In addition, typically only three doses are tested covering about a 50-fold range. This will make it impossible to assess the shape of the

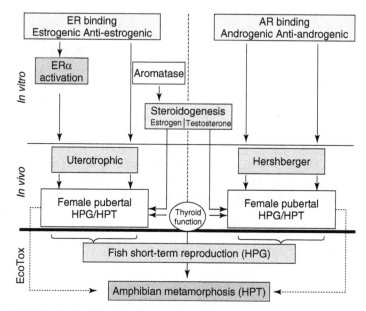

Figure 11.1 EDSP Tier I assays. Source: Adapted from Marty et al., 2011. Reproduced with permission of Oxford University Press.

dose–response curve, which cannot be assumed to be linear (monotonic) (Zoeller et al., 2012).

In 2009, the manufacturers of 67 chemicals – 58 pesticide active ingredients and 9 high-production-volume chemicals used as pesticide inert ingredients, received test orders for EDSP Tier 1 screening, based on their potential for human exposure. While USEPA is evaluating data submitted by them, it has finalized the second list of 109 chemicals for Tier 1 screening in June 2013 for their potential to affect estrogen, androgen, and thyroid hormones (THs). The chemicals include substances that have been listed as priorities within USEPA's drinking water contaminants and pesticide active ingredients programs (USEPA, 2013).

11.2.2 EDSP Tier 2

Chemicals that go through Tier 1 screening and found to have the potential to interact with the estrogen, androgen, or TH systems will proceed to the next stage of the EDSP. The USEPA intends to use a weight-of-evidence (WoE) approach to evaluate Tier 1 results and will determine which, if any, of the Tier 2 tests are necessary based on the available data (USEPA, 2010). Tier 2 testing is intended to confirm and characterize the effects observed in Tier 1 tests and to establish a quantitative relationship between the dose and that endocrine effect. The USEPA is still in the process of developing and validating Tier 2 tests. The proposed EDSP Tier 2 methods include mammalian toxicity tests, such as mammalian two-generation reproduction (rat), extended one-generation reproduction (rat), and ecological toxicity tests such

TABLE 11.2   USEPA's Assays in the EDSP Tier 1 (USEPA, 2009)

Screening Assays	Test Guideline OCSPP[b]	Test Guideline OECD	Receptor Binding E	Receptor Binding Anti-E	Receptor Binding A	Receptor Binding Anti-A	Steroidogenesis E	Steroidogenesis A	HPG Axis	HPT Axis
In vitro										
ER binding (rat uterine cytosol)	890.1250		X	X						
ER transcriptional activation (human cell line HeLa-9903)	890.1300	455	X							
AR binding (rat prostate cytosol)	890.1150				X	X				
Steroidogenesis (human cell line H295R)	890.1550						X	X		
Aromatase (human recombinant microsome)	890.1200						X			
In vivo										
Uterotrophic – rat	890.1600	440	X							
Hershberger – rat	890.1400	441			X	X	X[a]			
Pubertal male – rat	890.1550				X	X		X	X	X
Pubertal female – rat	890.1450		X	X			X		X	X
Fish short-term reproduction	890.1350	229	X	X	X	X	X	X	X	
Amphibian metamorphosis –frog[a]	890.1100	231								X

Abbreviations: OCSPP, Office of Chemical Safety and Pollution Prevention; OECD, Office of Economic and Cooperative Development; HPG, hypothalamic–pituitary–gonadal; HPT, hypothalamic–pituitary–thyroidal.

EDSP test guidelines assays are at http://www.epa.gov/ocspp/pubs/frs/publications/Test_Guidelines/series890.htm.

[a]5α-Reductase inhibition only.

[b]The name changed from OPPTS (Office of Prevention, Pesticides and Toxic Substances) to OCSPP (Office of Chemical Safety and Pollution Prevention) in April 2010. The test methods carry the tag of OPPTS. However, the name change does not affect the test methods.

as avian two-generation reproduction (Japanese quail), larval amphibian growth and development (*Xenopus laevis*), fish multigeneration reproduction (Medeka), and invertebrate multigeneration reproduction (Mysid shrimp and Copepod).

USEPA's listing of a substance for EDSP screening and testing is based only on its exposure potential, and it is not an indication that the substance is a potential endocrine disruptor. Also, positive results in Tier 1 screening are not evidence that a substance is an endocrine disruptor. Tier 1 screening determines whether a substance may interact with the endocrine system, and does not necessarily provide evidence of an adverse effect. Tier 2 is designed to determine adverse effects.

11.3 ASSAYS FOR THE DETECTION OF CHEMICALS THAT ALTER THE ESTROGEN SIGNALING PATHWAY

The Tier 1 *in vitro* assays for estrogenic activity include an estrogen receptor (ER) binding assay using rat uterine cytosol, human ERα transcriptional activation using a human cell line (HeLa-9903) stably transfected with human ERα, and an assay for the enzyme aromatase activity using human recombinant microsomes. In addition, there is a fish short-term reproduction assay, female rat pubertal assay, and rat uterotrophic assay (Table 11.1).

11.3.1 The ER Binding Assay (USEPA OPPTS 890.1250)

The ER binding assay is based on a competitive reaction in which a test compound displaces a radiolabeled ligand that is bound to the ER. The ER binding assay measures the ability of a radiolabeled ligand ($[^3H]$-17β-estradiol) to bind to rat uterine cytosolic ER in the presence of increasing test material concentrations (Fig. 11.2). A compound is considered positive for ER binding if it effectively competes with $[^3H]$-estradiol binding in a concentration-related manner, and an inhibitory concentration that decreases radioligand binding by 50% (IC_{50}) is obtained (Marty et al., 2011).

The ER competitive binding assay quantifies the number of specific binding sites, but cannot distinguish agonists from antagonists. Competitive binding assay provides relative binding affinities compared to positive controls (usually E2 or diethylstilbestrol, DES) and therefore enable a ranking and prioritization of compound series tested.

11.3.2 ERα Transcriptional Activation Assay (USEPA OPPTS 890.1300; OECD 455)

The ER transcriptional activation assay identifies chemicals that bind and activate the ER *in vitro*. The interaction of estrogens with ERs can affect transcription of estrogen-regulated genes, which could lead to the initiation or inhibition of cellular processes. The stably transfected ERα transcriptional activation (ER STTA) is an

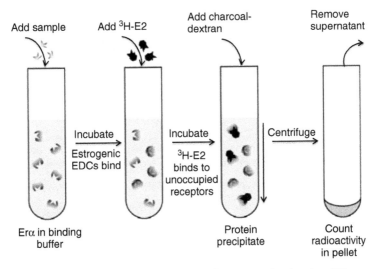

Figure 11.2   The competitive radio ligand-binding assay for *in vitro* ERα screening. Source: From Murk et al., 2002. Reproduced with permission of John Wiley & Sons.

in vitro screening assay to detect substances that bind to human estrogen receptor-α (hERα) and activate the transcription of estrogen responsive genes.

Estrogen diffuses into the target cell and binds to the ER, resulting in the dimerization of two estrogen-bound receptors. This ligand-bound ER–dimer complex can then interact with and activate specific DNA sequences called *estrogen responsive elements* (EREs), which regulate the transcription of estrogen-responsive genes. *In vitro* transcriptional activation assays mimic this action by using cells that have been specially engineered to contain DNA constructs which contain an ERE promoter linked to a reporter gene, such as luciferase (the luciferase gene is what gives fireflies the ability to glow), that produces a gene product that can be easily measured.

One of the first versions of this assay used was the yeast estrogen screen (YES) (Routledge and Sumpter, 1996) that employed a recombinant yeast (*Saccharomyces cerevisiae*) strain into which hERs were integrated. When an estrogenic substance binds with the receptor, the yeast secretes an enzyme β-galactosidase which can be measured (Fig. 11.3) (Routledge and Sumpter, 1996).

The present assay makes use of the stably transfected human cervical cancer hERα HeLa-9903 cell line, which was stably transfected with plasmids containing hERα and an estrogen-responsive luciferase reporter gene. This cell line can measure the ability of a test chemical to induce hERα-mediated transactivation of luciferase gene expression. The transactivation assay is the classical reporter assay that demonstrates functional activation of a nuclear receptor by a specific compound. In this assay, estrogen (or an estrogenic test compound) enters the cell, binds the ER, and activates this signaling pathway leading to the production of a luciferase

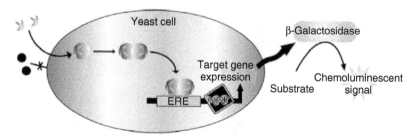

Figure 11.3 *In vitro* ERα screening assay: a schematic overview of the yeast estrogen screening (YES) assay. Source: From Murk et al., 2002. Reproduced with permission of John Wiley & Sons.

enzyme. The luciferase product is measured by the addition of the luciferase substrate, luciferin. This causes a light-emitting reaction to occur, which is quantified as relative light units using a luminometer. The amount of light emitted is proportional to the potency and/or the concentration of the estrogen (or estrogenic test compound).

The cells are exposed to seven noncytotoxic concentrations of the test chemical for 20–24 h to induce the reporter gene products. A test chemical is considered to be positive if the maximum response induced is equal to or exceeds 10% of the response of the positive control (1 nM 17β-estradiol) in at least two of two or two of three runs.

11.3.3 Aromatase Assay (USEPA OPPTS 890.1200)

The aromatase assay is an *in vitro* screening assay to detect substances that inhibit aromatase – the catalytic activity of cytochrome *P*450 enzyme complex (CYP 19), responsible for the conversion of androgens to estrogens during steroidogenesis. Inhibition of aromatase enzyme activity alters the levels of circulating estrogens in males and females, which may lead to effects on reproductive organs and other targets such as mammary gland.

The aromatase assay examines the effects of the parent compound on recombinant human aromatase activity. The assay is conducted by incubating human recombinant microsomes with increasing concentrations of test chemical, an aromatase substrate radiolabeled $[1\beta\text{-}^3\text{H}]$-androstenedione, and an essential cofactor nicotinamide adenine dinucleotide phosphate (NADPH) for 15 min at 36 °C. Aromatase activity is measured by measuring the rate of production of tritiated water ($^3\text{H}_2\text{O}$) during the conversion of ^3H-androstenedione to estrone (Fig. 11.4). Compounds that competitively inhibit aromatase activity will decrease estrone production and consequently $^3\text{H}_2\text{O}$ levels in a dose-related manner. 4-Hydroxy-androstenedione, which binds the enzyme's catalytic site to prevent substrate from attaching, is used as a positive control.

Inhibition of aromatase may also be determined in the H295R steroidogenesis assay (Section 11.4.2). This assay detects substances that affect production of

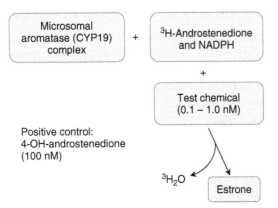

Figure 11.4 Aromatase assay process.

estradiol and testosterone but the steroidogenesis assay contains all the enzymes involved in steroidogenesis, from cholesterol to estradiol and testosterone. Aromatase is the final enzyme in this pathway. Chemicals causing aromatase inhibition will be detected in the steroidogenesis assay by causing reduced production of estradiol from the H295R cells, but as the assay is not specific for aromatase, it would not be possible to discern which enzyme(s) activity is altered. The H295R steroidogenesis assay, as an intact cell system, will also detect chemicals that induce aromatase enzyme activity whilst the aromatase assay itself is not capable of detecting inducers.

11.3.4 *In vivo* Uterotrophic Bioassay in Rodents (USEPA OPPTS 890.1600; OECD 440)

The uterotrophic bioassay is a short-term *in vivo* screening assay in female rodents with nonfunctional HPG axis for chemicals that interact with the ER. The uterus is the primary target organ for estrogens. The uterus responds to estrogens in two ways. An initial response is an increase in weight due to water imbibition. This response is followed by a weight gain due to tissue growth. The uterus responses in rats and mice are comparable, qualitatively. When the natural source of estrogen is not available, either because the animal is immature or because it has been ovariectomized, then the growth of the uterus becomes sensitive to external sources of estrogen. Thus, the administration of estrogen to immature and ovariectomized (whose ovaries had been removed) female rats results in the rapid growth of uterine tissue, imbibition of fluid, and increase in uterine weight. The primary end point in this assay is uterine weight, measured using one of two techniques: dry and wet weight. Thus, an increase in uterus weight in sexually immature/ovariectomized rats induced by a test chemical at a range of dose levels over 3 days dosing, compared with a negative control and 17β-estradiol as a positive control, constitutes a positive result and allows potency relative to estradiol to be calculated.

11.3.5   Pubertal Female Rat Assay (USEPA OPPTS 890.1450)

The pubertal female rat assay involves the use of weanling rats to screen for estrogenic and thyroid activity in females during sexual maturation via changes in steroidogenesis, gonadotropin secretion, prolactin, or hypothalamic function. This assay examines abnormalities associated with sex organs and puberty markers, as well as thyroid tissue. Sexual maturation is determined in females as vaginal opening (puberty), which is an estrogen-dependent event that follows the first period of ovarian follicular growth.

In this assay, Sprague–Dawley rats are dosed with the test chemical during period of sexual maturation starting from postnatal day (PND) 22 to PND 42 to 15 females per dose level. At PND 42, the rats are euthanized and the serum is collected. Some of the end points assessed in this assay include puberty onset, estrous cycle, and organ weights. The end points for thyroid disruption are serum total T4 and thyroid-stimulating hormone (TSH), and thyroid histopathology. Thyroid histopathology is evaluated subjectively using a five-point scale (Zoeller et al., 2012). Hydroxyatrazine is used as a negative control compound, as it has been found negative in both the male and the female pubertal assays.

11.3.6   Twenty-One-Day Fish Reproduction Assay (USEPA OPPTS 890.1350; OECD 229)

This assay screens for estrogenic and androgenic effects (function of the HPG axis). A minimum of 96 reproductively mature adult fathead minnows (*Pimephales promelas*) are exposed continuously for 21 days in a flow-through aqueous medium containing the test chemical at three concentrations and a control. It includes the measurement of parameters such as fecundity, fertility, gonadal histopathology, and sex steroid concentrations. In addition, adult survival, secondary sex characteristics (such as coloration patterns and tubercle scores), reproductive behavior, vitellogenin (VTG), and gonadal-somatic index are evaluated.

VTG is a yolk protein in female fish liver produced in response to estrogens and can be extracted from plasma and measured. Inhibition of VTG synthesis has been successfully used as a predictor of decreased fecundity (Kramer et al., 2010). However, fecundity is an indicator of general reproductive condition and not endocrine specific.

In contrast, male fish are known to have very low (often undetectable) levels of endogenous estrogens in their blood, and hence are not anticipated to have VTG in their blood (Sumpter and Johnson, 2008). Therefore, the production of VTG in male fish is predictive of ED.

11.4   ASSAYS FOR THE DETECTION OF CHEMICALS THAT ALTER THE ANDROGENIC SIGNALING PATHWAY

The Tier 1 assays to evaluate chemicals for their ability to interfere with androgen action are primarily in three parts: one *in vitro* androgen receptor (AR) binding assay (rat prostate) and two *in vivo* assays, the Hershberger assay (rat), and the male rat pubertal assay (Table 11.1). The concept of using these three assays is that, if a chemical that directly interacts with AR is identified in the binding study, and if it has functional consequence on the AR or testosterone biosynthesis, it will affect male reproductive organ weight in the *in vivo* assays (Zoeller et al., 2012).

11.4.1   AR Binding Assay (Rat Prostate Cytosol) (USEPA OPPTS 890.1150)

The binding assay uses the cytosol fraction from rat ventral prostate as a source of the AR in an *in vitro* displacement assay using the synthetic androgen [^{3}H]-methyltrienolone (R1881) with high affinity for the AR [similar to the natural androgen, dihydrotestosterone (DHT)] as the tracer. The assay determines the ability of a chemical to displace the radiolabeled ligand R1881 from AR (in a rat ventral prostate tissue homogenate) and provides a positive or negative result for the ability to bind to AR. The concentration–response curve allows the determination of potency, that is, IC_{50} (concentration at which 50% of radioligand is displaced by the test chemical), and relative binding affinity by calculating as

$$IC_{50} \text{ of R1881} \times 100 \div IC_{50} \text{ of the test chemical.}$$

11.4.2   H295R Steroidogenesis Assay (USEPA OPPTS 890.1550)

It is an *in vitro* screening assay to detect substances that affect the production of 17β-estradiol and testosterone by the H295R cells in the presence of test chemical in varying concentrations to identify alterations in steroid biosynthesis. As these cells have a limited metabolic capacity, the assay primarily examines the ability of the parent material to interfere with steroidogenesis. The human cell line (H295R cells) expresses all the key enzymes involved in steroidogenesis, from cholesterol to estradiol and testosterone. A positive or negative result for the ability of a chemical to induce or inhibit the production of estradiol and testosterone predicts interference with steroidogenesis. A positive result occurs if there is a significant difference in steroid production in the presence of less than 20% cytotoxicity (Marty et al., 2011).

11.4.3   Hershberger Bioassay in Rats for Androgenicity (USEPA OCSPP 890.1400; OECD 441)

The Hershberger assay is an *in vivo* screening assay for androgen agonists, antagonists, and 5α-reductase inhibitors using castrated adult male rats with a nonfunctional HPG axis. It detects the weight of androgen-sensitive accessory sex tissues (ASTs) (testes, prostate, epididymis, seminal vesicle, and levator ani-bulbocavernosus muscles) and is based on the premise that castrated, sexually mature male rats undergo regression of these tissues (Owens et al., 2007). These tissues are restored to their original weight upon treatment with testosterone, and that growth can be blocked by the concomitant administration of an anti-androgen.

To evaluate anti-androgenic potential, rats are given the test compound (oral gavage or subcutaneous injection) concurrent with 0.2 or 0.4 mg/(kg day) testosterone propionate subcutaneously for 10 days. If the test compound inhibits the testosterone-induced increase in AST weights, then the compound has potential anti-androgenic activity. Two or more organ weights must be significantly altered to yield a positive result. The Hershberger assay appears to perform well for the identification of potential androgens, anti-androgens, and 5α-reductase inhibitors.

The utilization of castrated or ovariectomized animals in the case of the Hershberger and uterotrophic assay, respectively, is to increase the sensitivity of these screens by avoiding the influence of endogenous hormones in the animals in obscuring possible effects of the test chemical. However, the ethics of a model where surgically castrated adult rats are required for the assay has been questioned. A stimulated weanling (noncastrated) male rat as an alternative to the castrated model in the Hersberger assay has been successfully evaluated (Tinwell et al., 2007). However, the weanling model did not detect weak anti-androgens as consistently as the castrated adult model (Freyberger and Schladt, 2009) and therefore it has not been included in either the USEPA or the OECD test guideline (Marty et al., 2011).

11.4.4   Pubertal Male Rat Assay (USEPA OPPTS 890.1500)

Puberty is the transitional period between the juvenile and the adult state, in which maturation of the HPG axis leads to the development of secondary sex characteristics and fertility. One of the strengths of the pubertal assays is that these assays look for changes in young animals during a dynamic period of endocrine activity.

The pubertal male rat assay involves the use of intact weanling rats to screen chemicals that interfere with androgen or thyroid function, or alter hypothalamic function, gonadotropin, or prolactin secretion in males during sexual maturation. This assay examines abnormalities associated with sex organs and puberty markers, as well as thyroid tissue. Preputial separation in the male is a marker of pubertal onset, and it has been used as the primary end point. During puberty, serum androgens change dramatically and reproductive organ weights grow rapidly in male rats. The male rat pubertal assay incorporates measures of androgen-dependent organ weights, age, and body weight at the time of preputial separation, testis histology, serum testosterone levels, T4, and TSH. In this assay, rats are dosed with test chemical during period of sexual maturation starting from PND 23 to PND 53 (31 days) to 15 males per dose level. At PND 53, the rats are euthanized and serum is collected (Stoker and Zorrilla, 2010).

11.4.5   Strengths and Limitations of Assays for Interference with Androgen Action

Despite the premise of these assays to detect chemicals that interfere with androgen action, these assays are not sensitive to chemicals such as phthalates, which do not act via the classic anti-androgenic mechanism of an antagonist with high affinity for the AR. The commonly used phthalates diethylhexyl phthalate (DEHP) and dibutyl phthalate (DBP) as well as their *in vivo* bioactive metabolites monoethylhexyl phthalate (MEHP) and monobutyl phthalate (MBP) disrupt male reproductive development in an anti-androgenic manner. However, AR binding assays or steroidogenic assays cannot predict their anti-androgenic action. Their ED activity is directed at early development of fetal testis, such that their exposure during gestation causes a significant reduction in fetal testosterone levels during the critical masculinization window between embryonic day 15 and 19. *In utero* exposure of phthalates causes malformation of reproductive tissues in male rats, which can only be ascertained by histological examination during testicular development (Zoeller et al., 2012).

One potential concern in male pubertal assay is the variability of testosterone measurements during the transition period.

11.5   ASSAYS FOR THE DETECTION OF CHEMICALS THAT ALTER THE HPT AXIS

For thyroid disrupting screening, Tier 1 has three *in vivo* assays that measure chemical effects on the thyroid system, namely, the male and female pubertal assays employing Sprague–Dawley rats, and the amphibian metamorphosis assay (Table 12.1).

11.5.1   Amphibian Metamorphosis Assay (OPPTS 890.1100)

This *in vivo* assay employing frog metamorphosis provides an environmental screen to detect compounds that have the potential to interfere with thyroid-dependent processes (function of the HPT axis). Because the tadpole (*X. laevis*) metamorphosis is obligatorily controlled by THs, amphibian metamorphosis is best characterized in anuran (tailed) amphibians, where tail resorption is perhaps the most dramatic manifestation of the morphological changes that THs can drive (Pickford, 2010). Thus, the amphibian model is used as a generalized model for vertebrate thyroid function in screening batteries for detection of thyroid disrupters.

X. laevis tadpoles are exposed in a flow-through test to aqueous test media containing the test chemical at three concentrations during an exposure period of 21 days starting at the larval stage 51 (i.e., late premetamorphosis) and examined for mortality, developmental stage, hind-limb length, snout-vent length, wet weight, and thyroid histopathology. In this process, thyroid histopathology is found to be the most sensitive end point and a reliable means to detect chemicals that depress circulating TH concentrations, either through decreased synthesis (e.g., perchlorate) or increased metabolism and clearance of TH (e.g., phenobarbitol) (Pickford, 2010).

11.5.2   Strengths and Limitations of Thyroid Disrupting Chemical Assays

One of the strengths of the male and female pubertal assays is that these assays look for changes in young animals during the prepubertal period, which is the dynamic period of endocrine activity and a very sensitive age for exposure to agents. These assays are capable of detecting EDCs that operate through a variety of modes of action (MOAs), that is, strong and weak (anti)estrogenic and (anti)androgenic compounds, steroid biosynthesis inhibitors, aromatase inhibitors, 5α-reductase inhibitors, thyroid-active agents, and compounds affecting the HPG or HPT axis. Other Tier 1 *in vitro* or mammalian assays do not detect some of these MOAs. Therefore, it may be difficult to dismiss a positive result in the pubertal assays even if there is some suspicion that the primary MOA is not endocrine mediated (Marty et al., 2011).

One limitation of pubertal assays is their performance criterion, that allows hormone measures in the range from about 4 to 30 µg/dl of serum total T4 and still be considered normal. As T4 levels are so variable, the chances of finding anything outside what the test mandates as within normal range are very unlikely. The Sprague–Dawley rats (untreated) are not known to have this range of serum T4 values, but it is likely that the intra-assay variability reported in the validation studies may have contributed to the adoption of the wide range of total T4 values (Zoeller et al., 2012).

Another limitation identified is the primary end point for consideration of thyroid hormone action being histapathological changes in the thyroid gland, which mostly reflect chemical-induced changes in serum TSH. Thus, the chemicals disrupting TH action at sites other than the thyroid gland through mechanisms that do not require changes in TSH are not considered. A typical example is that of PCBs, which reduce the levels of circulating total and free T4 but do not cause an increase in serum TSH or change elements of thyroid histapathology. If these chemicals were to undergo Tier 1 testing today, they likely would not be flagged as EDCs for study in Tier 2 (Zoeller et al., 2012).

However, a combination of positive amphibian metamorphosis assay with reduction in circulating thyroxin (T4) in the pubertal assay will be able to detect the effect of PCB on the thyroid system.

11.6 THE USEPA's EDSP21 WORK PLAN

Traditionally, the toxicological evaluation of environmental chemicals has largely relied on animal models that have been used to extrapolate to potentially harmful events in humans. These models have been developed to evaluate specific toxicological end points such as oral, dermal, and ocular toxicity, immunotoxicity, genotoxicity, reproductive and developmental toxicity, and carcinogenicity. While these animal models have provided useful information on the safety of chemicals, they are relatively expensive, of low throughput, and sometimes inconsistently predictive of human biology and pathophysiology (Hartung, 2009). However, using the current EDSP process to continue to identify chemicals for screening, having them screened, and making decisions about more definitive testing has not been found sustainable to evaluate the tens of thousands of chemicals that fall within the purview of USEPA. With the exponential increase in the number of chemicals, exceeding the current *in vivo* testing capacities by several hundred folds, it has led to a situation similar to that in the pharmaceutical industry where the use of combinatorial chemistry and increased availability of natural compounds stimulated the development of novel instrumentation and software tools for high throughput screening (HTS) of potential drug candidates (Seiler et al., 2011).

The US National Research Council (NRC) in their report *Toxicity Testing in the 21st Century: A Vision and a Strategy* has envisioned an approach that relies on a shift in toxicology research by moving away from traditional high-dose animal studies toward an understanding of the direct interactions of chemicals with a broad spectrum of potential toxicity targets comprising specific molecular entities and cellular phenotypes using well-designed *in vitro* assays. The ultimate goal being to use HTS assays to rapidly and inexpensively profile the bioactivity of chemicals of unknown toxicity and make predictions about their potential for causing various adverse endpoints (Dix et al., 2007). Following this vision, USEPA has proposed an Endocrine Disruptor Screening Program for the 21st Century (EDSP-21). Its work plan envisages incremental transition to incorporate and integrate computational toxicology methods or *in silico* models and molecular-based *in vitro* HTS to replace present *in vitro* assays for prioritizing and screening chemicals for Tier 1 screening. Combinations of HTS assays, measuring competitive ligand binding, reporter gene activation, and enzyme inhibition, can be used to characterize a chemical's potential for ED. Computational toxicology combines data from HTS, chemical structure analyses, and other biological domains (e.g., genes, proteins, cells, tissues) with the goals of predicting and understanding the underlying mechanistic causes of chemical toxicity and predicting the toxicity of new chemicals and products.

The proposed EDSP21 work plan has a near-term goal (<2 years) to use existing data, *in silico* models, and molecular-based *in vitro* HTP assays to prioritize chemicals for EDSP Tier 1 screening. The intermediate-term goal (2–5 years) is to replace current validated *in vitro* screening assays by incorporating computational or *in silico* models and molecular-based *in vitro* HTS assays into EDSP Tier 1 screening. The long-term goal (>5 years) is to consider full replacement of the EDSP Tier 1 screening battery with validated *in vitro* HTP/*in silico* assays and eliminate the use of animals for screening purposes (USEPA, 2011).

In this regard, USEPA through its ToxCast program, together with the associated multiagency Tox21 screening collaboration, seeks to develop ways to predict potential toxicity and to develop a cost-effective approach for prioritizing the thousands of chemicals that need toxicity testing (Collins et al., 2008).

11.6.1   The USEPA ToxCast Program

USEPA's ToxCast or "toxicity forecaster" program, launched in 2007, is using a battery of *in vitro* HTS assays to develop activity signatures predicting the potential toxicity of environmental chemicals (Dix et al., 2007; USEPA, 2012a, 2012b). ToxCast uses cellular tests rather than whole-animal tests to simulate and predict how processes in the human body may be impacted by exposure to chemicals and may determine which chemical exposures are most likely to lead to adverse health effects. The goal of the program is to use computational approaches to build predictive models of *in vivo* toxicity using *in vitro* HTS data and associated chemical and biological data. It proposes to acquire sufficient information on a range of chemicals so that "bioactivity profiles" or "*in vitro* signatures" can be discerned that predict patterns of toxic effects or phenotypes observed in traditional animal toxicity testing. The predictive bioactivity signatures are being developed on the basis of physicochemical properties, biochemical activities from HTS and cell-based phenotypic assays, gene expression analyses of cells *in vitro*, and physiological responses in non-mammalian model organisms (Kavlock et al., 2012).

The ToxCast assays examine various aspects of the estrogen (six assays), androgen (five assays), and thyroid (five assays) signaling pathways, as well as a number of other nuclear receptor (NR) pathways (e.g., glucocorticoid receptor, peroxisome-proliferator-activated receptor, pregnane X receptor; 36 assays), cytochrome P450 enzyme inhibition, G-protein-coupled receptors, and cell signaling pathway readouts–mechanistic information (Reif et al., 2010).

ToxCast is being developed in phases. ToxCast phase 1 (proof of concept) (2007–2010) focused on the molecular and cellular pathways that are the targets of chemical interaction and tested 309 well-characterized chemicals using a battery of 467 *in vitro* HTS assays. Assay included both cell-free (biochemical) and cell-based measures, largely using human cells or cell lines covering a wide spectrum of biological targets or effects. Toxicity-testing results were already available from conventional animal testing of chemicals screened during this phase. The purpose was to compare the results of the toxicity predicted by ToxCast with the toxicity data from the animal studies. This comparison is helping to determine which ToxCast assays can accurately predict different types of toxicity and disease. Phase II of ToxCast, launched in 2011, will serve to broaden the chemical diversity and provide data to evaluate the predictivity of the bioactivity signatures derived from Phase I data (Kavlock et al., 2012).

11.6.2 Tox21 HTS Programs

The US Tox21 robot-screening system (Fig. 11.5) unveiled in March 2011 (USEPA, 2011) represents a paradigm shift in toxicity testing of chemical compounds from traditional *in vivo* tests to less expensive and higher throughput *in vitro* robot-assisted methods. It has largely focused on human cellular and molecular targets to prioritize compounds for further in-depth toxicological evaluation, identify mechanisms of action, and, ultimately, develop predictive models for *in vivo* biological response (Shukla et al., 2010; Judson et al., 2010). The program shows great promise not only as a new and faster method but also for moving toxicology into a predictive science.

The HTS program represents a new paradigm in toxicological testing screens for mechanistic targets active within cellular pathways considered critical to adverse health effects such as carcinogenicity, reproductive and developmental toxicity, genotoxicity, neurotoxicity, and immunotoxicity in humans. In addition, it will allow toxicologists to better understand mixture and low-dose effects by testing both combinations of chemicals for additive damage, as well as how, for example, 15 different concentrations of a given chemical impact human cells.

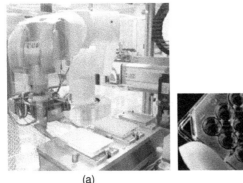
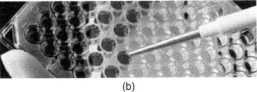

(a)   (b)

Figure 11.5   Tox21 Robotic tester (USEPA, 2011).

A chemical is tested in Tox 21 screening program by placing it on a 3 × 5 in. plate with 1536 tiny wells, each holding 1000–2000 different human or rodent cells. One well might contain liver cells, another brain cells, yet another skin cells, and so on. The robot puts the tray under a pin tool, which is the same size as the plate and has a corresponding pin that lines up above every well. The pin tool lowers and dispenses the chemical being testing simultaneously into each of the wells. The robot's arm then puts the tray in an imager, which scans for biological activity. Scientists can see how chemicals and cells interact on computer screens, with toxicity sometimes indicated by fluorescence. So, as a well glows, researchers can see which human body part would be affected. However, the effects of the chemical on an isolated cell may not be the same as when they are together. Thereafter, USEPA's computational toxicology figures out if, for example, the liver cell in a person will be affected by exposure to the chemical as it was in the test (USEPA, 2011).

The aim of Tox21 is to identify such *in vitro* assays that can detect perturbations in cellular pathways and establish relationships between *in vitro* perturbation (toxicity pathways) and *in vivo* outcomes (adverse outcome pathways). The initial focus will be on stress response and nuclear receptor signaling pathways. ED-related toxicity is a major concern for environmental chemicals, and nearly 3000 compounds have been screened in the pilot phase against 10 human nuclear receptors, namely ERα, AR, GR, TRβ, PPARδ, PPARγ, FXR, LXR, RXR, and VDR. With the Tox21 program using cell-based qHTS assays, the goal is to make better predictions of human toxicity using fewer animals in clinical studies.

Nevertheless, *in vitro* systems *per se* cannot fully mirror the integrated metabolic complexity of *in vivo* tests. While the design of *in vitro* systems can include key aspects of substance metabolism, these systems inherently fail to reflect tissue-specific coupling of phase-I or phase-II metabolism and the kinetics of substance absorption or distribution (Andersen and Krewski, 2010; Trosko, 2010). Also, the assessment of end points such as cytotoxicity, altered protein expression, or DNA damage mainly addresses acute adverse effects rather than subchronic or chronic organ toxicity.

11.7 CONCLUSIONS AND FUTURE PROSPECTS

The past two decades have witnessed a significant increase in efforts to improve and harmonize strategies and approaches to assess the risks of EDCs to humans and the environment. Regulatory structures have been established in the United States, Japan and Europe, and the first mandatory testing program, the EDSP, has been implemented by the USEPA. USEPA's listing of a substance for EDSP screening and testing is based on its exposure potential. Tier 1 testing screens for endocrine activity does not necessarily provide evidence of an adverse effect. Tier 2 is designed to determine adverse effects for evidence that a substance is an endocrine disruptor and, if endocrine-mediated adverse effects occur, then quantify the dose versus response.

The increasing requirements for testing and screening, however, have created new issues, and there are great concerns regarding the dramatic increase in use of live test organisms and huge costs associated with extensive testing. In response to these concerns, there is a growing demand for alternative testing strategies including priority setting, tiered screening, and the use of *in silico* systems and *in vitro* assays (Hecker and Hollert, 2011). The major reasons for the apparent lack of accepted cell-based *in vitro* reproductive and developmental assays are their failure with regard to tissue interactions in organs and developing embryos (Trosko and Chang, 2010). Close to 800 chemicals are known or suspected to be capable of interfering with hormone receptors, hormone synthesis, or hormone conversion. However, only a small fraction of these chemicals have been investigated in tests capable of identifying overt endocrine effects in intact organisms (UNEP/WHO, 2012). Thus, it is clear that laboratory testing alone will not provide insight into the endocrine-disrupting potential of these chemicals of interest. Among the promising approaches, statistical models and computational approaches may hold out the promise of helping to overcome this problem.

The use of stem cells offers a solution to many of these problems because these cell lines can differentiate into most cell types of human body in the test tube, thus creating the required functional microenvironments. Embryonic stem cell (ESC) differentiation assays are a particularly promising approach for replacing some of the *in vivo* tests because the differentiating cells display a variety of developmental processes suitable to monitor adverse effects of chemical exposure. The use of primary human stem cells is politically still surrounded by ethical debate. The molecular biology of cell differentiation, on the other hand, is evolutionarily highly conserved across vertebrates and invertebrates, suggesting that any chemical interference with shared essential signal transduction pathways for germ layer formation and subsequent organ differentiation will be highly predictive for human *in vivo* toxicity. Thus, the use of murine stem-cell assays allows for the first time to cross the species barrier, offering the possibility of toxicity testing truly relevant for the human system. Considering the current speed of stem cell research, it is conceivable that organ-specific *in vitro* assays will be available in the near future (Seiler et al., 2011; Pistollato et al., 2012).

REFERENCES

Andersen, M. E.; Krewski, D. The vision of toxicity testing in the 21st century: moving from discussion to action, *Toxicol. Sci.* **2010**, 117, 17–24.

Collins, F. S.; Gray, G. M.; Bucher, J. R. Transforming environmental health protection, *Science* **2008**, 319(5865), 906–907.

Dix, D. J.; Houck, K. A.; Martin, M. T.; Richard, A. M.; Setzer, R. W.; Kavlock, R. J. The ToxCast program for prioritizing toxicity testing of environmental chemicals, *Toxicol. Sci.* **2007**, 95(1), 5–12.

EPA, The future of toxicity testing is here: EPA Tox21 partnership taps high-tech robots to advance toxicity testing, *Science Matters*, August **2011**.

Freyberger, A.; Schladt, L. Evaluation of the rodent Hershberger bioassay on intact juvenile males—testing of coded chemicals and supplementary biochemical investigations, *Toxicology* **2009**, 262, 114–120.

Gelbke, H. P.; Kayser, M.; Poole, A. OECD test strategies and methods for endocrine disruptors, *Toxicology* **2004**, 205, 17–25.

Hartung, T. Toxicology for the twenty-first century, *Nature* **2009**, 460, 208–212.

Hecker, M.; Hollert, H. Endocrine disruptor screening: regulatory perspectives and needs, *Environ. Sci. Eur.* **2011**, 23, 15.

Judson, R. S.; Houck, K. A.; Kavlock, R. J.; Knudsen, T. B.; Martin, M. T.; Mortensen, H. M.; Reif, D. M.; Rotroff, D. M.; Shah, I.; Richard, A. M.; Dix, D. J. In vitro screening of environmental chemicals for targeted testing prioritization: the ToxCast project, *Environ. Health Perspect.* **2010**, 118(4), 485–492.

Kavlock, R.; Chandler, K.; Houck, K.; Hunter, S.; Judson, R.; Kleinstreuer, N.; Knudsen, T.; Martin, M.; Padilla, S.; Reif, D.; Richard, A.; Rotroff, D.; Sipes, N.; Dix, D. Update on EPA's ToxCast Program: providing high throughput decision support tools for chemical risk management, *Chem. Res. Toxicol.* **2012**, 25(7), 1287–1302.

Kramer, V. J.; Etterson, M. A.; Hecker, M.; Murphy, C. A.; Roesijadi, G.; Spade, D. J.; Spromberg, J. A.; Wang, M.; Ankley, G. T. Adverse outcome pathways and ecological risk assessment: bridging to population level effects. *Environ. Technol. Chem.* **2010**, 30(1), 64–76.

Marty, M. S.; Carney, E. W.; Rowlands, J. C. Endocrine disruption: historical perspectives and its impact on the future of toxicology testing, *Toxicol. Sci.* **2011**, 120(suppl. 1), S93–S108.

Murk, A. J.; Legler, J.; van Lipzig, H. H. M.; Meerman, J. H. N.; Belfroid, A. C.; Spenkelink, A.; Rijs, G. B.; Vethaak, D. Detection of estrogenic potency in wastewater and surface water with three in vitro bioassays, *Environ. Toxicol. Chem.* **2002**, 21(1), 16–23.

OECD, *Conceptual Framework for the Testing and Assessment of Endocrine Disrupting Chemicals*, Paris: OECD, **2002**. http://www.oecd.org/dataoecd/17/33/23652447.doc (accessed 23 Jan 2014).

OECD, *Guidance Document on Standardized Test Guidelines for Evaluating Chemicals for Endocrine Disruption, Version II*, Series on Testing and Assessment No. 150, Paris: OECD, **2012**.

Owens, W.; Gray, L. E. Jr.; Zeiger, E.; Walker, M.; Yamasaki, K.; Ashby, J., et al. The OECD program to validate the rat Hershberger bioassay to screen compounds for *in vivo* androgen and antiandrogen responses: phase 2 dose–response studies, *Environ. Health. Perspect.* **2007**, 115, 671–678.

Pickford, D. B. Screening chemicals for thyroid-disrupting activity: a critical comparison of mammalian and amphibian models, *Crit. Rev. Toxicol.* **2010**, 40(10), 845–892.

Pistollato, F.; Bremer-Hoffmann, S.; Healy, L.; Young, L.; Stacey, G. Standardization of pluripotent stem cell cultures for toxicity testing, *Expert Opin. Drug Metab. Toxicol.* **2012**, 8, 239–257.

Reif, D. M.; Martin, M. T.; Tan, S. W.; Houck, K. A.; Judson, R. S.; Richard, A. M., et al. Endocrine profiling and prioritization of environmental chemicals using ToxCast data, *Environ. Health Perspect.* **2010**, 118, 1714–1720.

Rotroff, D. M.; Dix, D. J.; Houck, K. A.; Knudsen, T. B.; Martin, M. T.; McLaurin, K. W.; Reif, D. M.; Crofton, K. M.; Singh, A. V.; Xia, M.; Huang, R.; Judson, R. S. Using *in vitro* high throughput screening assays to identify potential endocrine-disrupting chemicals, *Environ. Health Perspect.* **2013**,121, 7–14.

Routledge, E. J.; Sumpter, J. P. Estrogenic activity of surfactants and some of their degradation products assessed using a recombinant yeast screen. *Environ. Toxicol. Chem.* **1996**, 15(3), 241–248.

Seiler, A.; Oelgeschläger, M.; Liebsch, M.; Pirow, R.; Riebeling, C.; Tralau, T.; Luch, A. Developmental toxicity testing in the 21st century: the sword of Damocles shattered by embryonic stem cell assays? *Arch. Toxicol.* **2011**, 85, 1361–1372.

Shukla, S. J.; Huang, R.; Austin, C. P.; Xia, M. The future of toxicity testing: a focus on *in vitro* methods using a quantitative high-throughput screening platform, *Drug Disc. Today* **2010**, 15, 997–1007.

Stoker, T. E.; Zorrilla, L. M. The effects of endocrine disrupting chemicals on pubertal development in the rat: use of the EDSP pubertal assays as a screen, in *Endocrine Toxicology*, Eldridge, J. C.; Stevens, J. T., eds., New York: Informa Healthcare, **2010**, pp. 27–81.

Sumpter, J. P.; Johnson, A. C. 10th Anniversary perspective: reflections on endocrine disruption in the aquatic environment: from known knowns to unknown unknowns (and many things in between). *J. Environ. Monit.* **2008**, 10, 1476–1485.

Tinwell, H.; Friry-Santini, C.; Rouquié, D.; Belluco, S.; Elies, L.; Pallen, C.; Bars, R. Evaluation of the antiandrogenic effects of flutamide, DDE, and linuron in the weanling rat assay using organ weight, histopathological, and proteomic approaches, *Toxicol. Sci.* **2007**, 100(1), 54–65.

Trosko, J. E. Commentary on "Toxicity testing in the 21st century: A vision and a strategy": stem cells and cell–cell communication as fundamental targets in assessing the potential toxicity of chemicals, *Hum. Exp. Toxicol.* **2010**, 29, 21–29.

Trosko, J. E.; Chang, C. C. Factors to consider in the use of stem cells for pharmaceutic drug development and for chemical safety assessment, *Toxicology* **2010**, 270, 18–34.

UNEP/WHO, State of the science of endocrine disrupting chemicals—2012, Geneva, Switzerland: United Nations Environment Program/World Health Organization, 2012.

USEPA, Endocrine disruptor Screening Program (EDSP), Tier 1 screening battery, 2009. Available at: http://www.epa.gov/endo/pubs/assayvalidation/tier1battery.htm#assays (accessed 23 Jan 2014).

USEPA, Weight of evidence guidance: evaluating results of EDSP Tier 1 screening to identify candidate chemicals for Tier 2 testing, 2010. Available at: http://www.epa.gov/endo/pubs/EDSP_Draft_WoE_Paper_%20for_Public_Comments% 20_2010.pdf (accessed May 1, 2011).

USEPA, The future of toxicity testing is here: EPA Tox21 partnership taps high-tech robots to advance toxicity testing, *Sci. Matt. Newlett.* August, 2011. Available at: http://www.epa.gov/sciencematters/august2011/toxicity.htm (accessed 14 Jan 2014).

USEPA, ToxCast™: Screening chemicals to predict toxicity faster and better, United States Environmental Protection Agency, 2012a. Available at: http://www.epa.gov/ncct/toxcast/ (accessed 23 Jan 2014).

USEPA, Tox21 – Chemical testing in the 21st century, United States Environmental Protection Agency, 2012b. Available at: http://www.epa.gov/ncct/Tox21/ (accessed 23 Jan 2014).

USEPA, Endocrine Disruptor Screening Program; Final second list of chemicals and substances for Tier 1 screening, 2013. Available at: http://federalregister.gov/a/2013-14232 (accessed 23 Jan 2014).

Zoeller, R. T.; Brown, T. R.; Doan, L. L.; Gore, A. C.; Skakkebaek, N. E.; Soto, A. M.; Woodruff, T. J.; Vom Saal, F. S. Endocrine-disrupting chemicals and public health protection: a statement of principles from the Endocrine Society, *Endocrinology* **2012**, 153(9).

12

TRACE CONTAMINANTS: IMPLICATIONS FOR WATER QUALITY SUSTAINABILITY

12.1 INTRODUCTION

Water is fundamental to the quality of life, to economic growth, and to the environment. In the coming decades, availability of no natural resource may prove to be more critical to human health and well-being than water. However, global water challenges are also as much about quality as they are about availability. Water that is safe to drink, suitable to sustain agriculture, and available to maintain valued natural ecosystems constitutes a fundamental national and global need. Nevertheless, water quality is on the decline largely as a result of population growth, urbanization, industrial production, and environmental degradation. The availability of safe freshwater is diminishing at an alarming rate globally.

The burgeoning human population is stressing not only water resources but also food supplies, leading to rising demands for irrigation water and consequently to greater potential for water contamination by pesticides, fertilizers, and naturally occurring constituents. In a world in which only 2.5% of the water supply is fresh water – and unevenly distributed at that – this has serious implications. It is estimated that around 4 billion people worldwide have no or little access to clean and sanitized water supply (Malato et al., 2009). These statistical figures are expected to grow in the near future, as increasing water contamination occurs as a result of the presence of low levels of multiple unregulated chemical contaminants throughout the water supply (Wintgens et al., 2008; Suárez et al., 2008).

The revolution in synthetic chemistry has facilitated vast improvements in our quality of life; nonetheless, these benefits increasingly appear to have come with a hidden cost. This paradox of progress now mandates a reassessment of how our

Endocrine Disruptors in the Environment, First Edition. Sushil K. Khetan.
© 2014 John Wiley & Sons, Inc. Published 2014 by John Wiley & Sons, Inc.

consumption habits negatively impact our health. Today, nearly everything we buy, sell, and use depends on chemicals, and replacing the keystone ingredients of modern life would be challenging and require significant costs. Anthropogenic organic compounds used for many beneficial purposes in modern society commonly constitute contaminants when they are encountered in the environment (Halling-Sørensen et al., 2002). Persistent organic pollutants are prevalent among environmental contaminants because they are resistant to common modes of chemical, biological, or photolytic degradation. A contaminant is defined as "a substance that occurs in the environment at least in part as a result of man's activities and has a deleterious effect on living organisms" (Newman and Unger, 2003).

In the past decade, a great deal of interest and concern has been generated regarding trace contaminants (TCs) in water (Halling-Sorensen et al., 1998; Daughton and Terns, 1999; Snyder and Benotti, 2010; Sedlak et al., 2000; Drewes et al., 2002; Kolpin et al., 2002; Ternes et al., 2002; Westerhoff et al., 2005; Ternes and von Gunten, 2010, Richardson, 2011; Schwarzenbach et al., 2006). TCs are compounds that occur in small amounts in the environment. The term "emerging trace contaminants" is generally used to refer to substances that have no regulatory standard (Murray et al., 2010), and that have the potential to damage aquatic life and human health. They are pollutants not currently included in routine monitoring programs and may be candidates for future regulation (EPA, 2008). These pollutants include substances that have long been present in the environment but whose presence and significance are only now being elucidated (Daughton, 2004). In the literature, the terms "emerging trace contaminants" or "micropollutants" (Schwarzenbach et al, 2006) are usually used within the context of endocrine disrupting chemicals (EDCs) and pharmaceuticals and personal care products (collectively called PPCPs) (e.g., Ternes et al., 2004; Kasprzyk-Hordern et al., 2009).

Increasing sensitivity of analytical methods and growing scientific interest have resulted in the detection of a significant number of these contaminants of distinctly human origin in water supplies (Kolpin et al., 2002; Benotti et al., 2009). Many of these so-called contaminants of emerging concern have been, and will continue to be, detected in potable water supplies. It is also likely that the propensity for the contamination of fresh water will rise as human population continues to grow (Snyder and Benotti, 2010). As the power of analytical chemistry increases, the types of chemicals that can be detected also increase, and the limits of concentration at which they can be measured continually decrease. Thus, emerging contaminants (ECs) characterize the emerging awareness of the presence in the environment of many chemicals used by society and the concern over the risk that these chemicals may pose to humans and ecosystems (Daughton, 2001). Recent developments in analyzing the ECs have been reviewed (Richardson and Ternes, 2011).

12.2   TRACE CONTAMINANTS SOURCES IN WATER

Organic TCs are ubiquitous in the environment, especially in aquatic ecosystems, entering them largely through surface water runoff and through discharges of wastewater with chemical contaminants not completely removed by current treatment processes (Snyder et al., 2001; Kolpin et al., 2004; Voutsa et al., 2006). About 30% of the globally accessible renewable freshwater is used by industry and municipalities, generating together an enormous amount of wastewater containing numerous chemicals in varying concentrations. These wastewater discharges include household and industrial chemicals such as flame retardants, plasticizers, detergent metabolites, and commonly used PPCPs such as prescription and non-prescription drugs, fragrances, and antimicrobial cleaning agents. Thus, a major contribution to chemical contamination originates from wastewater discharges that impact surface water quality with incompletely removed organic contaminants (Kolpin et al., 2004; Snyder et al., 2001). Some of these compounds are known or suspected carcinogens, while others are estrogenic and have the potential to adversely affect the endocrine system of humans and aquatic organisms.

Additional contamination comes from diffuse agricultural activities, in which over 140 million tons of fertilizers and several million tons of pesticides are applied each year, and from atmospheric deposition. Leaching from septic tanks and municipal landfills and land application of biosolids (sludge) from wastewater treatment plants (WWTP) continue to be important sources of contaminants to groundwater (Clarke and Smith, 2011). Other potential routes of TCs include runoff from confined animal feeding operations, medicated pet excreta, aquaculture, spray-drift of chemicals used in agriculture, and the direct discharge of raw sewage (Fig. 12.1). Measurable concentrations of many of the TCs have been found in wastewater, surface waters, sediments, groundwater, and even drinking water (Petrovic et al., 2004; Benfenati et al., 2003, Petrovic et al., 2003; Snyder et al., 2003). These TCs affect the biological, chemical, and physical integrity of water, and could have profound effects on the flora and fauna that rely on clean waters. The variety of anthropogenic chemicals in the environment and the potential adverse impact on human health and the ecology of the natural environment are viewed with concern.

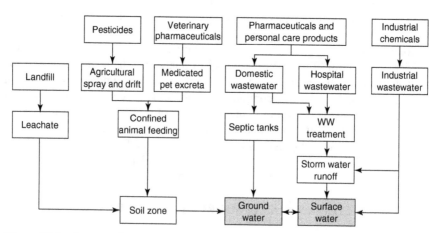

Figure 12.1   Sources of trace contaminants in water supply. Source: Adapted from Stuart et al. (2012). Reproduced with permission from Elsevier.

Many of the contaminants identified have the potential to cause an estrogenic response at very low concentrations (parts per billion to parts per trillion). Numerous examples of endocrine disruption identified in wildlife involve animals that are living in or closely associated with the aquatic environment. This is perhaps not surprising considering that surface water acts as a sink for both natural and anthropogenic chemicals discharged into the environment (Walker, 2009; Sumpter, 1997). The quantity of chemicals within the aquatic environment, together with the inherent susceptibility of aquatic life to the effects of EDCs, leads to significant impacts on the biota of aquatic ecosystems. In certain water bodies with large inputs of anthropogenic chemicals, aquatic life could be continually exposed to a range of EDCs, with some at concentrations that have been reported in the ranges of nanograms per liter.

12.3 WASTEWATER RECLAMATION PROCESSES

Global water sustainability depends in part upon effective reuse of water. As aquifers are depleted and global freshwater supplies continue to shrink, reuse of wastewater, directly or indirectly, becomes an attractive mechanism for supplementing the drinking water supply. The overarching goal for the future of reclamation and reuse of water is to capture water directly from nontraditional sources such as industrial or municipal wastewater and restore it. Use of surface water for potable water production is increasing, and in some places a significant share of this comprises wastewater effluent.

Once a WWTP discharges, natural attenuation occurs through microbial degradation, dilution, adsorption to solids, photolysis, or other forms of abiotic transformation. However, the natural processes are generally inefficient to reduce TCs to non-detect levels (Gerrity and Snyder, 2011). Biodegradation or biotransformation of TCs may take place only if a primary organic substrate is available for the bacteria to grow on. In the co-degradation scenario, the bacteria break down or partially convert the TC and do not use it as a carbon source. In another possible scenario, mixed-substrate growth takes place and the bacteria use the TC as a carbon and energy source and may mineralize it totally (Ternes et al., 2004).

Water utilities select a treatment train that is most appropriate for the contaminants found in the source water. The most commonly used processes include coagulation, sedimentation, filtration, and disinfection for surface water (Fig. 12.2).

12.3.1 Primary Treatment: Sedimentation/Coagulation

Chemical coagulation in water treatment employs aluminum sulfate or ferric chloride, which precipitate as metal hydroxides. Chemical lime softening removes dissolved calcium and magnesium, removing suspended solids (i.e., turbidity) from the water, and aid in removing dissolved organic carbon (DOC). However, coagulation alone is generally not effective in removing trace-level organic pollutants

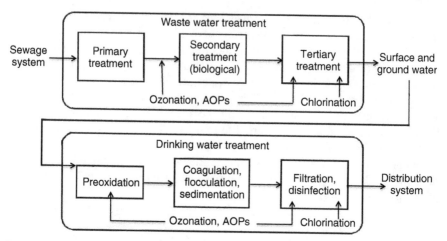

Figure 12.2   Possible applications of ozonation and advanced oxidation processes (AOPs) in treatment of wastewater and drinking water. Source: Adapted from Ikehata et al. (2006). Reprinted with permission from Taylor & Francis Ltd, http://www.tandf.co.uk/journals.

(Westerhoff et al., 2005; Snyder et al., 2007). For example, after aluminum sulfate coagulation, no removal of EE2 and only 5% and 2% elimination for E1 and E2, respectively, were observed (Westerhoff et al., 2005). A slightly higher efficiency of removals (20–50%) of natural estrogens and EE2 has been reported at a concentration of aluminum sulfate of 5 mg/l (Chen et al. (2007).

12.3.2   Secondary Treatment: Removal by Physical Methods or Biological Process

Filtration of water using traditional media (i.e., sand/anthracite) or activated carbon can help to remove some TCs. Rapid filtration through crushed anthracite-packed columns was observed to eliminate efficiently E1, E2, EE2 (95–99%), and E3 (84–93%) as a result of adsorption of these compounds to the layer of anthracite. Filtration of water containing these substances through sand-packed columns only removed 31–42% of the initial compound concentration (Chen et al., 2007). Membrane filtration (nanofiltration and reverse osmosis) has been shown to remove estrogens, with elimination rates between 60% and 85%, during drinking water treatment processes (Yoon et al., 2006; McCallum et al., 2008).

Adsorption using activated carbon has proven to be well suited to remove trace-level organic pollutants from water because of its high surface area and the combination of a well-developed pore structure and surface chemistry (Redding et al., 2009). It effectively removes many problematic organic pollutants, including a broad range of representative EDCs, such as steroid hormones, triclosan, bisphenol A, and so on (Westerhoff et al., 2005; Yoon et al., 2006; Liu et al., 2009). Granular activated carbon is used in a fixed-bed process such as granular media filtration whereas powdered activated carbon is added to water as a suspension, allowed to adsorb constituents from water, and then separated from the finished water. For example, powder activated carbon (5 mg/l with 4 h contact time) was able to remove 76%, 84%, 60%, and 77% of E1, E2, E3, and EE2, respectively (Westerhoff et al., 2005). However, disadvantage of physical methods is the need for post-treatment of the absorbent material or the generated waste, which increases their cost.

WWTPs typically employ biological processes for reduction of total suspended solids, dissolved organic matter (measured as biological oxygen demand), and nutrient loads prior to discharge into the receiving waters. The processes employed as secondary wastewater treatment include aerated conventional activated sludge (CAS) systems, or membrane bioreactors (MBRs), as a potential alternative (LeClech et al., 2006; Sahar et al., 2011). CAS process is a biological process that involves a mixed culture of suspended microorganisms for aerobic biodegradation of suspended and dissolved organics in wastewater. MBRs are a modification of the CAS process in which the secondary clarifier employing gravity settling has been replaced with membrane filtration. MBR and CAS systems remove micropollutants by either biological degradation or adsorption to the sludge, which is then physically removed from the wastewater. However, persistent polar metabolites and transformation products may survive the treatment processes and end up in drinking water sources.

12.3.3 Tertiary Treatment: Redox Processes

Redox processes supplement the aforementioned physical methods and have been widely investigated for treatment of secondary wastewater effluent, and in the pre-treatment and disinfection step of drinking water. Oxidation processes have shown satisfactory removal efficiency for EDCs, but present as the main drawback the formation of disinfection byproducts. Chlorination with chlorine dioxide and chlorine usually gives rise to both chlorination and oxidation products, in many cases with increased toxicity and biological activity relative to the parent compound.

Advanced Oxidation Processes (AOPs) developed for aqueous waste treatment and removal of TCs include ozonation, UV radiation, Fenton processes, hydrogen peroxide (H_2O_2), and catalysts such as titanium dioxide (TiO_2). Ozone can accomplish excellent removal of many compounds, but ozone-based AOPs such as ozone/UV and ozone/hydrogen peroxide can achieve higher removal of some compounds than ozone can by itself. These processes rely upon the formation of powerful radical species, primarily hydroxyl radicals ($\cdot OH$), and are rapidly gaining in use for the oxidation of many trace organic chemicals and industrial solvents (Esplugas et al., 2007). They have proven to effectively oxidize a broad variety of organic pollutants at both low and high concentrations. AOPs generally can achieve better removal than conventional oxidants and lead not only to the decomposition of target pollutants but also to complete mineralization if the treatment time is sufficient. However, it may not be necessary to operate the processes to this level of treatment. In those cases, the target pollutants can be degraded to the stage of biodegradable intermediates.

The enormous diversity of toxic and organic pollutants of different chemical composition eliminates the possibility of using a universal treatment method for water decontamination. Current disinfectants such as chlorine and ozone have the potential to generate toxic byproducts (e.g., trihalomethanes and bromide). Nanostructured crystalline TiO_2-based nanomaterials have gained significant recognition in environmental remediation of water. The findings suggest the possibility of employing TiO_2 nanoparticles as photocatalysts in solar-driven water treatment technologies as a sustainable approach for water contaminated with environmental contaminants of concern (Savage and Diallo, 2005).

12.4   INDIRECT WATER REUSE SYSTEMS

It is common in many of the US water systems to use water supply from a running source that receives treated wastewater discharges further upstream. This is a *de facto* reuse of treated wastewater to augment drinking water supplies. The use of treated wastewater (also known as reclaimed water) for drinking water augmentation, as well as for irrigation and industrial uses, is currently in practice in many areas as shortages of water supplies are becoming prevalent and severe with the ever-increasing population. Although this could significantly increase the total available water resources in the United States (NRC, 2012), the propensity of water contamination is greatly increased. Nevertheless, a risk analysis found that the risk of exposure to certain microbial and chemical contaminants from drinking reclaimed water is not any higher than that from drinking water from current water treatment systems – and in some cases may be orders of magnitude lower. Therefore, adjustments to the federal regulatory framework could enhance public health protection and increase public confidence in water reuse. In many urban areas that are under water stress (California, Australia, Singapore), direct or indirect potable or industrial reuse is practiced on large scales. Nonetheless, a concern remains on TC levels.

12.4.1   Removal of Trace Contaminants for Potable Water Reuse Applications

The relevance of EDCs as potential contaminants of drinking water is important, particularly in the reuse of wastewater. As discussed earlier, significant amounts of EDCs can be removed from wastewater via biological adsorption/oxidation processes in WWTPs, yet considerable quantities still remain in the effluents. These contaminants may be diluted, sequestered (e.g., in sediment), or degraded by physical or biological processes, but some are detected in the environment because of their persistence or relatively constant loading. Many EDCs have been frequently detected in wastewater-impacted surface waters in the United States (Bradley and Kolpin, 2013).

Reverse osmosis, in which clean water is driven through a membrane under pressure leaving a concentrated waste stream behind, and UV/H_2O_2 are the most common technologies for water reuse. However, concentrate discharge issues, chemical costs, and energy requirements hinder these options. The use of O_3 in water reuse applications is becoming an increasingly popular alternative because of its similar efficacy in reducing TCs concentrations with limited to no chemical addition and the potential for reduced energy requirements. The use of AOP appears to be favorable for reuse applications that require high-quality treated water, such as groundwater recharge and indirect potable reuse. A consequence of AOP is that total dissolved solids (TDSs), which can increase with AOP, have to be removed before reuse (Melcer and Klecka, 2011).

Futuristic direct reuse systems envisioned could integrate AOPs, including photocatalysis, using sunlight as the irradiation source and a biological single-stage MBR with an immersed nanofiltration membrane as part of a treatment train of biorecalcitrant pollutants, to provide an absolute barrier to pathogens and to destroy TCs that may pass the nanofiltration barrier (Shannon *et al.*, 2008; Malato et al., 2009; Oller et al., 2011). In Europe, the integrated use of conventional biological treatment with AOP has been applied to increase biodegradability and detoxification of effluent streams (Belgiorno et al., 2007; Ning et al., 2007).

In many potable water reuse systems, water is discharged after treatment to a natural system such as an aquifer, a reservoir, or a wetland, providing a buffer between water treatment and consumption (NRC, 2012). No regulatory limits have been established for TCs in drinking water. Nonetheless, recognizing that EDC effects on human health and aquatic life is still an evolving field and that regulatory requirements need to be based on best available science, a provision for monitoring was included in the Recycled Water Policy (2009) of the State of California's Water Resources Control Board (Anderson et al., 2010).

The California Department of Public Health (CDPH) specified in its Draft Groundwater Recharge Reuse Regulations that trace organics including PPCPs, EDCs, hormones, and other indicator compounds (caffeine and pharmaceuticals) need be monitored in recycled water used to recharge groundwater basins designated as domestic water supplies (CDPH, 2008). For water reuse in the United States, states can refer to the U.S. Environmental Protection Agency (EPA) guidelines for water reuse (EPA, 2004), CDPH Title 22 requirements (CDPH, 2008), or local standards for wastewater contaminants. For unrestricted urban reuse, states in the United States generally specify an acceptable treatment train in addition to turbidity and disinfection requirements.

12.5 LEACHING OF CONTAMINANTS IN WATER – THE CASE OF BOTTLED WATER

Concern for water quality has turned a large population to drink from bottled water. Bottled water is a unique conundrum in terms of regulation and the water's purity. In the United States, the Food and Drug Administration (FDA) regulates bottled water under the Federal Food, Drug, and Cosmetic Act, but the EPA regulates drinking water (tap water), and the two agencies' regulatory standards are not the same (Birnbaum and Jung, 2011). Mineral water bottled in polyethylene terephthalate (PET) and water in glass bottles or even tap water has been demonstrated to have some weak endocrine activity (Pinto and Reali, 2009; Wagner and Oehlmann, 2009). For example, additives such as bisphenol A, which are used as plasticizers in some packaging material, were shown to leach into the water. Seventy-eight percent of all samples from PET bottles bought in Germany showed estrogenic potentials with concentration equivalents of up to 75 ng 17β-estradiol per liter (Wagner and Oehlmann, 2009). In Italy, 10% of the investigated samples showed estrogenic activity, with maximum concentration equivalents of 23 ng 17β-estradiol per liter (Hecker and Hollert, 2011). The rate of leaching increased with both temperature and contact time (Keresztes et al., 2009).

12.6 WATER QUALITY SUSTAINABILITY AND HEALTH EFFECTS

Sustainable development is a key demand in our world of finite resources and endangered ecosystems. Adapting the United Nations definition, sustainability is defined *meeting the needs of the present without compromising the ability of future generations to meet their own needs* (Bruntland, 1987). The key point of this approach is to avoid irreversible damages to natural capital in the long term in turn for short-term benefits. When talking about creating a product, process, or system, the primary goal needs to be met without causing adverse unintended consequences. Thus, many potential environmental problems can be avoided by intelligent choices. By choosing to pursue the goal of perfect sustainability, it will result in continuous improvements and an integrated and cohesive approach to solving the problems we understand. This involves integrating economic progress, environmental stewardship, and ethical/social equity criteria and encapsulates the important issues in water policy.

Interest in the significance of trace levels of contaminants in potable water in public health is increasing, particularly with regard to the effects of long-term, low-dose exposures. Possible health effects of long-term exposure to contaminants via drinking water could include endocrine disruption, including effects on reproduction or fetal/child development; birth defects; metabolic, immune, and neurodevelopmental disorders; enhanced predisposition to cancer, overall accounting for one-sixth of the total burden of disease (Gross, 2007). With more recent knowledge and advances, concern becomes greater regarding the potential for long-term adverse effects of low, continuous exposure to many chemicals (Frazzoli et al., 2009).

Animals (and humans) are exposed to endocrine disruptors at all stages of their life cycle, and the effects of such exposures are now known to be passed to subsequent generations. The understanding of the nature and extent of health effects produced on developing organisms, from the prenatal period to adolescence, by the exposure to environmental agents is still incomplete; even so, significant evidence-based literature reports have been accumulated on the role played by several environmental factors in determining disease in children and in inducing effects that may become manifest only in adult life (Gross, 2007). In addition, evidence suggests that prenatal environmental exposures can significantly increase the risk of developing chronic diseases later in life, including male infertility, pregnancy loss, diseases of the uterus (e.g., endometriosis), malformations of the reproductive system (e.g., hypospadia and cryptorchidism), increased susceptibility to cancer of the testis and other target tissues, diabetes, cardiovascular disease, obesity, and psychiatric and behavioral conditions such as schizophrenia and mood disorders (Bernal and Jirtle, 2010). Numerous studies report a relation between exposure to EDCs and diseases and developmental delays in children (WHO, 2002). Many environmental toxins are able to cross the placenta and produce developmental defects in maternally exposed offspring (Patisaul and Adewale, 2009). The extent of hazardous exposure occurring during intrauterine and early life creates a body burden that may reveal later in life up to adulthood (EFSA, 2005), thus generating a problem of health sustainability for next generation.

12.7 TOXICOLOGICAL IMPLICATIONS

Aquatic toxicity, a major environmental concern and one of the leading indicators of anthropogenic impacts to natural systems, is of particular interest because numerous industrial chemicals directly or inadvertently enter surface and ground water. Human health standards in food, water, and air are based on the fact that for the vast majority of chemicals there is a safe level of exposure below which no adverse health effects are expected to occur. Methods used for drinking water guidelines/standards are frequently based on health or toxicological data grounded on the concept of acceptable daily intake (ADI) or tolerable daily intake (TDI) assuming a lifetime exposure. For human use of water, the exposure to chemicals is based on a daily consumption of water of 2 l/day over a lifetime, typically 70 years with no toxicological effects. Presently, for unknown compounds in drinking water, a threshold of toxicological concern (TTC) is applied (0.1 µg/l for nongenotoxic compounds; 0.01 µg/l for genotoxic compounds (Schriks et al., 2010).

The detection of many ECs in drinking water and its environmental sources (surface water and groundwater) raises considerable public concern. Especially when human health-based guideline values are not available, it is questionable whether the detected concentrations affect human health. As the detection of many of TCs is recent, no robust methods for their quantification and toxicological data for interpreting potential human or ecosystem health effects are available. Also, the toxicological relevance of many other unknown compounds for humans is often unknown. Uncertainty exists about the potential health impacts of long-term exposure to PPCPs and EDCs present at trace levels in drinking water, including especially the input of multiple chemicals at the same time (Jones et al., 2005).

In most of the investigations, the efficiency of removal of TCs is determined by measuring the disappearance of the parent compound during water treatment and little attention paid for the transformation products formed. Information on metabolites formed biotically, such as human metabolites excreted into the environment or the microbial metabolites formed during environmental biodegradation of ECs, is important to make ecological risk assessment and fathom their potential long-term adverse effects on humans and wildlife. Similarly, other toxic derivatives that need examination include those formed during abiotic treatment (such as chlorination, ozonation, or ultraviolet, UV exposure) employed in disinfection or AOP in water treatment.

Recent advances in mixture toxicity contribute to a more holistic appraisal of the effect assessment in toxicology. For exposure assessment, the same holistic view is desirable, but it is obstructed by the limitation of analytical tools to elucidate the entire chemical universe including an unknown number of yet-to-be identified compounds. The new effects-based methods include cell-based and low-complexity *in vitro* bioassays that can help to overcome this shortcoming because they characterize the actual biological effect of a complex sample and thus integrate the effects of unidentified compounds and potential mixtures. These methods hold great promise for applications to water quality assessment.

12.8   REGULATORY STRUCTURES TO MAINTAIN WATER QUALITY

In United States, the Clean Water Act was enacted to restore and maintain the chemical, physical, and biological integrity of the nation's waters. The goal of the Act is to guarantee water quality, and provides for the protection and propagation of fish, shellfish, and wildlife and for recreation. It is perhaps the most promising of existing frameworks of regulatory mechanisms, which if implemented fully could both limit human exposure to waterborne EC pollution and protect aquatic environments and species from EC harm (Lopez, 2010).

Drinking water, or potable water, is water intended for human consumption, with no other ingredient except that it may contain safe and suitable disinfectants. In the United States, under the 1974 Safe Drinking Water Act (SDWA), the EPA regulates drinking water. Making certain that drinking water is safe will also require determining and implementing guidelines for maximum acceptable concentrations of known ECs and their mixtures in drinking water (Falconer et al., 2006). The EPA already regulates more than 90 contaminants and has listed in its third (water) contaminant candidate list (CCL-3) several pharmaceuticals, pesticides, estrogenic hormones, perchlorate, and perfluorooctanoic acid (PFOA), and perfluorooctane sulfonate (PFOS), to prioritize research and data collection (EPA, 2011a). These contaminants are frequently detected in the freshwater environment and pose a human health hazard at environmental concentrations and therefore have high priority for regulation and treatment (Murray et al., 2010).

In the European Union, the primary piece of legislation governing drinking water is the Water Framework Directive (WFD – 2000/60/EC), and each member state is responsible for its implementation and inspection (Kaika, 2003). WFD identifies "substances and preparations, or the breakdown products of such, which have been proved to possess carcinogenic or mutagenic properties or properties which may affect steroidogenic, thyroid, reproduction or other endocrine-related functions in or via the aquatic environment." WFD also establishes a corresponding "Indicative List of the Main Pollutants" of concern. The European Drinking Water Directive sets limits for a small number of organic micropollutants. Proposed revisions include the ECs such as α-ethinylestradiol, β-estradiol, and PFOS (ClickGreen, 2012). Their inclusion addresses the potential harmful effects of their presence in the aquatic environment.

Increasing demands for sources of clean water, combined with changing land use practices, growth, aging infrastructure, and climate change and variability, pose significant threats to the US water resources. EPA, which is responsible for protecting America's water resources under the Clean Water Act and for ensuring that the Nation's drinking water is safe under the SDWA, is integrating its Drinking Water and Water Quality research programs to establish a Safe and Sustainable Water Resources Research Program to seek sustainable solutions to the problems facing US water resources. The goal is to ensure safe and sustainable water quality and availability to protect human and ecosystem health, as well as to meet societal, economic, and environmental needs. Another goal is to provide the tools and technology for sustainable drinking water and wastewater infrastructure management for water reuse (EPA, 2011b).

12.9 CONCLUSIONS AND FUTURE PROSPECTS

Adequate water supply of sufficient quality is critical to support human health and aquatic ecosystems. Given the current knowledge base on EDCs, it is clear that ensuring the availability of safe and sustainable water supply will be increasingly challenging. Emerging TCs, such as EDCs and PPCPs, are commonly described as chemicals or materials that have a real or perceived threat to human health or the environment. The very nature of wastewater suggests that nearly any substance used or excreted by humans has the potential to be present at some concentration in the treated water.

The ability to detect chemical contaminants in drinking water at low, biologically relevant concentrations quickly can help in identifying emerging health threats. Even though the elimination of TCs is mostly achieved via chlorination, ozonation and AOPs, byproducts generated can be less biodegradable and/or more toxic than the parent compound. There is increasing need for more efficient and cost-effective methods for treatment of wastewaters and raw waters for human consumption because demand for clean water is steadily rising. The environmental hazard of TCs may be enhanced via association with complex mixtures of other contaminants, human metabolites, and degradation products, as well as other residues present in municipal wastewater.

In the long run, it is vital to society that the chemical industry and the environmental community establish a dialogue to better control TCs in reclaimed water. Thus, good integrated management practices and technologies are needed to prevent further deterioration of our water sources by stopping endocrine-disruptive pollutants from entering our waterways. It will be much easier to prevent the release of contaminants into the waste stream than remove trace levels of compounds that have unknown health consequences and are difficult to measure, biodegrade, and treat (Levine and Asano, 2004).

Many of the materials that get eventually classified as EDCs are undeniably useful when originally used. They protect our grapes from fungus, our leafy greens from pests, and our children from fire ants and flammable pajamas. They lubricate machinery in our factories, refineries, and power plants. Even so, there needs to be a balance between the benefits of these "emerging pollutants" for the quality of life and the risks to humans and the environment, and this will be a difficult social task. There is a need to distinguish between those chemicals that can have permanent effects in the exposed individuals and their descendants, even in the absence of further exposure, and those compounds that have transient effects that can be mitigated or reversed through education, decontamination, and therapeutic manipulations. It is crucial that people have adequate information regarding the many chemicals that are present in our drinking water, food, containers, plastics, detergents, and so on. Chemicals that individuals encounter and ingest in small doses every day could have potentially serious health consequences, both for current and future generations, including infertility, immune disorders, metabolic disorders, and cancer (Van der Mude, 2011). Therefore, there is an urgent need for research programs that elucidate potential risks posed by various contaminants of emerging concern to human health and the environment (Novak et al., 2011).

Smarter regulation alone will not change the fact that the science on chemicals and health – especially for complex endocrine disrupters – will likely never be clear-cut, no matter how many studies are carried out. The scientific disagreements arise because the researchers hail from different disciplines such as endocrinology, toxicology, epidemiology, and chemistry, and also because they work in different cultures such as academia, industry, government, and environmental health and safety advocacy. Therefore, protection of water resources would need the efforts of all stakeholders involved in the water cycle. Successfully engaging the public is critical for making meaningful progress toward sustainability. Manufacturers, users, consumers, governments, administration, water utilities, and waste water services must work together to protect water resources from these substances in order to minimize as well as prevent negative impacts in the long term. Also, a sea change in research is necessary, from simply trying to understand the specific molecular target of an EDC, to focusing instead on the consequences for the population.

In 2012, a liability claim for atrazine-contaminated water supplies was successfully fought against the Swiss crop protection firm Syngenta. The weed killer, used to control broadleaf and grassy weeds primarily to corn, gets into streams and rivers as runoff after rainstorms, where it can enter drinking water supplies and can cause low birth weight, birth defects, and other reproductive problems if ingested. The lawsuit claimed that the company knew that atrazine would enter the drinking water systems that provide water to 52 million Americans. Syngenta denied it did anything wrong, but reached a $105 million agreement to defray the cost of removing atrazine from drinking water (Bomgardner, 2012). This settlement, being the first of its kind related to an EDC for protection of health of the affected population, could be the forerunner for various TCs entering into environmental waters used as source for drinking water supplies. It is likely that producers of these chemicals might face similar liability claims once the science clearly pinpoints individual chemicals for adverse effect on human health.

Addressing sustainability issues such as water and food production cannot be a choice between resources and the environment. Instead, there have to be more innovative solutions. Water quantity will not dramatically increase, so water quality must be addressed. The US intelligence community believes that fresh water supplies are unlikely to keep up with global demand by 2040 and there is no technological "silver bullet" on the horizon to improve water management. A lot of contamination is due to human waste, and there is also a large amount of industrial waste containing persistent metals and organics that must be and can be avoided from the beginning. The most important step to address the problem would be more efficient use for agriculture, which accounts for 70% of global fresh water use (Quinn, 2012).

REFERENCES

Anderson, P.; Denslow, N.; Drewes, J. E.; Olivieri, A.; Schlenk, D.; Snyder, S. *Monitoring strategies for chemicals of emerging concern (CECs) in recycled water, Final Report*, State Water Resources Control Board, Scramento, California, June **2010**.

Belgiorno, V.; Rizzo, L.; Fatta, D.; Rocca, C. D.; Lofrano, G.; Nikolaou, A.; Naddeo, V.; Meric, S. Review on endocrine disrupting-emerging compounds in urban wastewater: occurrence and removal by photocatalysis and ultrasonic irradiation for wastewater reuse, *Desalination* **2007**, 215, 166–176.

Benfenati, E.; Barceló, D.; Johnson, I.; Galassi, S.; Levsen, K. Emerging organic contaminants in leachates from industrial waste landfills and industrial effluent, *Trends Anal. Chem.* **2003**, 22, 757–765.

Benotti, M. J.; Trenholm, R. A.; Vanderford, B. J.; Holady, J. C.; Stanford, B. D.; Snyder, S. A. Pharmaceuticals and endocrine disrupting compounds in U.S. drinking water, *Environ. Sci. Technol.* **2009**, 43, 597–603.

Bernal, A. J.; Jirtle, R. L. Epigenomic disruption: the effects of early developmental exposures. *Birth Defects Res. A: Clin. Mol. Teratol.* **2010**, 88, 938–944.

Birnbaum, L. S.; Jung, P. From endocrine disruptors to nanomaterials: advancing our understanding of environmental health to protect public health, *Health Affairs* **2011**, 30(5), 814–822.

Bomgardner, M. M. Syngenta settles atrazine suite, *C&E News* **2012**, 90(23), 7.

Bradley, P. M.; Kolpin, D. W. Managing the effects of endocrine disrupting chemicals in wastewater-impacted streams, in *Current Perspectives in Contaminant Hydrology and Water Resources Sustainability*, Bradley, P. M., ed.,Intech, **2013**, pp. 1–26.

Bruntland, G. H. *Our Common Future, United Nations World Commission on Environment and Development (WCED)*, Oxford University Press, Oxford, **1987**.

CDPH, *Groundwater Recharge Reuse Draft Regulation, Title 22*, California Department of Public Health, 2008; Available at: http://www.cdph.ca.gov/certlic/drinkingwater/ Documents/Recharge/ DraftRechargeReg2008.pdf (accessed on 10 Oct. 2013).

Chen, C. Y.; Wen, T. Y.; Wang, G. S.; Cheng, H. W.; Lin, Y. H.; Lien, G. W. Determining estrogenic steroids in Taipei waters and removal in drinking water treatment using high-flow solid-phase extraction and liquid chromatography, *Sci. Total Environ.* **2007**, 378, 352–365.

Clarke, B. O.; Smith, S. E. Review of "emerging" organic contaminants in biosolids and assessment of international research priorities for the agricultural use of biosolids, *Environ. Int.* **2011**, 3, 226–247.

ClickGreen staff, *Europe to target pharmaceutical pollution with new water quality rules*, January 31, 2012. Available at: www.clickgreen.org.uk/news/international-news/123110-europe-to-target-pharmaceutical-pollution-with-new-water-quality-rules.html (accessed on 10 Oct. 2013).

Daughton, C. G. Non-regulated water contaminants: emerging research, *Environ. Impact Assess. Rev.* **2004**, 24, 711–732.

Daughton C. G. Pharmaceuticals and personal care products in the environment: overarching issues and overview, In *Pharmaceuticals and Personal Care Products in the Environment: Scientific and Regulatory Issues*, Daughton C. G.; Jones Lepp, T. L., ACS Symposium Series 791, Washington, DC: American Chemical Society, **2001**, pp. 2–38.

Daughton, C. G.; Ternes, T. A. Pharmaceuticas and personal care products in the environment: agents of subtle change? *Environ. Health Perspect.* **1999**, 107(6), 907–938.

Drewes, J. E.; Heberer, T.; Reddersen, K. Fate of pharmaceuticals during indirect potable reuse, *Water Sci. Technol.* **2002**, 46(3), 73–80.

EPA, *Guidelines for Water Reuse, EPA/625/R-04/108*, Washington, DC: Office of Water, EPA, **2004**.

EPA, *Aquatic Life Criteria for Contaminants of Emerging Concern*, Washington, DC: Science Advisory Board, Emerging Contaminants Work Group, U.S. Environment Protection Agency, **2008**. Available at: http://www.epa.gov/waterscience/criteria/library/sab-emergingconcerns.pdf (accessed on 15 September 2013).

EPA, *Contaminant Candidate List 3 (CCL3)*; Washington, DC: United States Environmental Protection Agency, 2011a. Available at: http://www.epa.gov/ogwdw000/ccl/ccl3.html#ccl3

EPA, *Framework for an EPA Safe and Sustainable Water Resources Research Program*, Office of Research and Development Office of Water Region VI, U. S. Environmental Protection Agency, June 2011b. Available at: http://www.epa.gov/ord/priorities/docs/SSWRFramework.pdf

Esplugas, S. Bila, D. M.; Krause, L. G.; Dezotti, M. Ozonation and advanced oxidation technologies to remove endocrine disrupting chemicals (EDCs) and pharmaceuticals and personal care products (PPCPs) in water effluents, *J. Hazard. Mat.* **2007**, 149(3), 631–642.

Falconer, I. R.; Chapman, H. F.; Moore, M. R.; Ranmuthugala, G. Endocrine-disrupting compounds: a review of their challenge to sustainable and safe water supply and water reuse, *Environ. Toxicol.* **2006**, 21(2), 181–191.

Frazzoli, C.; Petrini, C.; Mantovani, A. Sustainable development and next generation's health: a long-term perspective about the consequences of today's activities for food safety, *Ann. Ist Super Sanità* **2009**, 45(1), 65–75.

Gerrity, D.; Snyder, S. Review of ozone for water reuse applications: toxicity, regulations, and trace organic contaminant mitigation, *Ozone Sci. Eng.* **2011**, 33, 253–266.

Gross L. The toxic origins of disease, *PLoS Biol.* **2007**, 5, e193.

Halling-Sørensen, B.; Nielson, S. N.; Lanzky, I. F.; Holten, L. J.; Jorgensen, S. E. Occurrence, fate, and effects of pharmaceutical substances in the environment — a review, *Chemosphere* **2002**, 35, 357–393.

Halling-Sorensen, B.; Nielsen, S. N.; Lanzky, P. F. et al. Occurrence, fate and effects of pharmaceutical substances in the environment–a review, *Chemosphere* **1998**, 36(2), 357–393.

Hecker, M.; Hollert, H. Endocrine disruptor screening: regulatory perspectives and needs, *Environ. Sci. Europe* **2011**, 23, 15.

Ikehata, K.; Naghashkar, N. J.; Gamal El-Din, M. Degradation of aqueous pharmaceuticals by ozonation and advanced oxidation processes: a review, *Ozone Sci. Eng.* **2006**, 28(6), 353–414.

Jones, O. A.; Lester, J. N.; et al., Pharmaceuticals: a threat to drinking water? *Trends Biotechnol.* **2005**, 23(4), 163–167.

Kaika, M. The water framework directive: a new directive for a changing social, political, and economic European framework, *Euro. Plan. Stud.* **2003**, 11(3), 299–316.

Kasprzyk-Hordern, B., Dinsdale, R.M., Guwy, A.J. The removal of pharmaceuticals, personal care products, endocrine disruptors and illicit drugs during wastewater treatment and its impact on the quality of receiving waters, *Water Res.* **2009**, 43, 363–380.

Keresztes, S.; Tatár, E.; Mihucz, V. G.; Virág, I.; Majdik, C.; Záray, G. Leaching of antimony from polyethylene terephthalate (PET) bottles into mineral water, *Sci. Total Environ.* **2009**, 407(16), 4731–4735.

Kolpin, D. W.; Skopec, M.; Meyer, M. T.; Furlong, E. T.; Zaugg, S. D. Urban contribution of pharmaceuticals and other organic wastewater contaminants to streams during differing flow conditions, *Sci. Total Environ.* **2004**, 328, 119–130.

Kolpin, D. W.; Furlong, E. T.; Meyer, M. T.; Thurman, E. M.; Zaugg, S. D.; Barber, L. B.; Buxton, H. T. Pharmaceuticals, hormones, and other organic wastewater contaminants in U.S. streams, 1999–2000: a national reconnaissance. *Environ. Sci. Technol.* **2002**, 36 (6), 1202–1211.

LeClech, P.; Chen, V.; Fane, T. Fouling in membrane bioreactors used in wastewater treatment, *J. Membrane Sci.* **2006**, 284, 17–53.

Levine, A. D.; Asano, T. Peer Reviewed: Recovering sustainable water from wastewater: society no longer has the luxury of using water only once, *Environ. Sci. Technol.* **2004**, 38(11), 201A–208A.

Liu, Z. H.; Kanjo, Y.; Mizutani, S. Removal mechanisms for endocrine disrupting compounds (EDCs) in wastewater treatment – physical means, biodegradation, and chemical advanced oxidation: a review, *Sci. Total Environ.* **2009**, 407, 731–748.

Lopez, J. Endocrine-disrupting chemical pollution: why the EPA should regulate the chemicals under the clean water act, *Sustainable Development Law & Policy* **2010**, 19–23.

Malato, S.; Fernandez-Ibanez, P.; Maldonado, M. I.; Blanco, J.; Gernjak, W. Decontamination and disinfection of water by solar photocatalysis: recent overview and trends, *Catal. Today* **2009**, 147(1), 1–59.

McCallum, E. A.; Hyung, H.; Do, T. A.; Huang, C. H.; Kim, J. H. Adsorption, desorption, and steady-state removal of 17β-estradiol by nanofiltration membranes, *J. Membr. Sci.* **2008**, 319, 38–43.

Melcer, H.; Klecka, G. Treatment of wastewaters containing bisphenol A: state of science review, *Water Environ. Res.* **2011**, 83(7), 650–656.

Murray, K. E.; Thomas, S. M.; Bodour, A. A. Prioritizing research for trace pollutants and emerging contaminants in the freshwater environment, *Environ. Pollut.* **2010**, 158(12), 3462–3471.

Newman, M. C.; Unger, M. A. *Fundamentals of Ecotoxicology*, 2nd ed., Boca Raton, FL: Lewis Publishers, **2003**, p. 458.

Ning, B.; Graham, N.; Zhang, Y. P.; Nakonechny, M.; El-Din, M. G.; Degradation of endocrine disrupting chemicals by ozone/AOPs, *Ozone: Sci. Eng.* **2007**, 29(3), 153–176.

Novak, P. J.; Arnold, W. A.; Blazer, V. S.; Halden, R. U.; Klaper, R. D.; Kolpin, D. W.; Kriebel, D.; Love, N. G.; Martinovic-Weigelt, D.; Patisaul, H. B.; Snyder, S. A.; vom Saal, F. S.; Weisbrod, A. V.; Swackhamer, D. L. On the need for a national (U.S.) research program to elucidate the potential risks to human health and the environment posed by contaminants of emerging concern, *Environ. Sci. Technol.* **2011**, 45, 3829–3830.

NRC, Water Reuse: Potential for Expanding the Nation's Water Supply Through Reuse of Municipal Wastewater, Washington, DC, Water Science and Technology Board, National Research Council, **2012**.

Oller, I.; Malato, S.; Sanchez-Perez, J. A. Combination of advanced oxidation processes and biological treatments for wastewater decontamination – a review, *Sci. Total Environ.* **2011**, 409, 4141–4166.

Patisaul, H. B.; Adewale, H. B. Long-term effects of environmental endocrine disruptors on reproductive physiology and behavior, *Front. Behav. Neurosci.* **2009**, 3, 10.

Petrovic, M.; Eljarrat, E.; Lopez de Alda, M.J.; Barceló, D. Endocrine disrupting compounds and other emerging contaminants in the environment: a survey on new monitoring strategies and occurrence data, *Anal. Bioanal. Chem.* **2004**, 378, 549–562.

Petrovic, M.; Gonzalez, S.; Barceló, D. Analysis and removal of emerging contaminants in wastewater and drinking water, *Trends Anal. Chem.* **2003**, 22, 685–696.

Pinto, B.; Reali, D. Screening of estrogen-like activity of mineral water stored in PET bottles. *Int. J. Hyg. Environ. Health* **2009**, 212(2), 228–232.

Quinn, A. U.S. intelligence sees global water conflict risks rising, Reuters, March 22, 2012. Available at: http://www.reuters.com/article/2012/03/22/us-climate-water-idUSBRE82L0PR20120322

Redding, A. M.; Cannon, F. S.; Snyder, S. A.; Vanderford, B. J. A QSAR-like analysis of the adsorption of endocrine disrupting compounds, pharmaceuticals, and personal care products on modified activated carbons, *Water Res.* **2009**, 43, 3849–3861.

Richardson, S. D.; Ternes, T. A. Water analysis: emerging contaminants and current issues, *Anal. Chem.* **2011**, 83, 4614–4648.

Schriks, M.; Heringa, M. B.; van der Kooi, M. M.; de Voogt, P.; van Wezel, A. P. Toxicological relevance of emerging contaminants for drinking water quality, *Water Res.* **2010**, 44(2), 461–476.

Schwarzenbach, R. P.; Escher, B. I.; Fenner, K.; Hofstetter, T. B.; Johnson, C. A.; von Gunten, U.; Wehrli, B. The challenge of micropollutants in aquatic systems, *Science* **2006**, 313(5790), 1072–1077.

Sedlak, D. L.; Gray, J. L.; Pinkstone, K. E. Understanding micro-contaminants in recycled water, *Environ. Sci. Technol.* **2000**, 34(23), 509A–515A.

Sahar, E.; Ernst, M.; Godehardt, M.; Hein, A.; Herr, J.; Kazner, C.; Melin, T.; Cikurel, H.; Aharoni, A.; Messalem, R.; Brenner, A.; Jekel, M. Comparison of two treatments for the removal of selected organic micropollutants and bulk organic matter: conventional activated sludge followed by ultrafiltration versus membrane bioreactor, *Water Sci. Technol.* **2011**, 63(4), 733–740.

Savage, N.; Diallo, M. S. Nanomaterials and water purification: Opportunities and challenges, *J. Nanoparticle Res.* **2005**, 7, 331–342.

Shannon, M. A.; Bohn, P. W.; Elimelech, M.; Georgiadis, J. G.; Mariñas, B. J.; Mayes, A. M. Science and technology for water purification in the coming decades, *Nature* **2008**, 452, 301–310.

Snyder, S. A.; Benotti, M. J. Endocrine disruptors and pharmaceuticals: implications for water sustainability, *Water Sci. Technol.* **2010**, 61(1), 145–154.

Snyder, S. A.; Wert, E. C.; Lei, H.; Westerhoff, P.; Yoon, Y. Removal of EDCs and pharmaceuticals in drinking water and reuse treatment processes, Denver, CO, Awwa Research Foundation, **2007**.

Snyder, S. A.; Westerhoff, P.; Yoon, Y.; Sedlak, D. L. Pharmaceuticals, personal care products, and endocrine disruptors in water: implications for the water industry, *Environ. Eng. Sci.* **2003**, 20, 449–469.

Snyder, S. A.; Villeneuve, D. L.; Snyder, E. M.; Giesy, J. P. Identification and quantification of estrogen receptor agonists in wastewater effluents, *Environ. Sci. Technol.* **2001**, 35(18), 3620–3625.

Stuart, M.; Lapworth, D.; Crane, E.; Hart, A. Review of risk from potential emerging contaminants in UK groundwater, *Sci. Total Environ.* **2012**, 416, 1–21.

Suárez, S.; Carballa, M.; Omil, F.; Lema, J. M. How are pharmaceutical and personal care products (PPCPs) removed from urban wastewaters? *Rev. Environ. Sci. Biotechnol.* **2008**, 7, 125–138.

Sumpter, J. P. Environmental control of fish reproduction: a different perspective, *Fish Physiol. Biochem.* **1997**, 17(1–6), 25–31.

Ternes, T. A.; Joss, A.; Siegrist, H. Scrutinizing pharmaceuticals and personal care products in wastewater treatment, *Environ. Sci. Technol.* **2004**, 38(20), 392A–399A.

Ternes, T.; von Gunten, U. Editorial to special issue in Water Research: emerging contaminants in water, *Water Res.* **2010**, 44(2), 351.

Ternes, T. A.; Meisenheimer, M.; Mcdowell, D. et al. Removal of pharmaceuticals during drinking water treatment, *Environ. Sci. Technol.* **2002**, 36(17), 3855–3863.

Van der Mude, A. Endocrine-disrupting chemicals: testing to protect future generations, *Boston College Environ. Aff. Law. Rev.* **2011**, 38, 509. Available at: http://lawdigitalcommons.bc.edu/ealr/vol38/iss2/13 (accessed on 15 October 2013).

Voutsa, D.; Hartmann, P.; Schaffner, C.; Giger, W. Benzotriazoles, alkylphenols and bisphenol A in municipal wastewaters and in the Glatt River, Switzerland, *Environ. Sci. Pollut. Res. Int.* **2006**, 13(5), 333–341.

Wagner, M.; Oehlmann, J. Endocrine disruptors in bottled mineral water: total estrogenic burden and migration from plastic bottles, *Environ. Sci. Pollut. Res. Int.* **2009**, 16(3), 278–286.

Walker, C. H. *Organic Pollutant: An Ecotoxicological Perspective*, 2nd ed. Boca Raton, Fla, USA: Taylor and Francis, **2009**.

Westerhoff, P.; Yoon, Y.; Snyder, S.; Wert, E. Fate of endocrine-disruptor, pharmaceutical, and personal care product chemicals during simulated drinking water treatment processes, *Environ. Sci. Technol.* **2005**, 39(17), 6649–6663.

Wintgens, T.; Salehi, F.; Hochstrat, R.; Melin, T. Emerging contaminants and treatment options in water recycling for indirect potable use, *Water Sci. Technol.* **2008**, 57, 99–107.

Yoon, Y.; Westerhoff, P.; Snyder, S.A.; Wert, E.C. Nanofiltration and ultrafiltration of endocrine disrupting compounds, pharmaceuticals and personal care products, *J. Membr. Sci.* **2006**, 270, 88–100.

WHO, Endocrine disruptors, Geneva, 2002. Available at: www.who.int/ipcs/publications/new_issues/endocrine_disruptors/en/index.html (accessed on 15 September 2013).

13

POLICY AND REGULATORY CONSIDERATIONS FOR EDCs

13.1 INTRODUCTION

Because of the vast use of organic chemicals in modern society, almost any wastewater stream from industrial processes or households likely contains endocrine disrupting chemicals (EDCs), which also widely exist in environmental waters. Therefore, disposal of these chemicals without proper treatment always results in exposure to humans and the environment. Some of these chemicals are widely distributed and can have serious effects on wildlife species and human health over a long period even when they are present at very low concentrations. In humans, the types of harm that one would expect to see from reproductive and development risks, such as breast, testicular and prostate cancers, reproductive problems such as some birth defects, low birth rates, infertility, and early puberty, and some neurodevelopmental disorders, are generally increasing, particularly in Europe and the United States (Gee, 2008). Thus, there is a need to have a policy for assessing the risk and to regulate the introduction and maintenance in the environment of potential EDCs.

Endocrine disruptors can be defined broadly as chemicals that interfere with some element of the endocrine system; or, they can be more narrowly defined as causing observable adverse health effects as a result of their endocrine-modulating properties. This has a significant potential to shift the burden of actions in the policy arena. Choosing a definition that refers to any chemical interference with the endocrine system could make it easier to classify agents as endocrine disruptors, thereby potentially placing the burden of proof on industrial manufacturers and users of those chemicals to show that their chemicals should not be regulated as

Endocrine Disruptors in the Environment, First Edition. Sushil K. Khetan.
© 2014 John Wiley & Sons, Inc. Published 2014 by John Wiley & Sons, Inc.

stringently as other endocrine disruptors. On the other hand, choosing a definition that requires evidence of adverse health effects could potentially place the burden of proof on consumer and public-health organizations to show that chemicals are actually harmful before they could be regulated as endocrine disruptors (Elliott, 2012).

Regulatory bodies around the world have been tasked with finding a workable system to identify and validate "endocrine active disruptive substances" and to assess their effects using appropriate risk-based approaches. The goal is a set of clearly defined, integrated, and globally harmonized test methods that minimize the need for animal testing. The current model of testing one chemical at a time on adult laboratory animals is problematic and has not been without controversy. Such methods miss critical windows of exposure during developmental periods such as *in utero* and puberty and do not consider exposures to chemical mixtures. Current methods also do not always accurately predict human health effects, and they are animal-intensive and time consuming.

Improved understanding of the unique characteristics and impacts of EDCs upends many tenets of risk assessment on which policies regulating chemicals are currently based. When exposures occur during critical periods of development, EDCs can produce lifelong, sometimes multigenerational, changes. This suggests that risk assessment should account for timing of exposure in addition to dose (Grandjean and Budtz-Jørgensen, 2007). Some EDCs are most potent at concentrations several orders of magnitude lower than those tested by toxicological methods commonly used for regulatory purposes. EDCs in combination can produce additive or synergistic effects (Carpenter et al., 2002) that cannot be predicted by assessing individual chemicals in isolation. Some hormone alterations caused by EDCs might appear slight in an individual but can have potentially large effects at the population level (Woodruff et al., 2008) by reducing intelligence, reproductive capacity, or disease resistance. A new European Union Plant Protection Products Regulation (1107/2009) has named endocrine disrupting properties as one of the cut-off criteria for the approval of pesticides, although it currently fails to provide specific science-based measures for the assessment of substances with such properties. The development of assessment and decision criteria is a key challenge concerning the implementation of this new EU regulation (Marx-Stoelting et al., 2011).

13.2   REGULATING PARADIGM SHIFT IN CONVENTIONAL TOXICOLOGY

Endocrine-disrupting action breaks a large number of rules and assumptions that have guided conventional toxicology, which had previously focused on a chemical's capacity to induce acute toxicity or to cause cancer via mutagenesis. EDCs present new and fundamental differences for the science underlying the regulatory paradigm. Thus, the current chemical regulatory paradigm may need radical revision to allow adequate regulation of EDCs (Vogel, 2005).

13.2.1 Downward Movement of Safe Thresholds

Historical records show that "safe thresholds" for known neurotoxicants have been continuously revised downward as scientific knowledge advanced. For example, the initial "safe" blood level of lead, which is known to damage many organs and interfere with children's neurological development, was set at 60 µg/dl in 1960. This was revised down to 10 µg/dl in 1990. Current studies suggest that lead may have no identifiable exposure level that is "safe" (Grandjean, 2010). The estimated "toxic threshold" for mercury has also relentlessly fallen and, like lead, any level of exposure may be harmful. Such results raise serious questions about the adequacy of the current regulatory regime, particularly for EDCs. The current regime, by design, permits children to be exposed up to "toxic thresholds" that rapidly become obsolete (Schettler et al., 2000).

Regulatory agencies test, or approve testing, of chemicals by examining high doses and then extrapolating down to determine safe levels for humans and/or wildlife. These extrapolations use safety factors that acknowledge exposures of vulnerable populations, interspecies variability, and other uncertainty factors. However, this way of declared safe levels are never in fact tested. Particularly, many chemicals of concern have never been examined at environmentally relevant low doses at which humans and wildlife are exposed.

A conceptual shift is necessary in assessing the risk to human health posed by EDCs and recognizing that susceptibility to disease persists long after exposure and that chemicals at low doses can act like hormones in the body to disrupt development. Also, the low dose effects of many EDCs mean that low-dose and transient exposure can be just as dangerous or more than high-dose and prolonged exposure.

13.2.2 Nonmonotonic Low-Dose Effects (Nonthreshold substances)

The traditional toxicological paradigm is based on a key assumption that responses are based on the monotonic dose–response curve, in which more of the chemical leads to a greater effect. This may not be applicable to assess the toxicity of EDCs. Although low-dose nonmonotonic dose–responses have been well accepted for hormones and neurotransmitters, they are just starting to be appreciated for EDCs. Because many EDCs have only moderate relative binding affinities to nuclear receptors, these were believed to have weak endocrine activity, and resulted in the majority of earlier scientific studies about them at very high concentrations (µM–mM). Because of the nonmonotonic nature of their responses, many of the tested effects may have missed the concentration ranges in which these compounds are the most effective (Watson et al., 2011).

Low concentrations of many xenoestrogens are common in the environment, and without this information about low-concentration-induced responses, we are incorrectly assuming that xenoestrogens are ineffective and harmless. Therefore, it would only be prudent that animal testing protocols include testing of chemicals over a wide dose range, including doses experienced by typical human exposures (Myers, et al., 2009). Extrapolation of results from very high doses to predict lowest effective doses is no longer tenable in light of our latest understandings of mechanisms of the above (Watson et al., 2011).

13.2.3 Sensitivity of Development Periods

In humans and animals, there are critical windows of development, both for the reproductive organs and the brain, when sensitivity to hormones and EDCs is heightened. Chemicals with endocrine-disrupting activity are widely dispersed in our environment, often at levels plausibly associated with biological effects; exposure to humans is widespread. It seems clear that it is more the timing of the dose rather than the dose itself which, *inter alia*, distinguishes harmful from harmless exposures to reproductive and developmental toxicants. Such harm is often irreversible and sometimes multigenerational, causing lifetime personal and societal costs that cannot be offset by any benefits to the individual from intrauterine exposures (Grandjean et al., 2008). Even extremely small doses have effects, in particular if the exposure to theses doses occurred during the growth or gestation period. For example, there was no minimal dose for the phenomenon of gender inversion within turtle embryo caused by estradiol (Sheehan et al., 1999). This study illustrates quite well the limits of the idea that smaller levels of exposition eliminate the risks.

There is also the recognition that the placenta is not impenetrable to EDCs; on the contrary, most EDCs likely reach the developing fetus. Maternal estrogens are effectively sequestered by α-fetoprotein but most estrogen-like compounds only weakly or fail to bind to α-fetoprotein and can, therefore, enter fetal circulation relatively unimpeded (Patisaul and Adewale, 2009). Thus, it is now widely accepted that development is a window of exceptional vulnerability to EDC exposure. Chemicals such as thalidomide and DES proved tragic for those exposed to them while in their mothers' wombs. The implication is that exposure of pregnant women to toxins could be detrimental to their progeny in their adult life.

This calls for assessment of endocrine-disrupting effects with the most sensitive and appropriate methods currently available and particularly including exposures during periods of heightened susceptibility in critical life stages. Also, toxicological tests need to identify relevant hazards, such as the long-term functional development of progeny and the specific effects of exposure in the peripubertal stages (Mantovani, 2006). Until better tests become available, hazard and risk identification must rely also on epidemiological approaches. Normal endocrine signaling during development involves very small changes in hormone levels, yet these changes can have significant biological effects. That means subtle disruptions of endocrine signaling are a plausible mechanism by which chemical exposures at low doses can have effects on the body (Birnbaum, 2010).

13.2.4 Cumulative Exposures to Multiple EDCs (Exposures can be Additive)

Virtually all contamination is in the form of mixtures, and therefore, the potential deleterious impact of simultaneous exposure to multiple common EDCs and other environmental chemicals cannot be overestimated. With the exception of pesticides used on the food supply, current regimes regulate only one chemical at a time and do not take into account the potential for interactions. Since real-world exposures are to multiple chemicals, current regulatory standards, based on single chemical exposures, are inherently incapable of providing adequate margins of safety (Schettler et al., 2000). Empirical evidence exists on significant mixture effects from EDCs at or below individual no-observed-effect levels (NOELs). The concept of concentration addition (CA) model is often considered a general method for estimating mixture toxicity at the regulatory level. This CA as a default option is precautionary without implying massive and costly overprotection (Kortenkamp, 2007).

Over the last 10 years, evidence has accumulated on the basis of studies in lab animals and observations in wildlife on the potential for some chemicals and other environmental stressors, usually in combination, to produce reproductive and developmental harm. At the same time, evidence from human beings is beginning to accumulate, along with knowledge about mixtures of substances and about environmentally low but sometimes harmful doses. Exposure to these stressors via consumer products, water, and food is widespread (Gee, 2008).

Mixtures of endocrine disruptors can have additive or even synergistic effects (see for more details, Chapter 5). While synergism is a commonly demonstrated phenomenon in endocrinology, the work in this avenue on EDCs has been limited. A case in point is that of the herbicide S-metolachlor (0.1 ppb), which was found to have no adverse effect on its own in amphibians; however, in combination with atrazine, the harmful effects of atrazine, such as retarded larval development and growth, were multiplied (Hayes et al, 2006). In practice, these two herbicides are often mixed together in commercial products. Faced with this challenge, the most coherent approach may be to not limit research to effects of pure substances, but to start from the combinations that are the most often found in nature, that is, the ones organism are exposed to in their natural environment.

13.2.5   Long Latency Between Exposure and Effect (Delayed Effects)

Exposure to EDCs at very sensitive stages of development can result in profound changes in physiology and function which may not emerge clinically until much later in life. The exposure itself may cease, but the developmental impact and the subsequent adverse effect may have already been set in motion (Birnbaum, 2010). Epigenetic mechanism of EDCs can explain these latent effects of exposure-related changes in an individual's epigenetic status in one stage of their life affecting the health of the individual in later stages of their lifespan.

The concept of the "developmental origins of adult disease," as the term implies, suggests that there is a time lag between exposure and manifestation of the disease. Serious damage to health can be initiated in the early life stages of human and other species, but it may not become apparent until much later in their development. Harm that originates at the fetal stage can also appear in early life, causing birth defects, lifetime dysfunctions, such as lower IQ, or diseases of early adulthood, such as testicular and vaginal cancer and other damage to reproductive organs.

Therefore, new perspectives need to be incorporated into the regulatory approach that fetal exposure to environmental chemicals can lead to adult disease and that current test guidelines are not protective enough. Regulation can be improved by incorporating reliable "new" endpoints/tests more sensitive than what are already being measured and early diagnostic indicators for screening. Epigenetic marks may be important biomarkers both of exposures and of disease/dysfunction susceptibility, so these endpoints need to be assessed and their usefulness in predicting risk determined (Barouki et al., 2012).

13.3   POLICY OPTIONS FOR EDC REGULATION

Regulatory authorities have policy options available that can reduce the risks emanating through the exposure of EDCs in the environment. Some of these policy options listed here have already been adopted in the European Union.

13.3.1   Scientific Uncertainty and Precautionary Policy

Translating the emerging science of endocrine disruption into chemicals policy requires new toxicological tools and cumulative risk assessment methods (NRC, 2008). There is great uncertainty about which, how, and to what extent synthetic chemicals disrupt hormone systems. This uncertainty is not simply reducible by measuring a set of generally agreed upon biological parameters. Rather, it stems from limited knowledge about the ways that altered hormone function may be expressed at the cellular, organismic, and population levels. Scientific knowledge is especially limited in understanding both the exposure and variability of responses among populations and individuals. Thus, it demands a fundamentally new way of thinking about the risks associated with chemical exposures, one in which precaution informs the application of scientific evidence to public policy. This approach would acknowledge the scientific uncertainty and the potential to deliver as-yet unrecognized hazards to future generations (Gee, 2006).

While the limited evidence on the effects of endocrine disrupters may provide assurances of safety to some, this lack of evidence by no means indicates that these substances pose no risk to humans. It simply means that science has yet to fully study and understand the range of potential effects. Bisphenol A (BPA) is a poster child for this group of chemicals. Opinion may be divided on the potential health hazard of BPA, nevertheless the key question is whether unnecessary risks should be taken, especially with young children for whom exposure to these chemicals can mean increased health problems later in life. Too often, unreasonable delays in preventive responses have resulted from demands for detailed proof of causation and knowledge of mechanistic actions (Grandjean et al., 2004).

Scientific indicators are prompting that we need to do something, and we need to do it fast. Environmentalists think that the correct approach is to adopt the "precautionary principle," a better-safe-than-sorry approach favored in the European Union. This notion was first codified in the former West Germany in the late 1970s and early 1980s as *Vorsorgeprinzip*, and came to be known in English as the "Precautionary Principle" (Jordan and O'Riordan, 1999), defined at the 1992 Earth Summit at Rio de Janeiro as "where there are threats of serious or irreversible damage, lack of full scientific certainty shall not be used as a reason for postponing cost-effective measures to prevent environmental degradation." Changes in the regulatory process will protect future generations from preventable and potentially harmful exposures when conclusive evidence is lacking, but sound scientific studies indicate a strong possibility for adverse health effects.

Without the application of the precautionary principle, the regulatory system is decades behind the emergence of new pollutants that are continuously introduced into the consumer market place and ultimately continuously introduced to the environment with everyday consumer use. Scientific data about lead poisoning were present many years before the policies were changed and the chemical was banned. During that time, children's health continued to be harmed (Markowitz and Rosner, 2003). Use of the precautionary principle to ban or restrict chemicals in order to reduce exposure early, even when there are significant but incomplete data, would prevent significant and long-lasting harm. Precautionary approaches presume that an induced adverse response in animals is a reliable indicator of potential harm in humans, unless informed otherwise by multiple well-designed and well-conducted studies. The federal government has the responsibility to develop policies that protect people from the risk of exposure, or at the very least inform them of the risk to public health (Endocrine Society, 2009; Burger, 2003). In practical terms, this will require that producers to demonstrate the safety of a new chemical as a condition of its use, and that governments have the means of acting on early indications of harm.

13.3.2   Shifting the Burden of Proving Safe Products

The 1976 US Toxic Substances Control Act (TSCA), which covers chemicals other than medicines, cosmetics, and pesticides, essentially assumes that compounds introduced into the marketplace are safe until proven otherwise: potential risks to the environment or human health are acted upon only if the U.S. EPA can uncover and prove them. This assumes that science has the capacity to "prove" harm under the relevant scientific and legal standards, and creates an ethical position that prioritizes profit over human health by placing the burden of proof on public and environmental health advocates (Vogel, 2005). For EDCs, a new model is needed that shifts the burden.

One model might be the safety laws adopted by the European Union's Registration, Evaluation, Authorization, & Restriction of Chemical substances (REACH), which shift the burden of proof to industry, requiring chemical companies to prove that their products do not harm human health or the environment and to obtain special authorization for any chemicals of very high concern, before these can be used in commerce. In other words, the law put the onus on the chemical industry to show that a chemical is safe, rather than on regulators to prove that it is dangerous. The American chemical industry has reservations, citing the extra costs such testing would entail, but such a change could represent a long-overdue safety step (Walsh, 2010).

13.3.3   Need to Broaden the Risk Assessment

To prevent persistence and bioaccumulation/magnification, many synthetic compounds are readily metabolized to more polar forms often containing one or more hydroxy groups. This enhanced ability to undergo biotransformation also has increased the potential for the formation of more EDCs. Consequently, the additional and consistent testing of metabolites for endocrine-disrupting properties should be encouraged in the future in order to establish a better risk assessment process for these types of compounds.

The ability of several EDCs to affect the epigenome of both wildlife and humans could be potentially catastrophic to the welfare of future generations and requires careful attention by both toxicologists and endocrinologists. The epigenome is a very reactive system; its labile nature allows it to sense and respond to environmental perturbations to ensure survival during fetal growth. This pliability also leads to aberrant epigenetic modifications that persist into later life and induce numerous disease states. Epigenotoxicity could lead to numerous developmental, metabolic, and behavioral disorders in exposed populations. The heritable nature of epigenetic changes also increases the risk for transgenerational inheritance of the aberrant phenotypes. Thus, there is a need for the inclusion of epigenotoxic effects into the risk assessment process.

The investigation of nutritional supplementation as a parental preventive approach to counteracting environmental influences on the epigenome is another area that needs to be strengthened for arriving at possible solutions (Dolinoy et al., 2007). Some drugs in current clinical use influence DNA demethylation. Procainamide, a widely used antiarrhythmic drug, inhibits DNA methyltransferace (DNMT) activity and promotes DNA hypomethylation. Hydralazine, a peripheral vasodilator that is used to treat some types of hypertension, and valproic acid, a widely used antiepileptic and mood stabilizer, are now known to cause DNA demethylation. Because an effect on DNA methylation is one of the actions of these drugs, concerns that other drugs in current clinical use might also affect DNA methylation patterns have been raised. It would be prudent that future drug safety tests include measurement of DNA methylation/demethylation (Hochberg et al., 2011).

In the construction of the risk assessment, there is a need to choose animal species that are sensitive. For example, certain rats have exhibited high tolerances to the effects of endocrine disruptors. The choice of the breed of rat on which testing of chemicals is carried out is thus important to ensure meaningful data.

13.3.4   Cutting-Edge Bioassays Showing Developmental Endpoints

Regulatory bodies have generally relied on guideline studies conducted under what is known as "Good Laboratory Practice" (GLP), which provides a guarantee of reliability and cross-comparability for studies on chemical safety. However, research in laboratories around the world has produced many studies on lab animals, showing cognitive, developmental, and reproductive effects associated with exposure to

BPA, which seem to be triggered through BPA's hormone-mimicking qualities and its long-term epigenetic influence on gene expression. These effects are considerably subtler than the guideline studies designed for more clearly toxic substances. The cutting-edge biological techniques required for detecting these effects need validation and standardization in ways that make the result usable by regulators, who need to find faster ways to get the new techniques incorporated into guideline studies to evaluate and regulate properly (Anonymous, 2010).

Many environmental estrogenic EDCs can affect the development of the reproductive tract, including mammary gland development in experimental animals, and the effect can be especially significant if chemical exposure occurs during critical stages, such the gestational, neonatal, and peripubertal periods as well as pregnancy. The breast or mammary gland and uterus are target tissues for estrogen. There is growing evidence that the breast tissue is particularly vulnerable during development in the womb and puberty. During the peripubertal period, the mammary gland undergoes a rapid proliferative expansion, and its susceptibility to environmental exposures is known to affect breast cancer risk later in life (Fenton et al., 2012; Rudel et al., 2011; Yang et al., 2009). Therefore, testing of potential EDCs for effects on the mammary gland development would provide a sensitive endpoint (Enoch et al., 2007).

Reliable "in culture" bioassays are needed for several purposes. From a preventive viewpoint, chemicals that will be entering the food supply (such as those used in food packaging) or those that would be released massively into the environment (such as pesticides) need be tested for hormonal activity while still in the developmental stage of manufacturing. This would provide the means to avoid producing chemicals with unintended hormonal activity (Soto et al., 2006). Another use of bioassays is to discover markers of exposure: for example, testing water courses to find out whether they are contaminated with estrogenic substances. This will allow the detection of bioactivity without having to know *a priori* the chemical nature of all estrogens involved. This is important because only a very small list of chemicals has been tested for hormonal activity. This limited set precludes the use of chemical analysis to determine whether or not xenoestrogens are present in environmental samples (Soto et al., 2006).

Regulatory decisions that rely largely on toxicity testing in genetically similar animals under controlled laboratory conditions will continue to fail to reflect threats to the capacities and complexity of the human brain as well as important gene–environment interactions. The policy considerations need to include development and validation of animal model systems, which, when combined with detailed laboratory analyses of development and physiology, will accurately predict and quantify effects in humans (Endocrine Society, 2009).

There is also a need for consensus parameters (maximum residue limits, action levels, etc.) for various EDCs, as well as networks of reference laboratories providing validated analytical methods.

13.4   CONTROVERSY ON REGULATORY FRAMEWORK FOR EDCs

In the summer of 2013, a leaked draft document of the European Union proposing a regulation for endocrine-disrupting chemicals got mired in a controversy. The document has proposed that identification of an *in vitro* effect without a causal relationship to adversity in an intact organism may be sufficient to classify a substance as an endocrine disruptor. Traditional toxicologists, who favor traditional, specific approaches to toxicological testing, criticized the draft proposal. They took issue with the plans for special regulation of EDCs. In contrast, environmental scientists and others, who favor the precautionary intent of modern chemicals regulation in the face of multiplying indicators of harm, supported it.

Normally, chemical regulations are either hazard-based (the intrinsic potential for a substance to cause harm) or risk-based (the probability that they will actually cause harm), where risk is expressed by the equation

$$\underset{\text{(Probability of an adverse consequence)}}{\text{Risk}} = \underset{\text{(Effect)}}{\text{Hazard severity}} \times \underset{\text{(Time} \times \text{Concentration)}}{\text{Exposure}}$$

The risk-based approach implies that regulators should not be doing anything until they know for sure that the chemical is harmful, based on all the important facts from both sides of the above equation. This, "regulate a chemical only once it is proven dangerous" approach involves waiting until all the facts about a product are available. It means that later research might show that the early hints of hazard were right, and exposure has been harmful, some of which may be irreversible.

Hazard-based approach is acting at the first reasonable hint of hazard rather than continue to experiment on the public while research is done to get all the facts (similar to the precautionary principle; ban suspected hazards until they are proven safe). The precautionary principle is a legal concept for addressing scientific uncertainty and is enshrined in European Law in the EU Treaty (Bergman et al., 2013). This precautionary 'regulate a chemical till proven it is safe' approach protects against things that may turn out to be harmful. The negative side is the possible loss of the benefits of products that may turn out to be safe, or whose benefits outweigh the harm.

The two regulatory approaches and their different outcomes are portrayed in the controversy related to BPA. The FDA has not banned BPA in general because it says a Hazard × Exposure risk-based analysis finds that BPA is not dangerous at the doses to which we are exposed. The environmental scientists, focusing on the hazard side of the equation, say it is dangerous and should be regulated because birth defects were observed in infants who were exposed during fetal development *in utero* via the mother.

13.4.1   Diversity of Viewpoints of the Risk Assessors and the Endocrine Scientists

In toxicology, a correlation observation of harm by a chemical is followed up with a causation study to establish that the substance actually causes harm. Increasing harm from increasing concentration and/or time of exposure establishes the causation. It contrasts with endocrinology approach, which is based on finding mechanistic flags for concern (potential hazard rather than a specific approach emphasizing proof of harm) followed by having to prove the substance is safe before approval for use. Responding to mode of action (MOA) indicators of harm rather than proof from a definitive causation study can be expected to result in a proportion of the chemicals that would not in fact be EDCs. More traditional practitioners of toxicology are leery of this approach.

13.4.1.1 Traditional Toxicology Viewpoint Biological effects that have a homeostatic response should not be considered conclusive evidence of an EDC's activity. Toxicology argument is centered on the fact that endocrine disruption is not a toxicologically defined endpoint but a mode of action that may or may not result in adverse health effects, distinguishing between effects that occur within normal homeostatic limits (hormonally active) and those that can be described as harmful (an actual full-blown EDC). Normal endocrine functioning can be affected by ADME (absorption, distribution, metabolism, excretion) and other adaptive and protective mechanisms within animals (Chedrese, 2009). Against the continuously changing external environment of an organism, the homeostasis provides a level of protection for coping with xenobiotic exposures that are essential for the maintenance of life. For example, the hormone-like activity of chemicals can be neutralized within the balance of hormone homeostasis, precluding the adverse effects from occurring. Therefore, endocrine-active substances can interact directly or indirectly with the endocrine system, but otherwise do not create an adverse effect.

The healthy homeostasis of an organism results from an orchestrated network of myriad thresholds for a multitude of component substances. It is only above a certain threshold of exposure that the homeostasis and detoxifying mechanisms of the organism become overloaded and adverse effects can result. The crucial question, however, is at what level of exposure the response becomes adverse. Chemical risk assessment is built on this threshold of adversity, which is determined in regulatory toxicology on the basis of animal studies. Traditional toxicology also relies on a monotonically increasing dose–response relationship as evidence that the test agent causes the effect. It is the very constraint of assumed monotonicity that provides the statistical basis for sorting out significant trends from random statistical fluctuations.

13.4.1.2 Endocrinology Viewpoint EDCs are to be regarded as substances for which there are no practically identifiable safe threshold for adverse effects and adequate control of the risks. Endocrine systems have a programming role during development, and disruption of these programming events leads to irreversible effects (Bergman et al., 2013). EDCs have been shown to be capable of causing injury to the developing human brain and reproductive organs at the lowest levels detectable – levels far below those that harm adults, particularly if the exposure occurs during a critical developmental window.

Unlike traditional environmental toxicants in which the risk of adverse events increases as the exposure levels increase, endocrine disruptors may exert effects at both low doses and high doses. Further, an exposure dose for EDCs that may be considered safe cannot be reached because of the lack of monotonic dose–response curves; coexposures to a whole range of chemicals that may affect the same adverse outcome; irreversibility; exposure during critical stages of development; and early life exposure and onset of diseases later in life (Vandenberg et al., 2013).

It is opined that, because endogenous hormones already stimulate the endocrine system, the threshold for activation is already exceeded. Therefore, any potential hormonal activity that is introduced, no matter how slight, will increase (or decrease) this baseline activity. Because concentrations of endogenous hormones are low and fluctuate widely, small additions or subtractions of even a single molecule will result in altered hormonal responses (Hass et al., 2013).

13.4.2   A Debate on EU Regulatory Framework for EDCs

Disputes over chemical safety and trade-offs over risk have been long-standing, and much of the argument in this case centers on whether governments should require chemical manufacturers to clearly prove safety or whether safety should be presumed if dangers could not be shown definitively. The European Commission is trying to decide whether these chemicals are safe under certain threshold concentrations and pursuing a hazard-based cut-off criterion for ED properties for their approval for marketing and use. If no safe threshold can be determined, then to avoid a ban under Europe's REACH regulation adopted in 2006 which regulates industrial chemicals, industry would have to demonstrate that the economic benefits outweigh human health risks or that there are no alternatives. As companies worldwide that sell products in Europe would have to comply, the new rules would have wide ramifications.

Fueling the debate, the editors of journals of toxicology, endocrinology, and other related fields have published combative editorials about how endocrine-disrupting chemicals should be regulated (Cressey, 2013; Anonymous 2, 2013). In a coordinated set of identical editorials in 14 toxicology journals, their editors criticized the proposed EU regulations arguing that there is insufficient evidence to justify any new regulation regarding effects of chemicals on the endocrine system and advocating maintenance of the status quo in their regulation (Dietrich et al., 2013). The editorials also said that a threshold could be set for endocrine disruptors, and advocated distinguishing between the concentrations the hormonal system can adapt to and concentrations that result in actual adverse effects.

The editorials attracted robust rebuttal by a large group of endocrinologists and environmental and health scientists for ignoring scientific evidence and well-established principles of chemical risk assessment related to endocrine-disrupting chemicals (Anonymous1, 2013; Bergman et al., 2013; Vandenberg et al., 2013). Similar response came from an editorial in *Endocrinology*, signed by a large number of editors of endocrine, neuroendocrine, environmental, and other peer-reviewed journals, that the toxicologists' view neglects the well-established understanding that hormones act at extremely low dosages, the fundamental principles of how the endocrine system works, and how chemicals can interfere with its normal function, nor does it consider the consequences of that interference (Gore et al., 2013).

Risk assessment uses an extra set of data (exposure) over hazard assessment, but whether that makes it "more science-based" would depend on the quality of the science behind the extra data. As new evidence emerges about new developments unanticipated by risk assessment practices in the past, such as the possibility of low-dose effects, cumulative toxicity of mixtures, endocrine disruption and so forth, the accuracy of risk assessment in the face of knowledge gaps could start to appear questionable. And scientific standards of certainty may be impossible to attain when causes and effects are multiple, latent periods are long, timing of exposure is crucial, unexposed "control" populations do not exist, or confounding factors are unidentified. These knowledge gaps make even the hazard identification stage of risk assessment difficult enough. It could be argued that a hazard-based approach with no provision for factoring in estimates of exposure and consequent risk assessment is a pragmatic choice to nullify the risk of getting the risk assessment wrong, by eliminating hazard as much as possible.

13.5 CONCLUSIONS AND FUTURE PROSPECTS

EDCs pose an emerging threat to ecosystem health, illustrating the shortcomings in governance of the chemical enterprise with significant blind spots in characterizing EDCs. It is increasingly clear that, because of fetal sensitivity, the timing of exposures is critical, that exceedingly small doses of EDCs produced effects that can manifest later in life and can descend through generations, and that chemical mixtures produce compounded effects. It is often impossible to determine which plastics, cosmetics, toys, or other household items contain any of these compounds, so consumers have no adequate way to avoid them if desired. The thought that the mixture of chemicals a pregnant woman is exposed to during her pregnancy could affect not only her daughter's fecundity but also her granddaughter's is alarming and a major reason why the topic of endocrine disruption continues to receive global attention by scientists and the general public (Patisaul and Adewale, 2009).

Scientific certainties about the effects and the risks posed by EDCs could be decades away. Awareness of the systemic issues is a good start, but it remains to be seen whether regulations and regulatory institutions will change to adapt to these new types of toxins. To wait for conclusive scientific proof that these chemicals are adversely affecting human and wildlife populations before taking action could have devastating consequences for future generations. The adoption of the precautionary principle is one clear way forward, which can avoid these problems. Regulations cannot be "put on hold" until all the evidence has been collected. Development of policies and regulations must go hand in hand with ongoing research and any legislation must be able to adapt rapidly to advances in scientific knowledge (Bateson, 2000).

The European Union generally takes a precautionary approach to environmental risks, choosing restraint in the face of uncertainty. In the United States, lingering scientific questions justify delays in regulatory decisions. The self-regulating feedback systems of endocrine disruption cannot be expressed in terms of probabilities for adverse consequences along the dose-response curve, which makes it impossible to operationalize risk. And without risk, it is not possible for science to establish the kind of causation needed for regulatory purposes (Vogel, 2004). As the hazard concept is not fully applicable to EDCs, a shift toward acceptance of concern as a substitute (risk = concern × exposure) will enable the calculation of risk (Honkela et al., 2014). The notion of concern-based risk assessment could function as a pragmatic industry policy for working with materials with persistent uncertainties and likely risks. This will also operationalize precautionary processes, where cost considerations tend to overrule issues of precaution when quantitative estimates of data or exposure are not available (Honkela et al., 2014).

Regulatory testing of chemicals for endocrine-disrupting impacts lags behind the growing evidence of the compounds' health effects, particularly at levels to which people are routinely exposed. Low doses and windows of exposure are not currently captured in the regulatory testing regime for chemicals. There is a very large disconnect between regulatory toxicology and the modern science of endocrinology that is defining these issues. Policymakers have a lot of catching up to do in order to deal with the toxicology implications of EDCs (Deb, 2005). The fact that low-level exposures to EDCs cause multiple sexual organs to develop in some animals should raise grave concerns.

It is imperative that chemicals are used and produced in ways that lead to the minimization of significant adverse effects on human health and the environment. The US Congress need begin by reforming and strengthening the TSCA 1976 to require reviews of chemicals for safety, force manufacturers to provide adequate health data on any chemical under review, and empower agencies to restrict or ban the use of chemicals with clear evidence of harm. Chemicals policy reform, if done well, will support the market's movement to safer and greener alternatives to toxic chemicals. Introduction of Chemical Safety Improvement Act (CSIA) in the US Senate in 2013, which intends to bring crucial and necessary reforms to TSCA but considered badly flawed because of the complexity, costs, and delays it imposes on regulating chemicals (NY Times, 2013), has been a move in the right direction that could strengthen current chemical legislation.

Industry might be uncomfortable with the uncertainties, neither wanting to harm people nor to become embroiled in nonbeneficial technical and financial burdens. However, the environmental footprint of the chemical industry and its responsibility for implementing approaches for reducing and controlling chemical pollution in a sustainable manner have to be emphasized by regulatory enforcement. Major research and screening programs are under way around the world that could well lead to banning or curtailed use for many heavily used chemicals. Makers and users of chemicals can avoid the embarrassing surprises experienced with previous and new environmental issues and control programs by joining in the on-going issue-framing scientific, legislative, and regulatory processes (Jarrett, 2000). An important focus needs to be on reducing exposures by a variety of mechanisms. Regulatory actions to reduce exposures, while limited, have proven to be effective in specific cases (e.g., bans and restrictions on lead, chlorpyrifos, tributyltin, PCBs, and some other POPs) (UNEP/WHO, 2013). This has contributed to the decrease in the frequency of disorders in humans and wildlife. Given the importance of chemicals in modern societies, sustainable solutions can only be found through the active involvement of all stakeholders, including consumers, chemical manufacturers, politicians, and public authorities (Schwarzenbach et al., 2006).

The National Toxicological Program (NTP) is moving beyond the traditional approaches of testing one chemical at a time and is taking on the significant challenge of evaluating mixtures. EPA is gearing up to try to regulate chemicals, establishing a list of "chemicals of concern," which echoes a similar list developed by regulators in the European Union under a recent law requiring that chemicals be tested for safety before being sold.

Finally, the recently discovered phenomenon of transgenerational imprints by EDCs, such as vinclozoline and methoxychlor, on DNA regulatory mechanisms carried forward for four or perhaps more generations is a particularly worrying one. Therefore, simply cleaning up an environment and no longer using particular chemicals on a global level may have no ultimate effect as the damage is already done. In the given situation, to slow the rate and nature of environmental contamination by regulating better-known EDCs is the most that can be done for remediation (Gore and Crew, 2009). The effective reduction of people's exposures to EDCs has been far too slow given the gravity and irreversibility of the potential implications. To fully address the hazards of endocrine disruption, a comprehensive and sustainable chemicals policy is required, based on the green chemistry principles, green manufacturing methods, and precaution (Thornton, 2007). The aim of this policy need be that humans and the environment enjoy a high level of protection from the unacceptable risks associated with endocrine disruptors, before it is too little, too late, to avoid mistakes like those made with asbestos or lead.

The ongoing debate on the European regulation of EDCs provides an expose to the challenges regulators face trading between old science and new science, and societal interest on health and environment and corporate interests. Less enlightened groups stridently defend the status quo, denying that hazards exist with the chemicals they use, and question the plausibility of the science. Progressive groups see opportunities to create new value through safer alternatives.

REFERENCES

Anonymous, The weight of evidence, *Nature* **2010**, 464, 1103–1104.

Anonymous 1, Eight questions for toxicologists against proposals for new EU chemicals laws, *Health & Environment* **2013**, # 63 (22 September 2013).

Anonymous 2, Arguing about nothing? "Science-based" regulation of endocrine disruptors, *Health and Environment* **2013**, # 61 (21 July 2013).

Barouki, R.; Gluckman, P. D.; Grandjean, P.; Hanson, M.; Heindel, J. J. Developmental origins of non-communicable disease: Implications for research and public health, *Environ. Health* **2012**, 11, 42.

Bateson, P. *Endocrine disrupting chemicals (EDCs)*, Statement of the Royal Society, London , UK, 2000. Available at: http://royalsociety.org/uploadedFiles/Royal_Society_Content/policy/publications/2000/10070.pdf(accessed on 7 July 2012).

Bergman, A.; Andersson, A. M.; Becher, G.; van den Berg, M.; Blumberg, B.; Bjerregaard, P.; Bornehag, C. G.; Bornman, R.; Brandt, I.; Brian, J. V.; Casey, S. C.; Fowler, P.; Frouin, H.; Giudice, L. C.; Iguchi, T.; Hass, U.; Jobling, S.; Juul, A.; Kidd, K. A.; Kortenkamp, A.; Lind, M.; Martin, O. V.; Muir, D.; Ochieng, R.; Olea, N.; Norrgren, L.; Ropstad, E.; Ross, P. S.; Rudén, C.; Scheringer, M.; Skakkebaek, N. E.; Söder, O.; Sonnenschein, C.; Soto, A.; Swan, S.; Toppari, J.; Tyler, C. R.; Vandenberg, L. N.; Vinggaard, A. M. Science and policy on endocrine disrupters must not be mixed: a reply to a "common sense" intervention by toxicology journal editors, *Environ. Health* **2013**, 12, 68.

Birnbaum, L. *Endocrine disrupting chemicals in drinking water: risks to human health and the environment, Testimony before the subcommittee on energy and environment of the U. S. House of Representatives*, Feb. 25, **2010**. Available at: http://www.niehs.nih.gov/about/congress/docs/estimony birnbaum-feb252010.pdf. (accessed on 10 Sept. 2012)

Burger, J. Differing perspectives on the use of scientific evidence and the precautionary principle, *Pure Appl. Chem.*, **2003**, 75(11–12), 2543–2545.

Carpenter, D. O.; Arcaro, K.; Spink, D.C. Understanding the human health effects of chemical mixtures, *Environ. Health Perspect.* **2002**, 110 (suppl. 1), 25–42.

Cressey, D. Journal editors trade blows over toxicology, *Nature* **2013**, (20 September, **2013**).

Deb G. *Endocrine disruptors: A case study on atrazine.* 2005, Available at: http://www.temple.edu/law/tjstel/2005/fall/v24no2-Deb.pdf (accessed on 14 November 2013).

Dietrich, D. R.; Aulock, S. V.; Marquardt, H.; Blaauboer, B.; Dekant, W.; Kehrer, J.; Hengstler, J.; Collier, A.; Gori, G. B.; Pelkonen, O.; Lang, F.; Barile, F. A.; Nijkamp, F. P.; Stemmer, K.; Li, A.; Savolainen, K.; Hayes, A. W.; Gooderham, N.; Harvey, A. Scientifically unfounded precaution drives European Commission's recommendations on EDC regulation, while defying common sense, well-established science and risk assessment principles. *Chem. Biol. Interact.* **2013**, doi: 10.1016/j.cbi.2013.07.001.

Dolinoy, D. C.; Huang, D.; Jirtle, R. L. Maternal nutrient supplementation counteracts bisphenol A-induced DNA hypomethylation in early development, *Proc. Nat. Acad. Sci.*, **2007**, 104, 13056–13061.

Elliott, K. C. Ignorance, uncertainty, and the development of scientific language, In *Nichtwissenskommunikation in den Wissenschaften*, Janich, N., Nordmann, A., and Schebek, L., eds., Frankfurt am Main: Peter Lang , **2012**, pp. 295–315.

Endocrine Society, *Position Statement of Endocrine Society* (2009). Available at: http://www.endo-society.org/advocacy/policy/upload/Endocrine-disrupting-chemicals-position-statement.pdf (accessed on 10 March 2012).

Enoch, R. R.; Stanko, J. P.; Greiner, S. N.; Youngblood, G. L.; Rayner, J. L.; Fenton, S. E. Mamary gland development as a sensitive end point after acute prenatal exposure to an atrazine metabolite mixture in female Long-Evan rats, *Environ. Health Perspect.* **2007**, 115, 541–547.

Fenton, S. E.; Reed, C.; Newbold, R. R. Perinatal environmental exposures affect mammary development, function, and cancer risk in adulthood, *Ann. Rev. Pharmacol. Toxicol.* **2012**, 52, 455–479.

Gee, D. Establishing evidence for early action: the prevention of reproductive and developmental harm, *Basic Clin. Pharmacol. Toxicol.* **2008**, 102(2), 257–266.

Gee, D. Late lessons from early warnings: toward realism and precaution with endocrine-disrupting substances, *Environ. Health Perspect.* **2006**, 114, 152–160.

Gore, A. C.; Balthazart, J.; Bikle, D.; Carpenter, D. O.; Crews, D.; Czernichow, P.; Diamanti-Kandarakis, E.; Dores, R. M.; Grattan, D.; Hof, P. R.; Hollenberg, A. N.; Lange, C.; Lee, A. V.; Levine, J. E.; Millar, R. P.; Nelson, R. J.; Porta, M.; Poth, M. Power, D.M.;

Prins, G.S.; Ridgway, E.C.; Rissman, E.F.; Romijn, J.A.; Sawchenko, P.E.; Sly, P.D.; Söder, O.; Taylor, H.S.; Tena-Sempere, M.; Vaudry, H.; Wallen, K.; Wang, Z.; Wartofsky, L.; Watson C.S. Policy decisions on endocrine disruptors should be based on science across disciplines: A response to Dietrich et al. *Endocrinology* **2013**, doi: 10.1210/en.2013-1854

Gore, A. C.; Crews, D. Environmental endocrine disruption of brain and behavior, in *Hormones, Brain and Behavior*, Pfaff, D. W.; Arnold, A. P.; Etgen, A. M.; Fahrbach, S. E.; Rubin, R. T.; eds., 2nd ed., Vol. 3, San Diego: Academic Press, **2009**, pp. 1789–1816.

Grandjean, P. Even low-dose lead exposure is hazardous, *Lancet* **2010**; 375, 855–856.

Grandjean, P.; Bellinger, D.; Bergman, A.; Cordier, S.; Davey-Smith, G.; Eskenazi, B.; Gee, D.; Gray, K.; Hanson, M.; van der Hazel, P.; Heindel, J. J.; Heinzow, B.; et al. The Feroes statement: human health effects of developmental exposure to chemicals in our environment, *Basic Clin. Pharmacol. Toxicol.* **2008**, 102(2), 73–75.

Grandjean, P.; Budtz-Jørgensen, E. Total imprecision of exposure biomarkers: Implications for calculating exposure limits, *Am. J. Industr. Med.* **2007**, 50, 712–719.

Grandjean, P.; Bailar, J. C.; Gee, D.; Needleman, H. L.; Ozonoff, D. M.; Richter, E., Sofritti, M.; Soskolne, C. L. Implications of the Precautionary Principle in research and policy-making, *Am. J. ind. Med.* **2004**, 45(4), 382–385.

Hass, U.; Christiansen, S.; Axelstad, M.; Sørensen, K.D.; Boberg, J. *Input for the REACH-Review in 2013 on Endocrine Disruptors*, Danish Center on Endocrine Disrupters, Danish Environmental Protection Agency, **2013**.Available at: http://www.mst.dk/NR/rdonlyres/B865F94A-54C0-43DF-AB0F-F07A593E1FD0/0/Reachreviewra pportFINAL21March.pdf (accessed on 1 Feb 2014).

Hayes, T. B.; Case, P.; Chui, S.; Chung, D.; Haeffele, C.; Haston, K.; Lee, M.; Mai, V. P.; Marjuoa, Y.; Parker, J.; Tsui, M. Pesticide mixtures, endocrine disruption, and amphibian declines: are we underestimating the impact? *Environ. Health Perspect.* **2006**, 114 (Suppl. 1), 40–50.

Hochberg, Z.; Feil, R.; Constancia, M.; Fraga, M.; Junien, C.; Carel, J.-C.; Boileau, P.; Le Bouc, Y.; Deal, C. L.; Lillycrop, K.; Scharfmann, R.; Sheppard, A.; Skinner, M.; Szyf, M.; Waterland, R. A.; Waxman, D. J.; Whitelaw, E.; Ong, K.; Albertsson-Wikland, K. Child health, developmental plasticity, and epigenetic programming, *Endocr. Rev.* **2011**, 32(2), 159–224.

Honkela, N.; Toikka, A.; Hukkinen, J.; Honkela, T. Child health, developmental plasticity, and epigenetic programming, *Environ. Sci. Policy* **2014**, 38, 154–163.

Jarrett, R. E. Endocrine disruptor chemicals as a rising compliance issue, *Fed. Facil. Environ. J.* **2000**, 11(1), 25–39.

Jordan, A. and O'Riordan, T. The precautionary principle in contemporary environmental policy and politics, In *Protecting public health and the environment*, Raffensperger, C. and Tickner, J. A., eds., Washington, D.C.: Island Press, **1999**, pp. 15–35.

Kortenkamp, A. Ten years of mixing cocktails: a review of combination effects of endocrine-disrupting chemicals, *Environ Health Perspect.* **2007**, 115(S-1), 98–105.

Marx-Stoelting, P.; Pfeil, R.; Solecki, R.; Ulbrich, B.; Grote, K.; Ritz, V.; Banasiak, U.; Heinrich-Hirsch, B.; Moeller, T.; Chahoud, I.; Hirsch-Ernst, K. I. Assessment strategies and decision criteria for pesticides with endocrine disrupting properties relevant to humans, *Reproductive Toxicol.* **2011**, 31(4), 574–584.

Mantovani, A. Risk assessment of endocrine disrupters. The role of toxicological studies, *Ann. N Y Acad. Sci.* **2006**, 1076, 239–252.

Markowitz, G.; Rosner, D. *Deceit and Denial: The Deadly Politics of Industrial Pollution*, Berkeley/New York: University of California Press/The Milbank Memorial Fund, **2003**.

Myers, J.P.; Zoeller, R.T.; vom Saal, F.S. A clash of old and new scientific concepts in toxicity, with important implications for public health, *Environ. Health Perspect*, **2009**, 117(11), 1652–1655.

NRC, *Science and Decisions: Advancing Risk Assessment*, Washington, DC: National Academies Press, **2008**.

NY Times, An opening to strengthen chemical regulations, Editorial, *New York Times*, **2013**.

Patisaul, H. B., Adewale, H. B. Long-term effects of environmental endocrine disruptors on reproductive physiology and behavior, *Front. Behav. Neurosci.* **2009**, 3, 10.

Rudel, R. A.; Fenton, S. E.; Ackerman, J. M.; Euling, S. Y.; Makris, S. L. Environmental exposures and mammary gland development: state of the science, public health Implications, and research recommendations, *Environ. Health Perspect.* **2011**, 119, 1053–1061.

Schettler, T.; Stein, J.; Reich, F.; Valenti, M.; Wallinga, D. *In Harm's Way: Toxic Threats to Child Development*, Clean Water Fund, Greater Boston Physicians for Social Responsibility, **2000**. Available at: http://www.igc.org/psr/ (accessed on 10 March 2011).

Schwarzenbach, R. P.; Escher, B. I.; Fenner, K.; Hofstetter, T. B.; Johnson, C. A.; con Guntern, U.; Wehrli, B. The challenge of micropollutants in aquatic systems, *Science* **2006**, 313, 1072–1077.

Sheehan, D.M. et al., No threshold dose for estradiol-induced sex reversal of turtle embryos: how little is too much? *Environ. Health Perspect.* **1999**, 107(2), 155–159.

Soto, A. M.; Maffini, M. V.; Schaeberle, C. M.; Sonnenschein, C. Strengths and weaknesses of *in vitro* assays for estrogenic and androgenic activity, *Best Prac. Res. Clin. Endocrinol. Matab.* **2006**, 20, 15–33.

Thornton, J. W. What can we do about endocrine-disrupting chemicals? in *Endocrine-Disrupting Chemicals: From Basic Research to Clinical Practice*, Gore, A. C., ed., Totowa, NJ: Humana Press, **2007**, pp. 329–347.

UNEP/WHO, *State of the Science of Endocrine Disrupting Chemicals—2012*, Geneva, Switzerland: United Nations Environment Program/World Health Organization, **2013**.

Vandenberg, L. N.; Colborn, T.; Hayes, T. B.; Heindeld, J. J.; Jacobs Jr., D. R.; Lee, D. H.; Myers, J. P.; Shioda, T.; Soto, A. M.; vom Saal, F. S.; Welshons, W. V.; Zoeller, R. T. Regulatory decisions on endocrine disrupting chemicals should be based on the principles of endocrinology, *Reprod. Toxicol.* **2013**, 38, 1–15.

Vogel, J. Tunnel vision: the regulation of endocrine disruptors, *Policy Sci.* **2004**, 37(3–4), 277–303.

Vogel, J. M. Perils of paradigm: complexity, policy design, and the Endocrine Disruptor Screening Program, *Environ. Health* **2005**, 4, 1–11.

Walsh, B. The perils of plastic, *Time*, **2010**. Available at: http://www.time.com/time/specials/packages/article/0,28804,1976909_1976908_1976938-4,00.html#ixzz0jrmR4DaI (accessed on 1 Feb 2014).

Watson, C. S.; Jeng, Y. J.; Guptarak, J. Endocrine disruption via estrogen receptors that participate in nongenomic signaling pathways, *J. Steroid Biochem. Mol. Biol.* **2011**, 127 (1–2), 44–50.

Woodruff, T. J.; et al., Meeting report: Moving upstream-evaluating adverse upstream endpoints for improved risk assessment and decision-making, *Environ. Health Perspect.* **2008**, 116(11), 1568–1575.

Yang, C.; Tan, Y. S.; Harkema, J. R.; Haslam, S. Z. Differential effects of peripubertal exposure to perfluorooctanoic acid on mammary gland development in C57Bl/6 and Balb/c mouse strains. *Reprod. Toxicol.* **2009**, 27, 299–306.

14

GREEN CHEMISTRY PRINCIPLES IN THE DESIGNING AND SCREENING FOR SAFE CHEMICALS AND REMEDIATION OF EDCs

14.1 INTRODUCTION

The rising concern about the toxic properties of chemicals has given rise to the field of green chemistry – the science-based design of chemical products and processes that reduce or eliminate the use and generation of hazardous substances. Over the last two decades, the field of green chemistry has emerged around several visions as its focus and content. Many core ideas are commonly held, and several embody considerable tension. The quest of learning how to design chemicals for commerce that are free of toxic properties and other hazards is the consensus definitional mission and has been so all the way back to the early 1990s.

Green chemists find themselves trapped in the cold embrace of an understanding that certain everyday chemicals are militating against a sustainable future by disrupting the hormonal control of development. When one adds to this the recognition that certain endocrine disruptors (EDs) exhibit spectacular technical and cost performances in diverse product lines of the present day economy, the process finding escape route for the welfare of living things is forbidding indeed as it calls for massive change in the chemical enterprise. Bisphenol A (BPA), which is made from phenol and acetone and is the basic building block of polycarbonate plastic, is a case in point. It seems virtually inconceivable that any mimic will be able to match the cost and performance features of BPA, or occupy easily the locale in the existing supply of this >10 B lb/year product. Poly(vinyl chloride) (PVC) is another case in point where millions of tons are being added to the built environment each year.

Endocrine Disruptors in the Environment, First Edition. Sushil K. Khetan.
© 2014 John Wiley & Sons, Inc. Published 2014 by John Wiley & Sons, Inc.

The burning of PVC produces dioxins, which are exceptionally potent endocrine disruptors (EDs). Thus, PVC is incompatible with a sustainable civilization. The argument that green chemists can solve these problems given sufficient time is a *non sequitur* that distracts green chemistry from its authentic roles of addressing solvable problems of hazardous chemicals (Collins, 2013).

The quest for insight and tools to enable the design of safer and more sustainable chemical products and processes brings chemists face to face with toxicology, and especially with rapidly expanding insight into low-dose adverse effects associated with endocrine disruption endpoints. The understanding of endocrine disruption once acquired becomes a test of character. Thus, the unifying mission of green chemists is amalgamated with the commitment to acknowledge the limitations while proclaiming the promise of green chemistry. Despite the barriers, the inspiring news is that deep and growing understanding of the challenges that EDs place in path of sustainability is taking hold in our world. And in consequence, consumer-driven, regulatory, and technical solutions are becoming commonplace.

14.2 BENIGN BY DESIGN CHEMICALS

One of the green chemistry principles is that chemical products can be designed to preserve efficacy of function while reducing toxicity and other environmental hazards (EPA, 1993; Anastas and Warner, 1998). Endocrine disruption is a hazard that, to date, has been inadequately addressed by both industrial and regulatory science. Unlike pharmaceuticals or pesticides, the potential for new commercial chemicals to cause endocrine-disruption-related adverse health effects on people, wildlife, and the environment is not always considered upfront. But, the potential threat of chemicals with unintended human and environmental hazards has become increasingly clear. Phthalates – as plastic additives – are now known to disrupt hormonal balance. Other widely used plasticizers – such as BPA – can interfere with reproductive functions, as is increasingly shown from animal research.

Historically, chemists have aimed to make products that are effective and economical, and the toxic effects of new chemicals and materials did not receive much consideration in the design process. As synthetic chemists typically are not trained in toxicology, the task for evaluation of toxicity of chemicals has traditionally been left to toxicologists further down the commercialization line (Van Noorden, 2011). Decades of safety tests have generated enough data for researchers to learn how chemicals produce toxic effects. Computer models are now helping to identify the molecular properties that underlie these undesirable effects. Chemists are now expected to take the responsibility for the molecules they design for being safe to both human health and the environment (Voutchkova et al., 2010a). The growing understanding of toxicity puts the onus on chemists to upfront avoid making molecules that fall in the danger zone.

Knowledge of the mechanisms by which chemicals cause toxicity is important when contemplating the design of safer chemicals. Molecular designers need to consider the most likely reactivity of a chemical inside an organism, and to make efforts to minimize rationally its bioavailability (exposure), metabolic activation, or ligand-binding interactions with biomolecules. Particularly, consideration of the biotransformation of chemicals by metabolic pathways is important for minimizing the potential for bioactivation and resulting toxicity and maximizing the rapid oxidation and/or conjugation and elimination of the chemical (Osimitz and Nelson, 2012). An analysis that associates specific physical and chemical properties with toxicity, analogous to Lipinski's "Rule of Five" of drug-likeness describing various physical and chemical property ranges of successful pharmaceutical candidates (Lipinski et al., 1997), has not been reported. Nonetheless, there have been some advances in understanding the mechanisms of toxicity (Boelsterli, 2003).

Recently, property-based guidelines have been developed for the design of chemicals with reduced acute and chronic aquatic toxicity to multiple standardized species and endpoints by exploring properties associated with bioavailability, narcotic toxicity, and reactive modes of action, such as electrophilic interactions. Two simple properties, namely, n-octanol–water partition and ΔE, are predictive of a molecule being acutely toxic to fish and other aquatic organisms. These have emerged by analyzing data on hundreds of chemicals that have been tested by the U.S. Environmental Protection Agency (EPA) and the Japanese environment ministry for their acute toxicity to three diverse aquatic species. The aquatic species tested are the fathead minnow (*Pimephales promelas*) (LC_{50}, 96-h assay), Japanese Medaka fish (*Oryzias latipes*) (LC_{50}, 96-h assay), and the water flea *Daphnia magna* (EC_{50}, 48-h assay) (Voutchkova et al., 2011).

The acute aquatic toxicity caused by most industrial chemicals is predominantly the result of narcosis (a disturbance in the cell membrane permeability by hydrophobic chemicals), a nonspecific mechanism involving disruption of the cell membrane of an aquatic organism. The toxic potencies of chemicals that act by narcosis are related to their propensity to accumulate in the membranes. Octanol–water partition, which measures lipophilicity, is a well-established model parameter for bioavailability and narcotic toxicity in aquatic species. It has been found that the most toxic chemicals tend to be quite soluble in fat relative to water (n-octanol–water partition coefficient, log $P_{O/W}$), making it easier for a molecule to pass through a cell's membrane and that these chemicals are adept at ripping electrons from other molecules, a property that makes it more likely they will cause damage once inside a cell. Thus, compounds with low log $P_{O/W}$ values are more water soluble and are likely to be less bioavailable to fish than more lipid-soluble chemicals with higher log $P_{O/W}$ values (Voutchkova et al., 2010b). The compounds with higher log $P_{O/W}$ (up to ~7) are also more bioaccumulative.

Reactivity with biomolecules is associated with frontier orbital energies, especially with the energy of the lowest unoccupied molecular orbital (LUMO) and the difference between the LUMO and the highest occupied molecular orbital (HOMO) (ΔE) (Zvinavashe et al., 2009). LUMO and HOMO energies are computationally derived using quantum mechanical calculations, such as density functional theory (DFT) methods, which calculate the molecular electron probability density (ρ) and from that the molecular electronic energy. The LUMO energy is a good predictor for electrophilic reactivity, which is necessary for reaction with basic macromolecules, such as DNA or protein residues. Lower LUMO energies are related to higher electrophilic reactivity, one of the major modes of action in aquatic toxicity. The compounds of low or no concern for acute aquatic toxicity have higher LUMO energies. The HOMO energy, on the other hand, is a predictor for nucleophilic reactivity. The difference in energies between the energy of the LUMO (E_{LUMO}) and the HOMO (E_{HOMO}) is called the band gap (i.e., $\Delta E = E_{LUMO} - E_{HOMO}$). The smaller the band gap of a molecule, the more likely it is to be a reactive compound (Fleming, 2010). Since most chemicals are not both nucleophilic and electrophilic, either a low LUMO or a high HOMO orbital energy usually causes the difference between the two (ΔE) to become smaller, and is thus associated with higher chemical reactivity. This measure of chemical reactivity (ΔE) was highly correlated to chronic and acute toxicity, particularly when standardized endpoints in these common model organisms were considered (Voutchkova-Kostal et al., 2012).

Combining the data on all species, a range of values for variables relating to these two properties were quantified. The analysis indicated that 70–80% of the compounds with low or no acute aquatic toxicity concern by EPA guidelines to the three species had a defined range for log $P_{O/W}$ values of less than 2 and ΔE values greater than 9 eV (Table. 14.1), compared to compounds that were of high acute toxicity concern and did not meet these criteria. When these rules were applied to chemicals that had been tested on the model organism green alga *Pseudokirchneriella subcapitata* (EC_{50}, 72-h), it was found that 23 out of 29 low-concern compounds fell inside the range. It could be, therefore, concluded that staying within the safer range increases the chances of designing a compound with very low acute aquatic toxicity by 2–5 fold (Voutchkova et al., 2011).

Unlike acute aquatic toxicity, which is predominantly due to narcosis, chronic aquatic toxicity often involves specific ligand–receptor interactions, such as endocrine disruption endpoints. Nevertheless, the property-based guidelines for acute aquatic toxicity have been found to generally extend for common standardized chronic aquatic toxicity endpoints with model organisms (Voutchkova-Kostal et al., 2012). That these guidelines are a work in progress is reflected in some chemicals being found exceptions. Some were classified as of low chronic concern, but fell in the likely toxic space, such as phthalates, which is attributed to the hydrolysis of the esters to phthalic acid, or formation of emulsions in the aquatic

TABLE 14.1   Design guideline of chemicals for reduced acute and chronic aquatic toxicity

Property	Value
Log $P_{O/W}$ (A measure of lipophilicity and bioavailability)	>2
ΔE (HOMO–LUMO) (A measure of reactivity with biomolecules)	>9 eV

environment. Others fell into low toxicity concern, but were found to have high acute toxicity, such as hydrazine (Voutchkova-Kostal et al., 2012).

14.3   CHEMICAL ENDOCRINE DISRUPTION SCREENING PROTOCOL

Chemists generally lack the expertise or predictive tools to detect endocrine-disruption toxicity when they set out to design a molecule focusing on functionality, efficacy, and cost. Green chemistry research has aimed at identifying and developing chemicals that do not have endocrine-disrupting activity. For achieving this goal, a suite of peer-reviewed assays for synthetic chemists, the great majority of whom are not trained in biology, endocrinology, or toxicology, is required to be produced. To be effective at detecting endocrine-disrupting activity, an assay would have to take into account potential low-dose and nonlinear effects of chemicals and the many possible interactions such chemicals can have with genetic receptors. A collaboration of a multidisciplinary team consisting of experts in biology, toxicology, and chemistry has created a design tool to address this problem through a process to eliminate potentially harmful chemicals early in development that are less likely to elicit hormonal responses in humans and animals. The endocrine disruption testing protocol for use in the design of new materials is designed to address concerns that newly developed green chemicals may not be much better for the endocrine system than the existing chemicals. It has been developed to help chemists move toward a new generation of inherently safer materials.

It could be argued that there are already enough assays on EDCs and enough educational materials existing, so no additional work on this area is needed. However, chemists who work on designing new chemicals cannot negotiate the thicket of information around all available assays on EDCs. They need a vetted and reliable shortcut for navigating through available tools and a clearly delineated suite of tests that would be necessary and/or sufficient to establish confidence that a new compound is not an EDC. Moreover, there is a need for clear scientific principles by which companies and chemists can evaluate the reliability of assays and tools as well as the practices of the many research and testing companies offering these services.

14.3.1   Tiered Protocol for Endocrine Disruption

A Tiered Protocol for Endocrine Disruption (TiPED), which stems from a cross-disciplinary collaboration among scientists, has been proposed to determine potential endocrine-disrupting activity of a new chemical (Schug et al., 2013). The protocol involves a five-tiered approach, starting from the simplest and least expansive assays and working through more specialized tests to a whole animal lifetime assessment to determine whether a new chemical has endocrine-disrupting characteristics. The five-tiered phases include computational and quantitative structure–activity relationship (QSAR) modeling (Tier 1), high-throughput *in*

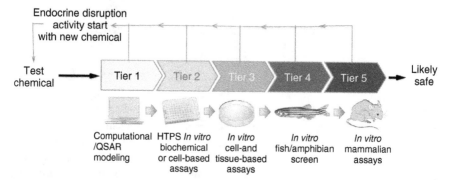

Figure 14.1 Tiered testing protocol for identifying ED characteristics in designing new materials goes through the process of selecting assays during design or redesign phases (Source: Modified from O'Brien and Myers, 2011).

vitro screening (HTS), and biochemical or cell-based assays (Tier 2) to quickly weed out problem chemicals. These tests are followed by more specific *in vitro* cell-based screening assays (Tier 3) with a focus on refining, reducing, and replacing animal testing as much as possible. The final two tiers involve use of *in vivo* fish/amphibian screen (Tier 4) and *in vivo* mammalian assays (Tier 5) (Schug, 2011; Schug et al., 2013). Each tier increases the complexity and cost, but also potentially the reliability of results (Fig. 14.1).

In trying to head off potentially harmful endocrine disrupters before they reach the market place, the rationale of this approach were provided by Schug and colleagues (2013). A positive result at any step in the process is an indication of potential ED activity and thus provides the chemist an opportunity to modify the chemical under development. TiPED's initial two phases rely on predictive computer modeling and HTS to quickly weed out problem chemicals.

Tier 1 is a computational assessment that encompasses statistical and mathematical models to predict endocrine-disrupting properties based on physical properties and the chemical reactivity of a molecule. A molecule that is run through Tier 1 without detecting ED activity implies that the chemical being developed, based on its structure, does not fit into a receptor-binding pocket or possess structural characteristics or physicochemical properties associated with toxicity. In Tier 2, *in vitro* screens using biochemical assays and cell-based assays allow direct testing of a compound's ability to modulate biological signaling pathways. The tests serve to confirm information from Tier 1 that a chemical actually does not bind to any of the known receptors probed.

Tier 3 then incorporates cell- and tissue-based assays that assess whether a chemical activates signaling pathways that lead to cell division, differentiation, cell death, or endocrine-mediated processes. A negative EDC activity in Tier 3 provides additional assurance that, at the subcellular level, integrative genomic pathways were not disrupted. This tier also allows the assessment of metabolism using human liver cells, providing some insight into potential EDC activity by metabolites. Thus working a compound through the first three tiers without detecting EDC activity mostly reduces the likelihood that the molecule is working as an EDC via well-studied mechanisms.

The final two phases involve the use of fish/amphibian and mammalian *in vivo* models. In Tier 4, the risks of false negatives are further reduced through *in vivo* whole-animal experiments, which includes fish and amphibians assays, allowing examination of the impact of a chemical for multiple endpoints involving multiple hormones and EDC effects that work through mechanisms integrating different elements of the endocrine system. Finally, Tier 5 involves testing in mammalian models that are often required to verify the lack of EDC properties necessary for extrapolation to humans. In this Tier, primarily rodents provide focused assessment of endpoints/tissues/diseases/pathways that may have been missed by earlier tiers because they lack the complexity of mammalian development (Schug et al., 2013).

The protocol advises industrial chemists on how to screen newly synthesized compounds for endocrine-related effects, how to test at very low doses, and how to look for nonmonotonic dose–response curves (Fagin, 2012). The idea behind the protocol is that the designer of a new molecule can use current existing science to predict endocrine disruption characteristics early in the design phase of developing materials. If the tests reveal EDC characteristics, the chemist has a choice of either starting all over or redesigning the molecule. Chemists can design molecules to not act like hormones; the truth is that they just have not been focused on these aspects earlier. The use of this approach decreases the chances that a lot of money and time will be spent developing a material that might turn out to be detrimental in the future. However, TiPED remains a scientific framework in progress, as it is unlikely to detect all possible mechanisms of endocrine disruption, because scientific understanding of these phenomena is still advancing (Ritter, 2012).

Considering the complexity of hormone action and the known complexity of EDC effects on hormone action, the goal of identifying all EDCs in a rapid animal-based screen is impossible to achieve. The EPA has developed the initial two technologies to assist in rapid screening. HTS is a faster and more efficient high-volume testing strategy to identify interactions between chemicals and estrogen, androgen, and thyroid receptors (Knudsen et al., 2011). The other approach is based on computer modeling and simulates chemical behavior based on its structure (QSAR) and is largely dependent on factors such as data quality, molecular descriptors, and statistical algorithms employed to build the model. Both of these approaches are useful to quickly weed out problem chemicals, but limited, because they test only for hormone–receptor binding (Vogel, 2005). Predictive toxicology has many advantages in terms of throughput and cost, but reliability and robustness are two major concerns preventing it from being widely applied to risk assessment.

14.4 GREEN OXIDATIVE REMEDIATION OF EDCs

Low levels of EDCs in water are a major concern for society because EDCs exert physiological effects at very low concentrations that can translate into human impairment. Precautionary thinking ordains that drinking water should be free from trace EDC contaminants to minimize unpredictable long-term risks. A prudent course is to treat EDCs in the water as an urgent issue with the strategic intent of protecting human health and the environment.

Drinking water treatment primarily relies upon adsorptive and oxidative processes to remove or transform organic materials (see Chapter 12 for more details). Persistent trace contaminants can be removed by membrane filtration (nanofiltration and reverse osmosis) or filtration over activated carbon. However, the absorption or retention capacity of both approaches decreases with operation time as natural organic matter builds up and interferes. For chemical oxidation, oxidants such as chlorine, chlorine dioxide, and ozone are frequently employed, with ozone tending to be the most reactive.

An area of focus of green chemistry is remediation of trace contaminants, such as EDCs, where the intent is on reducing or eliminating the use and generation of hazardous substances. Environmental endocrine activity is dependent on the presence of an aromatic ring structure with an extended carbon backbone. All natural and synthetic hormones are aromatic compounds and the EDCs generally share this characteristic. Several green chemical methods have been employed for the degradation of bioactive aromatic compounds, including ozonation (redox potential: 2.07 V), advanced oxidation processes (AOPs) such as H_2O_2/UV and O_3/H_2O_2, and a catalytic oxidation process employing Fe-TAML/H_2O_2 (Khetan and Collins, 2007). AOPs are employed where ozone treatment alone does not oxidize. Chemical oxidation for complete mineralization is generally expensive because the oxidation intermediates formed during treatment tend to be more and more resistant to their complete chemical degradation. One attractive alternative is partial oxidation of the biologically persistent part to produce biodegradable reaction intermediates. For example, an AOP based on ozone, by increasing the pH value and by addition of hydrogen peroxide involving highly reactive hydroxyl radicals, is used to destroy or reduce the concentration of targeted environmental contaminants to acceptable level.

14.4.1 Catalytic Oxidation Processes

Selective catalytic reagents offer numerous green chemistry benefits including lower energy requirements. They are superior to stoichiometric reagents for remediation of pollutants by replacing the need for large quantities of reagents otherwise needed to carry out the transformations and contribute to the waste stream. However, heavy-metal-based catalysts are typically extremely toxic. Reduction of EDCs in water by an environmentally benign method is an important green chemistry goal. Therefore, a catalyst that avoids toxic components and functional groups, as well as efficiently mimics the action of natural enzymes, will be ideally suited for remediation of EDCs. Solid water-soluble redox catalysts, such as iron(III)-tetraamido macrocyclic ligands (Fe-TAMLs) (Fig. 14.2), that activate hydrogen peroxide provide an environmentally friendly method for breaking down toxic compounds that contaminate water, including EDCs.

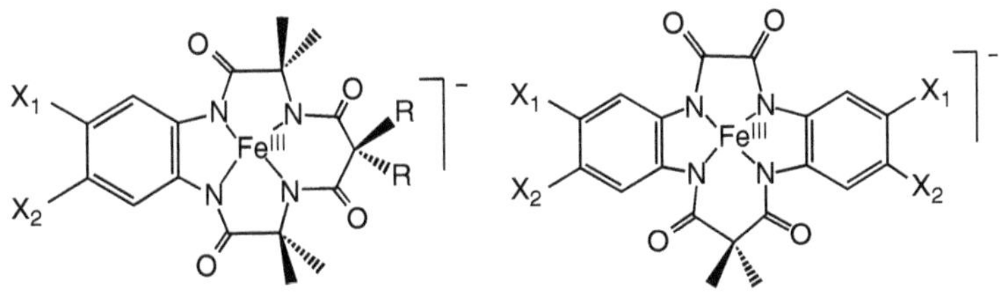

a   b

A_1; $X_1 = X_2 = H$; R = H B_1; $X_1 = X_2 = H$

A_2; $X_1 = X_2 = H$; R = F B_2; $X_1 = NO_2$; $X_2 = H$

Figure 14.2 Two structures of iron(III)-tetraamido macrocyclic ligand (Fe-TAML) – fluorinated and nonfluorinated.

Synthetic Fe-TAMLs mimic peroxidase enzymes, but are far more stable and reactive than natural enzymes, as these do not have steric limitations imposed by the protein component of enzymes. These oxidation catalysts have shown reactivity reminiscent of short-circuited catalytic cycles of the cytochrome-P450 enzymes and have been found useful in pollution remediation (Collins et al., 2009). Although many other biomimetic oxidation catalysts exist, their applications require non-aqueous conditions or they achieve fewer turnovers (Meunier, 2000).

The catalytic activity of Fe-TAMLs varies depending on the substituents. The basic Fe-TAML (Fig. 14.2a), where R, X_1, and X_2 positions are occupied by hydrogen, is of modest activity and the fluorinated version at R positions is relatively more aggressive. As halogenated compounds are generally found to be environmentally more persistent, a new generation of Fe-TAMLs (Fig. 14.2b) without halogen substituents has also been developed to ameliorate their activities, which have equal or more aggressive activity than fluorinated Fe-TAMLs (Ellis et al., 2010).

Fe-TAML catalysts have been shown to function at very low concentrations, both in the amount of catalyst required and with trace quantities of EDCs. At concentrations typically used for decontaminating water, Fe-TAMLs were also found to be devoid of endocrine disruption capability of their own, as verified by a Tier 4 TiPED test exposing zebrafish embryos (Truong et al., 2013). Zebrafish is an extremely useful model for understanding how cells respond to environmental chemicals during early development in vertebrates, including humans.

Several known EDCs, such as E2 and EE2 (Shappell et al., 2008; Chen et al., 2012), fenitrothion (Chanda et al., 2006), and chlorpyrifos (Kundu et al., 2012), are reported to undergo facile degradation employing this process. Catalytic oxidation of the strong estrogenic compound EE2 with Fe-TAML (A_1)/H_2O_2 resulted in the epimeric intermediates 17α-ethynyl-1,4-estradiene-10α,17β-diol-3-one, and 17α-ethynyl-1,4-estra-diene-10β,17β-diol-3-one (Fig. 14.3), displaying a slightly higher estrogenicity than EE_2 itself, as determined by the YES assay. Both the epimers were further degraded to unidentified products, which showed no estrogenicity (Chen et al., 2012; Shappell et al., 2008).

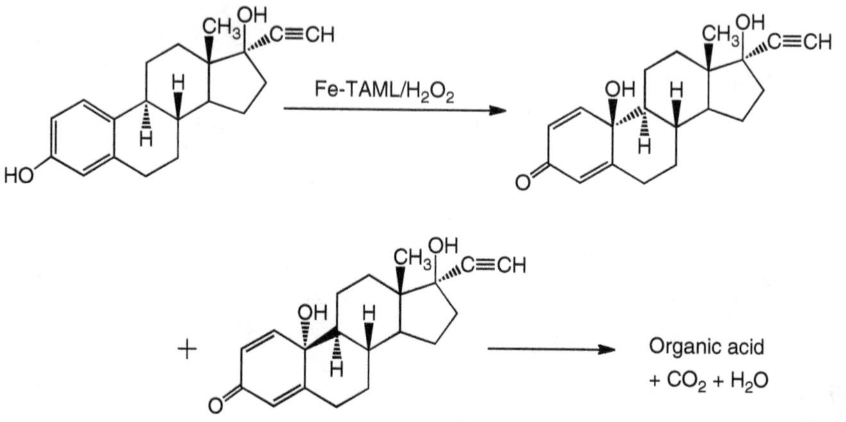

Figure 14.3   EE2 oxidative degradation using Fe-TAML/H_2O_2 (Chen et al., 2012).

Treatment of an anti-androgenic organophosphorus pesticide fenitrothion with Fe-TAML (A_2)/H_2O_2 resulted in partial mineralization and formation of nontoxic small molecules as end products (Fig. 14.4) (Chanda et al., 2006).

Some of the EDCs such as BPA, tetrabromo-BPA (TBBPA), and tetrachloro-BPA (TCBPA) in environmentally relevant conditions were also effectively oxidized by Fe-TAML/H_2O_2 system, where oxidation products showed reduction in toxicity (BPA) or no observed toxicity (TBBA) (Collins et al., unpublished results).

14.5   CONCLUSIONS AND FUTURE PROSPECTS

One can ban BPA, but if there are no better materials, another equally bad chemical will take its place. What are needed are win–win solutions (Walsh, 2010). It is unlikely that any substitute will be able to match the cost and performance features of BPA, or occupy easily the locale in the existing supply. The possibility that green chemists would be able to solve all such chemical issues is also unrealistic. Therefore, this argument should never serve as a distraction from the important regulatory role of government in protecting the public and future generations in real time.

Any biological activity of chemicals is undesirable in the commercial chemical industry. However, the task of developing a rational strategy for the design of chemicals with reduced toxicological hazard is exceptionally challenging and requires a collaborative effort from chemists and toxicologists. This challenge is further complicated by the fact that most chemists receive little or no formal training in the design of chemicals that have reduced toxicity. Some progress has been made for the development of property-based guidelines for the design of safer chemicals with reduced acute and chronic aquatic toxicity to multiple standardized species and endpoints. When new chemicals are designed to reduce the intrinsic toxicity, workers

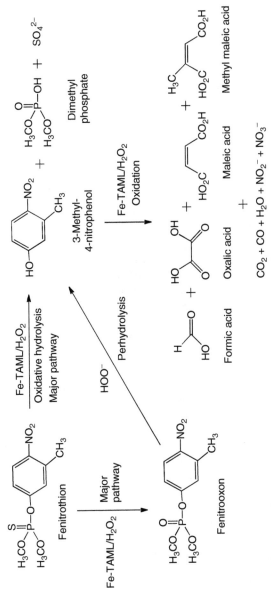

Figure 14.4 Catalytic oxidative degradation of fenitrothion, an anti-androgen, by Fe-TAML/H_2O_2 (Chanda et al., 2006).

and the general population will benefit. Additionally, a tiered protocol has been proposed for screening of new chemicals that a chemist can use current existing science to test for endocrine disruption early in the design phase of developing materials. These protocols, which remain a work in progress, will in all likelihood be refined and simplified with improved understanding of identifying and detecting endocrine activity. Also, biomimetic oxidation processes for treatment of toxic chemicals at the end of the pipeline have been developed that reduce or eliminate toxicity by degradation/transformation into biodegradable small molecules or mineralization without producing any residual toxicity of their own. All these parallel processes, which are in early phases, will result in reduced presence of toxic chemicals in the environment and, consequently, improvement in human health. Participation of the chemical industry in the developments of green products and degradation technologies will also help protect it from future potential liabilities.

REFERENCES

Anastas, P. T.; Warner, J. C. *Green Chemistry: Theory and Practice*, New York: Oxford University Press, **1998**.

Boelsterli, U. A. *Mechanistic Toxicology: The Molecular Basis of How Chemicals Disrupt Biological Targets*, New York, NY: Taylor & Francis, **2003**.

Chanda, A.; Khetan, S. K.; Banerjee, D.; Ghosh, A.; Collins, T. J. Total degradation of fenitrothion and other organophosphorus pesticides by catalytic oxidation employing Fe-TAML peroxide activators, *J. Am. Chem. Soc.* **2006**, 128, 12058–12059.

Chen, J. L.; Ravindran, S.; Swift, S.; Wright, L. J.; Singhal, N. Catalytic oxidative degradation of 17α-ethinylestradiol by Fe^{III}-TAML/H$_2$O$_2$: Estrogenicities of the products of partial, and extensive oxidation, *Water Res.* **2012**, 46(19), 6309–6318.

Collins, T. J. *In a conversation with Sushil Khetan*, **2013**.

Collins, T. J.; Khetan, S. K.; Ryabov, A. D. Chemistry and applications of iron-TAML catalysts in green oxidation processes based on hydrogen peroxide, in *Handbook of Green Chemistry – Green Catalysis, Vol. 1: Homogeneous Catalysis*, Anastas, P. T. and Crabtree, R. H., eds., Weinheim, Germany: Wiley-VCH, **2009**, pp. 39–77.

Ellis, W. C.; Tran, C. T.; Roy, R.; Rusten, M.; Fischer, A.; Ryabov, A. D.; Blumberg, B.; Collins, T. J. Designing green oxidation catalysts for purifying environmental waters, *J. Am. Chem. Soc.* **2010**, 132(28), 9774–9781.

EPA, The 12 Principles of Green Chemistry, Washington, DC: United States Environmental Protection Agency, **1993**. Available at: http://www.epa.gov/gcc/ pubs/principles.html (accessed on 16 October 2012).

Fagin, D. Toxicology: the learning curve, *Nature* **2012**, 490, 462–465.

Fleming, I. *Molecular Orbitals and Organic Chemical Reactions*, Fleming, I., ed., 1st ed., New York: John Wiley and Sons, **2010**.

Khetan, S. K.; Collins, T. J. Human pharmaceuticals in the aquatic environment: a challenge to green chemistry, *Chem. Rev.* **2007**, 107(6), 2319–2364.

Knudsen, T. B.; Kavlock, R. J.; Daston, G. P.; Stedman, D.; Hixon, M.; Kim, J. H. Developmental toxicity testing for safety assessment: new approaches and technologies, *Birth Defects Res. B Dev. Reprod. Toxicol.* **2011**, 92, 413–420.

Kundu, S.; Chanda, A.; Espinosa-Marvan, L.; Khetan, S. K.; Collins, T. J. Facile destruction of formulated chlorpyrifos through green oxidation catalysis, *Catal. Sci. Technol.* **2012**, 2(6), 1165–1172.

Lipinski, C. A.; Lombardo, F.; Dominy, B. W.; Feeney, P. J. *Adv. Drug Delivery Rev.* **1997**, 23, 3–25.

O'Brien, K. P.; Myers, P. *Catalyzing green chemistry innovation through key collaborations*, Webinar, **2011**. Available at: https://migreenchemistry.org/wp-content/uploads/2011/09/Webinar_6-29-2011_OBrien-and-Myers.pdf (accessed on 10 Dec. 2012).

Osimitz, T. G.; Nelson, J. L. Understanding mechanisms of metabolic transformations as a tool for designing safer chemicals, in *Handbook of Green Chemistry Vol. 9: Designing Safer Chemicals*, Boethling, R. and Voutchkova, A., eds., Wiley-VCH Verlag GmbH, **2012**, pp. 47–75.

Ritter, S. K. Designing away endocrine disruption, *C&E News* **2012**, 90(51), 33–35.

Schug, T. *NIEHS scientists join forces with green chemists*, *Environmental Factor*, **2011**. Available at: http://www.niehs.nih.gov/news/newsletter/2011/april/science-scientists/index.cfm (accessed on 15 Nov. 2012).

Schug, T. T.; Abagyan, R.; Blumberg, B.; Collins, T. J.; Crews, D.; DeFur, P. L.; Dickerson, S. M.; Edwards, T. M.; Gore, A. C.; Guillette, L. J.; Hayes, T.; Heindel, J. J.; Moores, A.; Patisul, H. B.; Tal, T. L.; Thayer, K. A.; Vandenberg, L. N.; Warner, J. C.; Watson, C. S.; vom Saal, F. S.; Zoeller, R. T.; O'Brien, K. P.; Myers, J. P. Designing endocrine disruption out of the next generation of chemicals, *Green Chem.* **2013**, 15, 181–198.

Shappell, N. E.; Vrabel, M. A.; Madsen, P. J.; Harrington, G.; Billey, L. O.; Hakk, H.; Larsen, G. L.; Beach, E. S.; Horwitz, C. P.; Ro, K.; Hunt, P. G.; Collins, T. J. Destruction of estrogens using Fe-TAML/peroxide catalysis, *Environ. Sci. Technol.* **2008**, 42, 1296–1300.

Truong, L.; DeNardo, M. A.; Kundu, S.; Collins, T. J.; Tanguay, R. L. Zebrafish assays as developmental toxicity indicators in the green design of TAML oxidation catalysts, *Green Chem.* **2013**, 15(9), 2339–2343.

Van Noorden, R. How to design a safer chemical, *Nature*, 29 July **2011**.

Vogel, J.M. Perils of paradigm: complexity, policy design, and the endocrine disruptor-screening program, *Environ. Health* **2005**, 4(2), 11.

Voutchkova-Kostal, A. M.; Kostal, J.; Connors, K. A.; Brooks, B. W.; Anastas, P. T.; Zimmerman, J. B. Towards rational molecular design for reduced chronic aquatic toxicity, *Green Chem.* **2012**, 14(4), 1001–1008.

Voutchkova, A. M.; Kostal, J.; Steinfeld, J. B.; Emerson, J. W.; Brooks, B. W.; Anastas, P.; Zimmerman, J. B. Towards rational molecular design: derivation of property guidelines for reduced acute aquatic toxicity, *Green Chem.* **2011**, 13(9), 2373–2379.

Voutchkova, A. M.; Osimitz, T. G.; Anastas, P. T. Toward a comprehensive molecular design framework for reduced hazard, *Chem. Rev.* **2010a**, 110(10), 5845–5882.

Voutchkova, A. M.; Ferris, L. A.; Zimmerman, J. B.; Anastas, P. T. Toward molecular design for hazard reduction—fundamental relationships between chemical properties and toxicity, *Tetrahedron* **2010b**, 66, 1031–1039.

Zvinavashe, E.; Du, T. T.; Griff, T.; van den Berg, H. H. J.; Soffers, A. E. M. F.; Vervoort, J.; Murk, A. J.; Rietjens, I. M. C. M. Quantitative structure-activity relationship modeling of the toxicity of organothiophosphate pesticides to *Daphnia magna* and *Cyprinus carpio*, *Chemosphere* **2009**, 75, 1531–1538.

INDEX

www.ingramcontent.com/pod-product-compliance
Lightning Source LLC
Chambersburg PA
CBHW072111250125
20788CB00003B/30